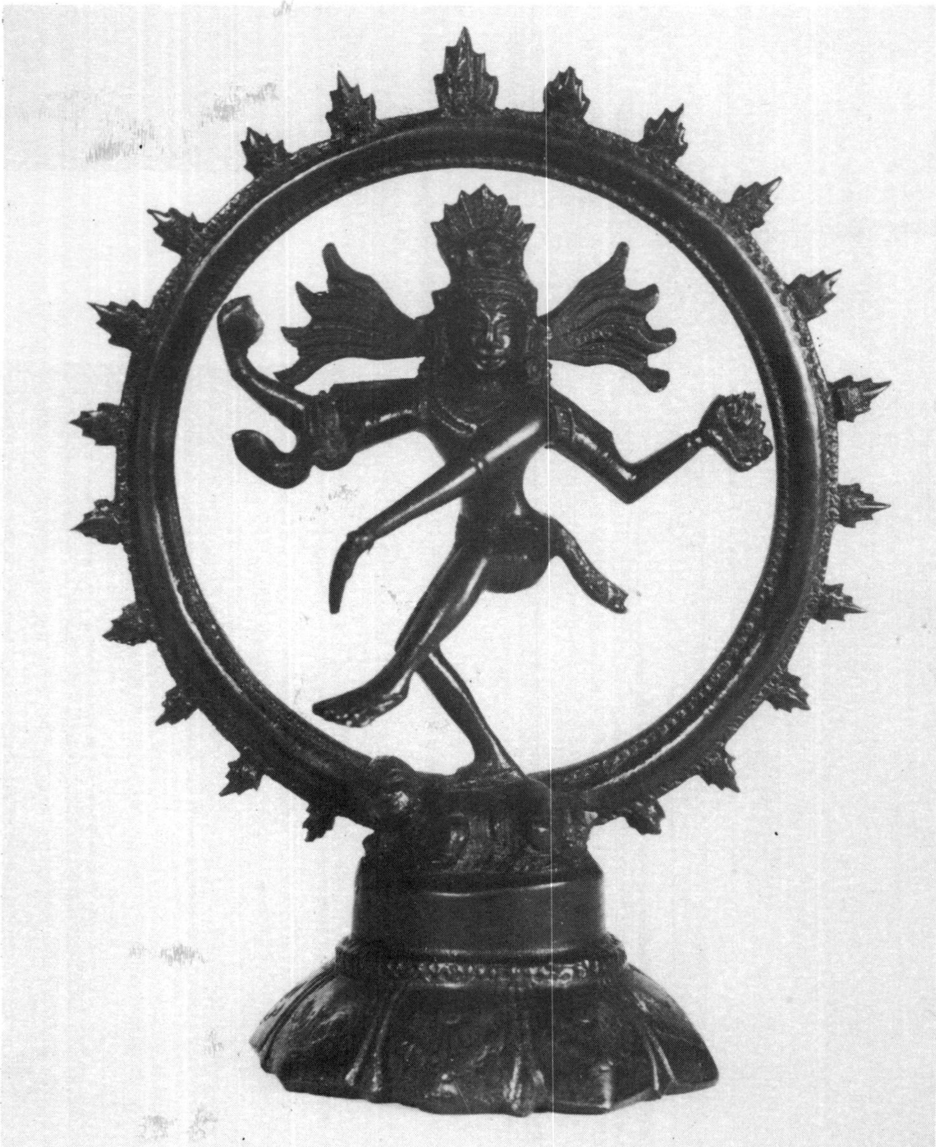

Shiva: the god of destruction and of creativity symbolizes both the destructive power of schizophrenia and the creativity of many of its sufferers.

The Biological Basis of Schizophrenia

The Biological Basis of Schizophrenia

Edited by
Gwynneth Hemmings
The Schizophrenia Association
of Great Britain

and

W. A. Hemmings
University College of North Wales
Bangor, Gwynedd,
Wales

MTP PRESS LIMITED *International Medical Publishers*

Published by
MTP Press Limited
Falcon House
Lancaster, England

ISBN: 0 85200 233–5

Printed in Great Britain by The Blackburn Times Press,
Northgate, Blackburn, Lancs. B82 1AB

Contents

SECTION 4: TREATMENT

SECTION 5: DIETARY FACTORS

SECTION 6: IMMUNOLOGICAL FACTORS

SECTION 7: ALCOHOLISM

List of Contributors

H. BARUK
5 Quai de la République,
94410 Saint-Maurice,
Paris,
France

D. A. BENDER
Courtauld Institute of Biochemistry,
Middlesex Hospital Medical School,
London,
England

E. D. BIRD
Department of Neuropathology,
McLean Hospital,
Belmont,
Massachusetts 02178,
USA

G. A. BUSCAINO
Universita' di Napoli,
2a Faculta di Medicina e Chirurgia,
Clinica Neurologica,
Napoli,
Italy

M. W. P. CARNEY
Northwick Park Hospital,
Watford Road,
Harrow,
Middlesex,
England

D. N. CHALLACOMBE
Children's Research Unit,
Musgrove Park Hospital,
Taunton,
Somerset,
England

J. R. COCKRELL
Department of Basic and
Clinical Immunology and
Microbiology,
Medical University of South Carolina,
Charlestown,
S. Carolina 29403,
USA

T. J. CROW
Division of Psychiatry,
Clinical Research Centre,
Northwick Park Hospital,
Watford Road,
Harrow,
Middlesex,
England

J. W. T. DICKERSON
Department of Human Nutrition,
University of Surrey,
Guildford,
Surrey,
England

F. C. DOHAN
Eastern Pennsylvania Psychiatric Institute,
Henry Avenue and Abbotsford Road,
Philadelphia,
Pennsylvania 19129,
USA

W. P. FAULK
Department of Basic and Clinical
Immunology and Microbiology,
Medical University of South Carolina,
Charlestown,
S. Carolina 29403,
USA

J. GRUZELIER
Department of Psychiatry,
Charing Cross Hospital,
London,
England

W. Th. J. M. HEKKENS
Academische Zeinkenhuis,
Laboratorium voor Gastroenterologie,
gebouw 26 Rijnburgerse,
10 Leiden,
Holland

W. A. HEMMINGS
ARC Immunology Group,
Zoology Department,
University College of North Wales,
Bangor,
Gwynedd,
Wales

LIST OF CONTRIBUTORS

D. A. HUDSON
Institute of Child Health,
Virology Department,
Children's Hospital,
Birmingham,
England

D. RICHTER
IBRO Secretariat,
41 Queen's Gate,
London,
England

S. B. ROSALKI
St. Mary's Hospital,
Harrow Road,
London,
England

M. SANDLER
Bernhard Baron Memorial Research
Laboratories,
Department of Clinical Pathology,
Queen Charlotte's Hospital for Women,
Goldhawk Road,
London,
England

M. M. SINGH
University of Tennessee Center for the
Health Sciences,
Schizophrenia Research Programme,
Veterans Administration Hospital,
1030 Jefferson Avenue,
Memphis,
Tennessee 38104,
USA

J. A. SMITH
Department of Pharmaceutical Chemistry,
School of Pharmacy,
University of Bradford,
Bradford,
England

M. TAYLOR
Department of Psychology,
Ulster College,
The Northern Ireland Polytechnic,
Jordanstown,
Newtown Abbey,
Co. Antrim,
N. Ireland

K. E. WEBSTER
Department of Anatomy,
King's College,
London,
England

L. WETTERBURG
Department of Psychiatry,
Karolinska Institute,
St Göran's Hospital,
Box 12500,
S11281 Stockholm,
Sweden

R. J. WURTMAN
Laboratory of Neuro-endocrine Regulation,
Department of Nutrition and Food Science,
Massachusetts Institute of Technology,
Cambridge,
Massachusetts 02139,
USA

N. J. YORKSTON
Bethlem Royal, Maudsley and
Friern Hospitals,
London,
England

Preface

For years lip service has been paid to a belief in a biological basis for schizophrenia, but nevertheless psychosocial and psychodynamic "theories" of schizophrenia have been promulgated, and these have detracted from the all important biological work. Eclecticism has ruled the day and has caused considerable confusion. As a result research in schizophrenia has not progressed as fast as it should have done and treatment has been less effective than it could otherwise have been. This book is devoted to a wholly biological approach to the problem of schizophrenia, in the hope that many more workers will enter this exciting field of research. A wide variety of topics is covered, including brain structure; the genetics, pathogenesis and treatment of schizophrenia; a consideration of dietary and immunological factors and finally a chapter on alcoholism as it seems possible that the problems of schizophrenia and addiction are linked.

We are grateful to all our contributors and to MTP Press for their enthusiasm for this book.

Gwynneth P Hemmings
William A Hemmings

SECTION 1:
Structure

1
The brain stem reticular formation

K. E. WEBSTER

There can be no question that the brain stem reticular formation no longer exercises the same fascination for neurologists that it did a quarter of a century ago. And there can be only little doubt that interest has ebbed partly because of the central importance claimed for it in explaining a multitude of neurological phenomena: the reticular formation was well on the way to becoming the seat of the soul and a good deal else besides. The recent, if restricted, revival of interest has so far either ignored the daunting accumulation of information – second only to that of the 'limbic system' in its exasperating obscurantism and self-contradiction – or acknowledged it with varying degrees of criticism.

A prominent feature of the received way of discussing the reticular formation – a feature which, if not the worst, is certainly the most facile, and one which few, if any, investigators can claim never to have employed – is the way in which the formation is so often used as a convenient explanation for anything found difficult in terms of known neurology – its use, to put it bluntly, as a neurological tipping ground. For example, stimulation of the reticular formation is known to affect skeletal muscle tone in ways varying from inhibition or facilitation to the production of walking movements (Figure 1, see Lindsley *et al.*, 1949; Grillner and Shik, 1973; Kuypers, 1973). Thus to explain the motor effects of the forebrain basal nuclei or subthalamus, it is often thought unnecessary to do more than to lead the pathways into the reticular formation and there to desert them. Similarly, the pathways to and from the hypothalamus controlling the autonomic outflow, and those apparently mediating 'instinctive' behaviour patterns such as fear and rage, are routed into and through the reticular formation (Zanchetti, 1967). Mechanisms concerned with respiration are also to be found here. A sensory function for the reticular formation was first proposed 70 years ago by Kohnstamm and Quensel (1908). There is no doubt that the reticular formation 'samples' sensory information of most kinds – but what it does with these 'samples' is another matter. With the exception of the experience of pain, it is difficult to find evidence which more than *implicates* the reticular formation in sensory processing, to discover observations of the kind that allow a statement of some explicit, well-defined functional role for the reticular formation as opposed to other parts of the nervous system (see, e.g. Hernández-Peon, 1955; Lindsley, 1961). For example, Scheibel and Scheibel (1967) can suggest a description no more precise than '. . . a major function of the (reticular) core is to describe not the pageantry

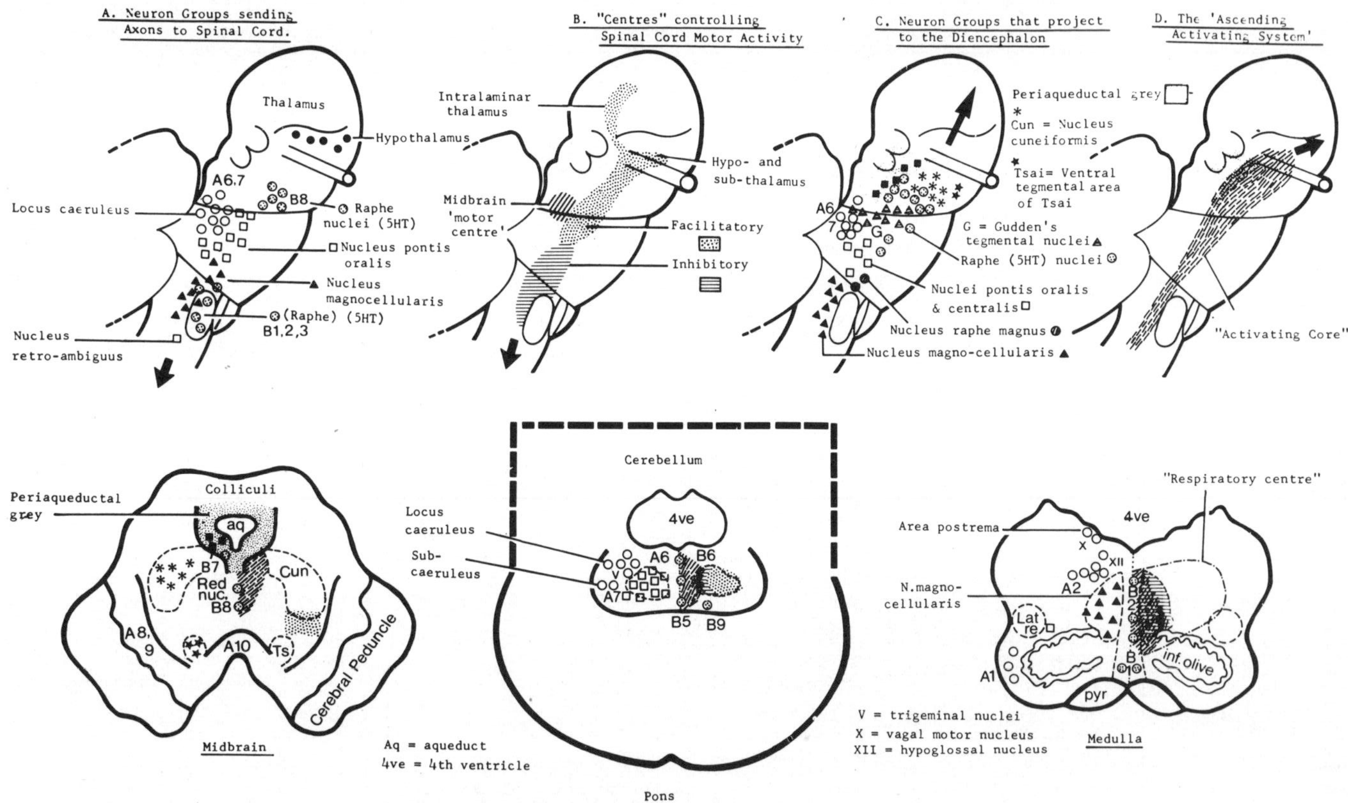

Figure 1 Schematic representation of various features of the reticular formation projected on the lateral aspect of the human brainstem (upper row) and representative cross-sections (lower row).

and colour of the passing parade, but the loudness of the shouting that accompanies it.' It must not be overlooked, of course, that the brain controls its own sensory input, and the reticular formation probably plays some part in this.

The observations which have perhaps become a paradigm of reticular formation studies are those of Moruzzi and Magoun (1949), who described the phenomenon of 'ascending activation'. They proposed there to exist, throughout the length of the brain stem, a polysynaptic core (i.e. a neuronal network, in which interaction passes from cell to cell by multiple routes of varying length) responsible for maintaining the animal awake. Later, this concept was extended to embrace a mechanism not only to keep one awake, but to maintain selective attention to features in the environment. Both these functions would clearly require the multiplicity of sensory inputs mentioned above. Further work showed the critical (but not exclusive) region associated with 'ascending activation' to lie in the midbrain or upper pons (Lindsley *et al.*, 1949; Demetrescu *et al.*, 1965; Jouvet, 1967; and Moruzzi, 1972). *Prolonged* activation is elicited most easily from this region. In its simple form, the general hypothesis was that in the reticular formation the brain possesses some general *positive* mechanism which martials its activity into a state of active awareness, without which the organism lapses into unconsciousness, even though its specific sensory and motor pathways are still functioning. It may be as well here to mention some problems that accompany work of this kind, quite apart from the formidable problems of language. First, it was (and sometimes still is) assumed that electrical changes in the brain (desynchronization of the massed electrical discharges of the forebrain as recorded through the scalp – the electroencephalogram or EEG) following stimulation of the 'ascending activating system' are a neurophysiological sign of behavioural wakefulness. This is not the case: for example, the unresponsive and often stuperose-seeming animal with bilateral destruction of the substantia nigra and neighbouring reticular formation has an EEG usually associated with waking. (Such animals may well pass through waking periods without being able to *express* a response.)

The reverse situation also exists: desynchronization (i.e. 'electrical waking') also occurs during one phase of behavioural sleeping (v.i.). I take it to be sensible to regard 'waking' as meaning *behavioural* waking; and similarly with being unconscious. Clearly the underlying brain mechanisms are more complicated than the simple 'activation' hypothesis might suggest (see Jouvet, 1967). A further (and more technical) problem arises from the very structure of the reticular formation (v.i.), which makes it difficult, if not impossible, either to destroy or to stimulate particular regions without involving others. As pointed out by Ramón-Moliner and Nauta (1966), one other cause of confusion has been the common use of the terms 'reticular formation', 'reticular system', 'ascending activating system' and the like, both as synonyms and as terms requiring no precise definition, as in the question: 'Do flies have a reticular formation?'

It may seem, however, that these are not real problems. A semantic exercise will correct the last confusion; and as for the multiplicity of functions – the reticular formation is not alone in this. In fact, the semantic exercise is not as simple as might be imagined: even 'reticularists' admit that it is difficult to define the characteristics of the reticular formation (Ramón-Moliner and Nauta, 1966). And against the second argument one can point out that we know relatively little of the internal organization of the reticular formation – it remains substantially a 'black box' – and, more seriously, unlike most other parts of the brain concerned with perception (the 'specific pathways'), where functional activities are held in spatial isolation and brought together in a readily discernible, orderly manner, all the activities so far mentioned are ascribed to territories that at least overlap considerably, and often coincide. The term 'non-specific pathway' presupposes organization of this sort.

The differences between the 'specific' and 'non-specific' can be emphasized by a brief examination of some sensory pathways in the brain. The visual, somatosensory (body sensibility) and auditory systems all comprise well-defined pathways made up of clearly demarcated nuclei (collections of neuronal cell bodies) each linked to the other by readily discernible tracts of axons. Each system, although subject to descending influence, makes a steady progress upwards and 'ends' in the cerebral cortex, where an ordered progression of convergent pathways links the information from diverse senses, directing it into the labyrinthine circuitry of the so-called limbic system – brain regions concerned with memory, recall, emotion, response, etc. (Powell, 1973). At the same time, these specific sensory pathways are said to divert information into the polysynaptic thicket of the non-specific reticular formation, where, as we shall see, cells and their processes present a bewildering mixture, and information converges and diverges in all directions. There, the information is said to serve in some ill-specified way functions related to consciousness, attention, body posture and the like (Scheibel and Scheibel, 1967).

What are the results of applying the techniques that have produced so clear a picture of the specific sensory systems to the reticular formation itself? One of the first and relatively simple exercises is to attempt a division into nuclei, i.e. spatially separate collections of nerve cells, each group with a distinctive morphology (including its connections with the rest of the nervous system), implying an identifiable function. To a medical student, making his first acquaintance with the subject the reticular formation usually appears to be and is often (half-facetiously) described as: 'What is left in the brain stem when everything else has been identified'. Perhaps the most vigorous opponent of this view has been Olszewski. He and his colleagues have identified more than 40 nuclei in the mammalian brain stem (e.g. Olszewski and Baxter, 1954; see also Brodal, 1957). Moreover, not only is it impossible to deny that such sub-divisions are visible in simple histological preparations, but also that, in some cases at least, their connections are quite precise, e.g. those of the medullary lateral reticular nucleus with the spinal cord and cerebellum (see Corvaja *et al.,* 1977); or of the midbrain tegmental nuclei of Gudden with the limbic system (Nauta and Haymaker, 1969).

It must be admitted, however, that considerable difficulties are posed for those who hold this more or less conventional mosaic view of the reticular formation. Consider, for example, the arrangement of dendrites, which processes comprise up to 95% of the receptor surface of a nerve cell (Sholl, 1953). In the reticular formation, dendrites extend over long distances: those from the cells of one nucleus interdigitate with the dendrites of another, overlapping by distances measured in millimetres (Ramón-Moliner and Nauta, 1966; Scheibel and Scheibel, 1967). Further, these dendrites weave their way through the profusion of fibre bundles that comprise the central tegmental fasciculus of Forel. These bundles are a major source of input to reticular cell dendrites, and are themselves made up, to a large extent, of reticular cell efferents. Such an arrangement scarcely encourages credence in the notion of well-demarcated nuclei. Mannen (1960) after studying the architecture of the reticular formation, introduced the terms 'open' and 'closed' nuclei, the former made up of neurons with dendrites arranged as just described (the 'isodendritic' configuration of Ramón-Moliner and Nauta, 1966); and the latter with dendrites which are short, much branched, and curved and re-entrant at the boundary of a nucleus, producing a sharp interface with the surroundings (the 'idiodendritic' configuration). Idiodendritic neurons, or something like them, are found, for example, in cranial nerve nuclei, the olivary complexes, and the basilar pons and nuclei of the specific sensory pathways. They are also found in other 'specifically connected' brain stem nuclei such as the lateral reticular nucleus, and Gudden's nuclei (v.s.). The remainder make up the 'isodendritic' core of the brainstem, extending from the spinal cord to at least the subthalamic region of the forebrain (Leontovich and Zhukova, 1963; Ramón-Moliner and Nauta, 1966). Apart from the dendritic characteristic already mentioned, one of the few readily recognizable signs of morphological regularity is the flattening of the dendritic trees, so that they are arranged across the brain stem, radiating from their cell bodies like the spokes of rimless wheels, crossing the afferent fibre bundles at right angles (Scheibel and Scheibel, 1967). At first sight this arrangement is not unlike that found in the cerebellum between the Purkinje cell dendrites and their afferent parallel fibres. Indeed, it incorporates one of its essential features – one axon contacts many neurons. However, in the reticular formation, instead of each fibre making a localized, single contact, many of the axons give off collateral branches that run *along* the dendrites, presumably establishing many separate contacts, and certainly crossing nuclear boundaries. Only the spatial separation across the brain stem of the principal sources of input (e.g. the spinal cord, the cerebral cortex, the inferior and superior colliculi, the cerebellum, other parts of the reticular formation) may tend to produce a bias of input in any one region – which will, however, contain dendrites from more than one nucleus (Valverde, 1962; Scheibel and Scheibel, 1967). This accords well with the observation that many neurons in the reticular formation are polysensory (i.e. they may be activated by more than one type of stimulus). Indeed, both this physiological observation and the morphology so far discussed are compatible with notions of non-specific function. The description of reticular neurons such as those of the magnocellular nucleus in the medulla, each sending branches of one and the same axon into the spinal cord as well as up to the diencephalon of the forebrain, adds strength to this, as does the finding that the brain stem in the region of this nucleus takes part in the control of skeletal muscle tone, of respiration as well as in 'ascending activation' and therefore, presumably, in the phenomena of consciousness (see Figure 1). This 'diffuse network' hypothesis would retain the nuclear nomenclature only for descriptive convenience, but would admit that in real terms no more than a general sub-division seems possible. This sub-division admits of a medial column, containing mostly large cell bodies scattered on either side of the medially placed raphe nuclei, and a lateral column containing most of the smaller neurons. The medial sub-division is that which gives rise to most of the efferents that reach the forebrain, whereas the lateral division, apart from a projection of pontine origin to the spinal cord, and projections from certain special cell groups (v.i.), appears to be more intrinsic in its connections (Nauta and Kuypers, 1958; Kuypers, 1973; Kuypers and Maisky, 1975).

One way of attempting to push the analysis of the reticular formation further whilst accepting wholeheartedly the 'diffuse' concept (including the notion that the formation acts to give 'general tone' to activity in different parts of the nervous system, whether they be concerned with movement, sensation or processes as complex as those of cognition and memory), is to regard it as a mosaic of *individual neurons*, rather than of nuclei. This mosaic is to be treated as a statistical network to which one applies some form of computer analysis (e.g. Magoun quoted by Scheibel and Scheibel, 1967). One problem with this approach is that 'network theory' can be applied to any part of the nervous system, and it is easy to lose sight of the specific characteristics of the immediate problem (e.g. Burns, 1968). The other is that many investigators are not properly equipped either to understand what is being proposed or to appraise its value.

Another approach is more traditional. Let us suppose the reticular formation to be a collection of more or less specific neuron populations, but populations that are to a large extent mixed together rather than separated into spatially isolated groups. The problem then becomes one of finding a clearly distinguishing feature to identify each population. Recently introduced techniques now make this possible, since they enable one to trace out and identify neuronal pathways on the basis of the particular transmitter substances they contain. The most successful of these to date has been the application of the Falck-Hillarp technique, by means of which various monoamine compounds found in some neurons can be made to fluoresce under ultraviolet light. (As it turns out, many of these cells in the reticular formation had been recognized as forming distinct and unusual groups by virtue of their containing the pigment neuromelanin.) On this basis, neurons can be divided into two groups: those that exhibit a greenish fluorescence and which contain catecholamines (dopamine and noradrenaline), and those that fluoresce a weak yellow colour due to the presence of the indolealkylamine compound serotonin (5-hydroxytryptamine, 5HT). Details of these cell groups are given in Tables 1 and 2, and Figures 2–7. (Our knowledge is derived largely from studies of laboratory animals, including rat, cat and monkey (see, for example, Dahlström and Fuxe, 1964; Pin *et al.*, 1968; Felton

Table 1 Locations of monoamine-containing cell groups

Group	*Nucleus with which cells are associated*
A1	Anterior to lateral reticular nucleus
A2	Nucleus commissuralis (part)
A3	Dorsal accessory olive (part)
A4	Nucleus pigmentosus tegmentocerebellaris
A5	Deep to subcaeruleus
A6	Locus caeruleus
A7	Nucleus subcaeruleus
A8	Substantia nigra lateralis
A9	Substantia nigra compacta
A10	Nucleus linearis, nucleus parabrachialis pigmentosus, interstitial nucleus of ventral tegmental decussation
A11	Substantia grisea periventricularis (IIIrd ventricle), around fasciculus retroflexus
A12	Hypothalamus nucleus arcuatus, nucleus periventricularis anterior)
A13	Zona incerta (medial)
B1	Nucleus raphe pallidus } + paramedian nucleus
B2	Nucleus raphe obscurus } + paramedian nucleus
B3	Nucleus-raphe pallidus + nucleus raphe magnus
B4	Periventricular grey (IVth ventricle)
B5	Nucleus raphe pontis
B6	Central pontine grey
B7	Nucleus raphe dorsalis + periaqueductal grey
B8	Nucleus raphe medianus
B9	Lateral to interpeduncular nucleus

Table 2 Projections of catecholamine pathways

Cell group	*Proposed distribution of projection fibres*
A1 (NA) A2 (NA)	Spinal cord
A1–A5 (NA)	Hypothalamus, preoptic area
A3 (NA) A4 (NA) A5 (NA)	
A6 (NA) A7 (NA)	Thalamus, neocortex, hippocampus, amygdala, septum, cerebellum, spinal cord
A8 (DA)	Striatum
A9 (DA)	Striatum. Anterior cingulate cortex
A10 (DA)	Mesolimbic region (nucleus accumbens, olfactory tubercle, interstitial nucleus of stria terminals): Frontal cortex: Entorhinal cortex; Septum
A11 (DA)	?Medial hypothalamus; midline thalamus; habenulae; pretectum
A12 (DA)	Median eminence
A13 (DA)	?Caudal thalamus; zona incerta; dorsal and anterior hypothalamus

[NA = Noradrenaline; DA = Dopamine]

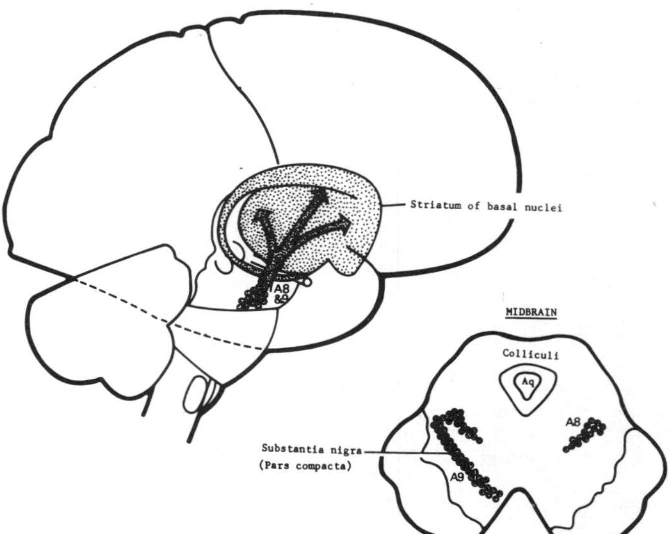

Figure 2 The nigro-striate pathway in schematic lateral view of the human brain. The lower figure illustrates the position of the substantia nigra pars compacta (cell group A9) and pars lateralis (A8). Circles represent cell bodies

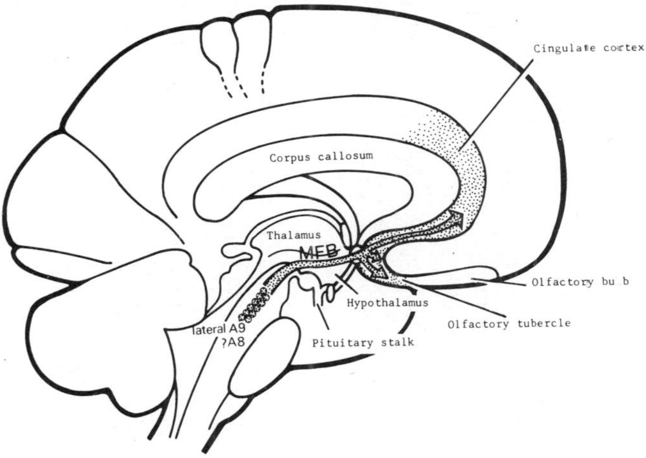

Figure 3 Scheme of the additional pathways thought to arise from the substantia nigra pars compacta. MFB = Median forebrain bundle

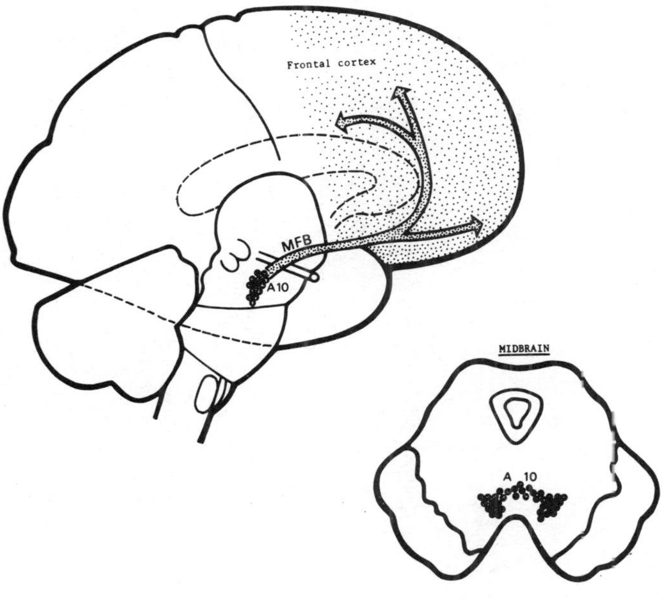

Figure 4 Probable distribution of fibres from cell group A10 (see also Figure 5). The hatched line outlines the position of the corpus callosum. MFB = Median forebrain bundle

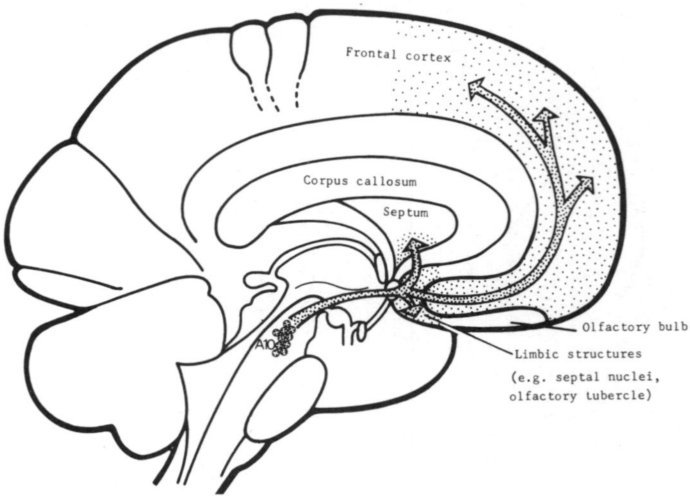

Figure 5 Additional projection fields of cell group A10

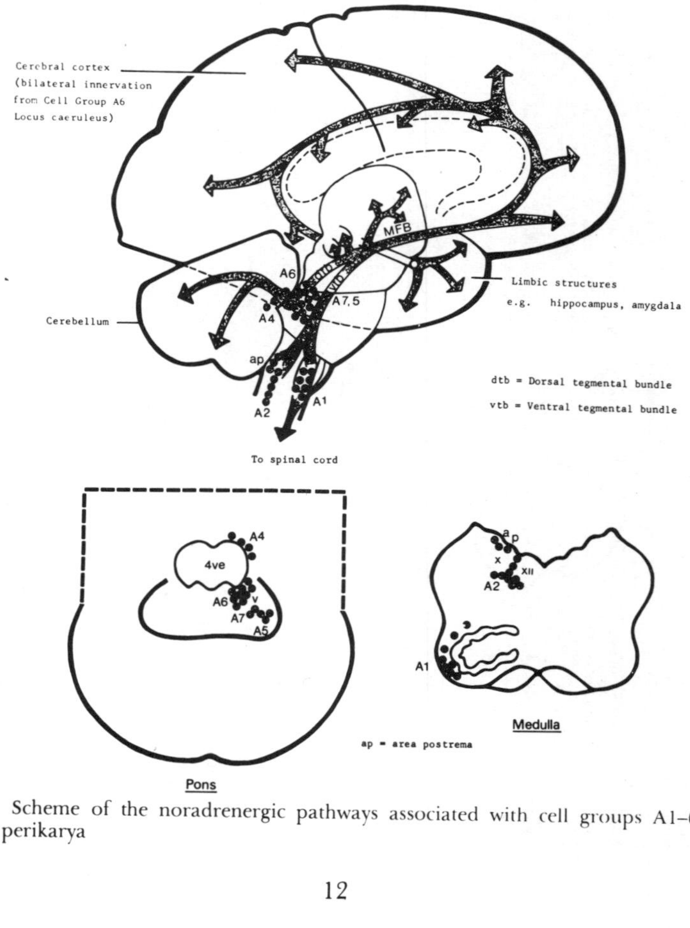

Figure 6 Scheme of the noradrenergic pathways associated with cell groups A1–6. Circles represent perikarya

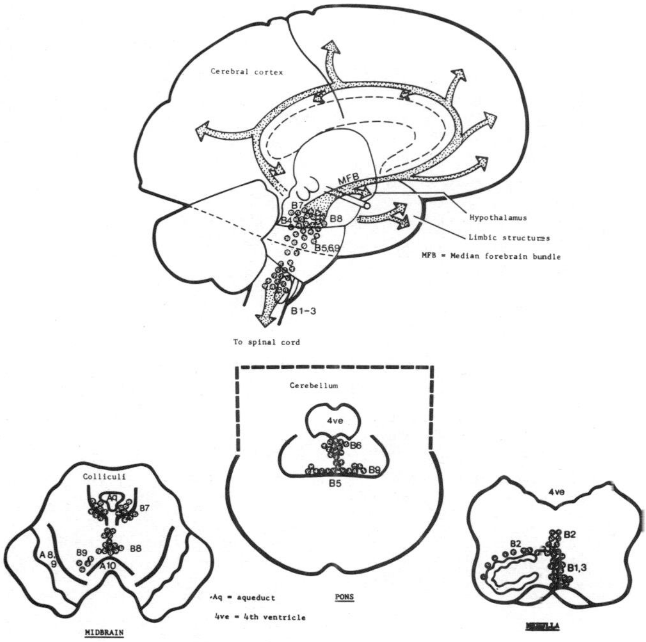

Figure 7 Serotonergic pathways illustrated as in other figures

et al., 1974; Jacobowitz and Palkovits, 1974; Palkovits and Jacobowitz, 1974; Lindvall *et al.*, 1974) but the illustrations use the human brain on the assumption that it is more familiar to non-specialists. The broad accuracy of the figures is supported by the observations of Nobin and Björklund, 1973, and Olson *et al.*, 1973a,b, on adult and fetal human brains.) Some of these findings have been challenged and it is possible that some of the projections have been postulated as a result of excessive enthusiasm. For example, there is evidence that the *dendrites* of these neurons contain transmitter and have morphologies in some ways not unlike their axons (v.i.). Areas like the inferior olivary complex, which is close to monoamine cell groups, may therefore have no more than the appearance of a catecholamine innervation, due only to dendrites passing through its substance (Sladek and Bowman, 1975; Sladek and Parnavelas, 1975).

Catecholamine-containing cells (the A groups of Dahlström and Fuxe, 1964) tend to lie away from the mid-line. None of the dopamine-containing cells (groups A8–13) are found in the hindbrain: most of these cells (groups A8–10) are found in the midbrain (Figures 2–5), where the most striking collection forms the pars compacta of the substantia nigra (A9). Groups A11–13 are in the diencephalon, where group A12 is associated with the median eminence. Noradrenergic groups (A1–7) (see Figure 6) occur in the hindbrain, and their projection fibres lie in the central tegmental fasciculus where they form two rather poorly demarcated bundles: the dorsal tegmental bundle (associated with group A6 – the locus caeruleus) and the ventral tegmental bundle running throughout the brain stem (Ungerstedt, 1971). In the upper brain stem the fibre systems of the two sides exchange axons and finally, as they approach the hypothalamus, join the median forebrain bundle to enter the forebrain. (A full description of the extremely complex trajectories of these and the other catecholamine fibres is given by Lindvall and Björklund, 1974). The distribution of fibres from the locus caeruleus has been especially well studied (see Maeda *et al.*, 1973; Jones and Moore, 1977): these cells distribute axons to widespread regions of the brain (Table 2). Much of this projection, including that to the cerebral (neo)cortex, is bilateral (Freedman *et al.*, 1975; Kievit and Kuypers, 1975; Gatter and Powell, 1977). Fibres from midbrain cell groups A8–10 gain the forebrain by running through the lateral hypothalamus and medial subthalamus and reach the corpus striatum through the ansal system. Some of these fibres, however, run forwards in the company of the median forebrain bundle and innervate the granular frontal cortex, as well as the anterior cingulate cortex and other 'mesolimbic' and limbic structures (Ungerstedt, 1971; Lindvall and Björklund, 1974; Lindvall *et al.*, 1974; Fuxe *et al.*, 1974; Beckstead, 1976; Berger *et al.*, 1976; Carter and Fibiger, 1977).

Serotonin-containing cells (see Figure 7) were named groups B1–9 by Dahlström and Fuxe. They are found almost exclusively close to or within the midline raphe nuclei. As with the catecholamine A groups, these cells do not necessarily constitute the whole population of a nucleus, e.g. the cells of group B3 found in the nucleus raphe magnus are relatively few and lie scattered among neurons that contain no monoamines. Catecholamine-containing fibres have been seen ramifying among the serotonin cells and perhaps synapsing with them (Dahlström and Fuxe, 1964). The associated serotonin projection fibres are found in the central tegmental fasciculus, close to the midline.

That monoamine fibres innervate extensive regions of the brain is apparent from the illustrations and tables, but it should not be assumed that the distribution in a given region is uniform. For example, the noradrenergic cells of the locus caeruleus (A6) projecting to the occipital lobe of the cerebral cortex are relatively fewer in number than those to the paracentral region (Gatter and Powell, 1977). Also, in the cortex, the endings of noradrenergic fibres are said to concentrate in layer 1; serotonin fibres in layers 4, 5 and 6; and dopamine fibres in layers 5 and 6 (Emson and Lindvall, 1976). (Note that those of intralaminar or 'non-specific' thalamic origin, representing the classical reticular pathway, end in layers 1, 2 and perhaps 3 (Jones and Leavitt, 1974; T. R. Price and K. E. Webster – unpublished observations.)

The axons of monoamine-containing cells are peculiar in several ways. They are extremely thin (less than 1 μm in diameter), lack myelin sheaths, and remained largely undiscovered by conventional methods (Moore, 1970; Moore *et al.*, 1971). Their very wide distribution seems to be brought about by extensive collateral branching. (It is remarkable that the few thousand cells that make up the locus caeruleus should innervate such widely scattered regions.) The branching often becomes more intense once a target area is reached. Another striking characteristic of these axons is the occurrence of numerous varicosities along their length. These swellings contain dense-cored vesicles (presumably the immediate source of the amine transmitter) but most lack the membrane thickenings visible by electron microscopy which would be expected to relate the axons to the surfaces of target sites (Hökfelt, 1968; Descarries and Lapierre, 1973; Lapierre *et al.*, 1973; Tennyson *et al.,* 1974; Descarries *et al.,* 1975). Such thickenings are characteristic of the usual functional (synaptic) junction between nerve cells: they indicate regional membrane specialization where two cell processes are literally bound together. It is presumed that they also label sites to which the action of transmitter substance, and therefore the passage of information across the junction, is limited. It has been suggested that in the case of monoamine systems, transmitter may be released from *any* varicosity, perhaps producing something akin to a 'lake' of transmitter rather than localized 'puddles'. This suggests a humoral mechanism akin to that of hormones, but it must be borne in mind that the absence of electron-dense membrane specializations does not necessarily indicate that localized receptor specializations are absent from the postsynaptic membrane. Nor does it automatically follow that the transmitter could act generally upon *any* neuron in the vicinity, and through any part of its surface. With that qualification, it is certainly difficult to see how, other than in some quasi-hormonal fashion, one other most curious feature of these fibres could operate: some serotergic axons thrust their way between ependymal cells lining the brain cavities (especially the third and fourth ventricles) where they appear to terminate quite freely in the cerebrospinal fluid (Lorez and Richards, 1975; Chan Palay, 1975). It has been suggested that the varicosities may not be a stable structural/functional feature, but may vary in number and position, waxing and waning over relatively short periods of time (Descarries *et al.*, 1975). They are certainly capable of considerable growth in the adult (Moore *et al.,* 1971; Emson *et al.,* 1977). This could well imply that any function of the monoamine pathways could vary, at least in effectiveness, with time. The prospect of so labile a morphology is a challenging one which awaits investigation and exploitation. The characteristics of the projections from these cell groups therefore appear to fit them for some general, 'controlling' role, rather than the conveying of highly specified information.

A discussion of possible functions of these pathways must be prefaced with a word of warning. First, the experimental procedures used are often subject to the criticisms levelled against investigation of the reticular formation in general (v.s.). Secondly, it must be admitted that much of the evidence of the functional significance of these neurons is circumstantial and involves a great deal of extrapolation from a test-tube experiment to generalized phenomena such as the overall behaviour of laboratory animals and the effects of drugs on patients. Interpretation of both these latter in terms of *specific neuronal mechanisms* is notoriously difficult, and subject to major revisions from time to time, as the history of our knowledge of the essential immediate pathology of Parkinson's disease shows. There is, of course, a well-established relationship between the proper functioning of the dopamine cells (group A9) of the substantia nigra and the performance of movement. This is probably an expression of the relationship of the neurons with the basal nuclei, malfunction of which can produce motor disturbances of many kinds, including the release of repetitive, stereotyped behaviour patterns (see Webster, 1975; Yahr, 1977). Note, however, that nigral cells also project to 'mesolimbic' areas (Figure 3 and Table 2). Disappearance of these (and possibly other) monoaminergic neurons is the essential lesion of Parkinson's disease. (Only a few years ago some primary disturbance of a *cholinergic* mechanism could be and commonly was held to be responsible, on the basis of techniques fundamentally similar to those now used to investigate the monoamine systems. That should perhaps give us pause.) There is good experimental evidence that hypokinesia (failure to move), adypsia (failure to drink), and aphagia (failure to eat), and a general lack of responsiveness to the environment, previously ascribed to damage to the lateral hypothalamus is in fact a consequence of destruction of the ascending fibres from the substantia nigra and perhaps the ventral tegmental region (group A10) (Ungerstedt, 1974; see also Kelly, 1975). To ascribe some precise function to this latter collection of cells is difficult, but the distribution of its projection fibres (to limbic structures and granular frontal cortex – Figures 4 and 5; Table 2) suggests that its disruption would have considerable behavioural consequences. Group A10 also lies within the 'reward area' found by self-stimulation experiments – that is the region in which stimulation seems to yield a feeling of 'pleasure' or 'well-being' – although the interpretation of such findings is extraordinarily difficult (Crow, 1972).

It is well-established that many of the powerful drugs used in the treatment of psychosis (e.g. phenothiazine derivatives) interfere with dopamine-based transmission. Some of these produce parkinsonian-like side effects, presumably because of their effects on the nigro-striatal system: interestingly, those drugs that do not, tend to have additional, inherent anticholinergic properties (Fuxe *et al.,* 1970; Iversen, 1975). There is also evidence that some hallucinogenic drugs (amphetamine derivatives) act through dopaminergic receptors and therefore possibly upon these systems. Whether one can ascribe psychotic illness at least in part to pathology of all or some of these systems remains a fascinating but still unproven hypothesis. It seems likely to be at least a 'final common path'. The few reports of *morphological* postmortem findings in the brains of schizophrenics have not so far been encouraging in comparison with those from the brains of patients suffering from Parkinson's disease (Olson *et al.,* 1973b).

In general the noradrenergic pathways are assumed to play a role in the mechanisms of drive and aggression (Fuxe, *et al.,* 1970). Again, the ventral (noradrenergic) tegmental bundle lies within the 'reward' area of Olds (Ritter and Stein, 1974). Tricyclic antidepressant drugs appear to be effective through interfering with noradrenergic transmission. Of these drugs, imipramine is also thought to influence serotoninergic pathways, as are some hallucinogenic compounds. The latter observation raises the possibility of some involvement of serotonin neurons in the symptomatology of psychosis, but this link is very much weaker than that of the dopamine systems (but see Ellison, 1975 for a different view).

Findings of such a generalized nature are clearly compatible with the widespread distribution of the monoamine pathways in the forebrain (Table 2). Indeed, in the absence of these far-flung projections it would be difficult to account for such effects. For example, temporal lobe stimulation also produces hallucinations, whether by involvement of its supplementary visual or auditory cortices or its limbic-system components. Few would suggest, however, that psychosis is *specifically* a temporal-lobe disturbance; but temporal lobe activities can easily be invoked under the umbrella of malfunction of such diffuse systems as those making up the monoamine pathways.

The suggestion of some involvement in the pathologies of depression and psychosis is interesting not only in itself but in relation to the well-known disturbances of sleep that accompany these afflictions. Normal sleep has two phases: a stage of light sleep (when body muscle tone is high), referred to as 'slow wave sleep' (SWS) because of the characteristic pattern of electrical discharge as recorded in the EEG; and a stage of deep sleep when muscles are relaxed. These two phases alternate throughout sleeping hours. The latter phase occupies some 25% of the total sleep period, and is the phase during which dreaming occurs (Jouvet, 1967, 1972, 1974). It is known as 'rapid eye movement sleep' (REMS) or 'paradoxical sleep' (PS). The former description is self-explanatory: it is interesting to note that the discharge patterns of the lateral geniculate body and occipital cortex (parts of the specific visual pathway) also change during REMS. The term 'paradoxical sleep' refers to the observation that the 'brain wave' pattern closely resembles that found when the animal is awake.

The upper parts of the raphe system (nuclei raphe dorsalis et raphe medianus containing B7 and 8) appear to control SWS, which is abolished by their destruction, whilst PS is unaffected. PS can be suppressed by destruction of the lower raphe nuclei (nuclei raphe pontis et magnus, with which groups B3, 4, 5 are associated). In this case, however, SWS is also reduced, but not eliminated. Pharmacological studies suggest the crucial cells in the raphe to be those containing serotonin, but other neurons are also involved in regulating sleep. After bilateral destruction of the locus caeruleus area (probably of the noradrenergic cell groups A6, 7) the animal falls into continuous slow wave sleep, from which it does not really waken. All signs of paradoxical sleep are absent. Thus the raphe system appears to be involved in the mechanisms of falling asleep and the production of both SWS and PS; and the locus caeruleus in the mechanisms of PS and waking. Coma following extensive damage in the upper part of the midbrain might be regarded as due to the severance of the forebrain from these mechanisms controlling waking and sleeping, together with the added effects of interruption of the nigral projection system. The normal function of sleep is unknown, but there appears to be a relationship between the occurrence of a normal sleep cycle and the effective laying down of memory traces (see Fishbein and Gutwein, 1977). Again, the proposed widespread distribution of the monoamine systems to the forebrain is in keeping with the functional observations. Additionally, the changes in muscle tone during PS could be attributed to the known projection of the locus caeruleus to the spinal cord.

The relationship to waking raises the possibility that we are here dealing with the substrate of the 'ascending activating system', and much evidence supports this correlation. The dorsal tegmental bundle and the locus caeruleus appear to be the strongest contenders for the title (Bonvallet and Newman-Taylor, 1967; Shellenberger and Gordon, 1975), but a general identity of areas producing 'cortical activation' and the location of catecholamine pathways cannot be ignored. However, the monoamine pathways are not the only contenders for this role.

It has been proposed that the responsible pathways are in fact cholinergic. The histochemical method for acetylcholinesterase has enabled maps of the distribution of cells containing this enzyme to be produced (Shute and Lewis, 1967; Jacobowitz and Palkovits, 1974; Palkovits and Jacobowitz, 1974). A rough distribution is indicated in Figure 8. Cholinesterase-positive neurons in the midbrain nucleus cuneiformis and in the pontine parabrachial nucleus appear to project upon the forebrain through the ventral tegmental bundle (Palkovits *et al.*, 1974). The proposed distribution of their axons in the forebrain overlaps considerably with those of monoamine cells, and includes limbic structures and cerebral cortex. A serious disadvantage of this method is that acetylcholinesterase is not of necessity associated with the presence of acetylcholine *as a transmitter*. For example, the occurrence of histochemically identified acetylcholinesterase in the cell bodies of the locus caeruleus is entirely unexplained (Lewis and Schon, 1975).

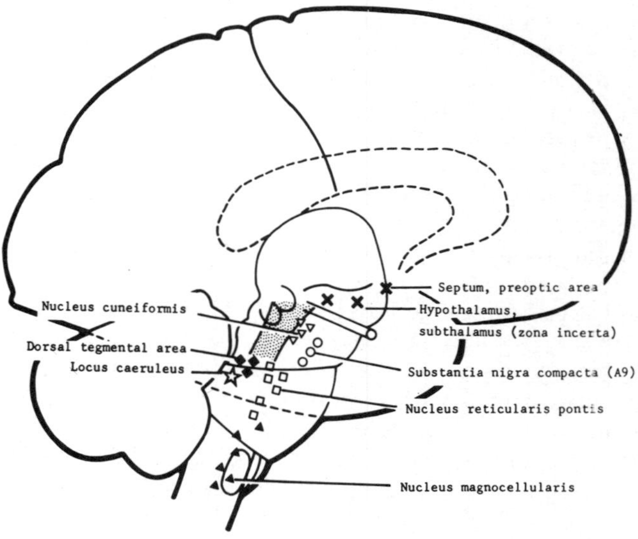

Figure 8 A scheme of the general distribution of histochemically identified cholinesterase-containing cell groups. The shaded area represents the periaqueductal grey. N.B. All cranial nerve motor nuclei are cholinesterase positive

On the other hand 'ascending activation' with cortical desynchronization is accompanied by increased release of acetylcholine from the cerebral cortex.

Other possible transmitter anatomies are now being mapped out; the distribution of the peptides known as substance P, and the enkephalins (Hughes and Kosterlitz, 1977), as well as the location of opiate receptor sites, have received special attention. This work is still at an early stage, and although the distribution of enkephalin-containing fibres and terminals in the forebrain shows remarkable similarity to that of the monoamines (the basal nuclei, septum, hypothalamus, amygdala, cerebral cortex all contain enkephalins, see Simantov *et al.*, 1977), no very wide distribution of possible parent cells has so far been established. According to Hökfelt *et al.* (1977), met-enkephalin cells occur in the periaqueductal grey of the midbrain, the nuclei raphe magnus et pallidus (cf. cell groups B2, 3), and in the nucleus caudalis of the trigeminal nerve and spinal cord dorsal horn laminae I, II and V. There is a close relationship between these and the substance P distribution which appears to link this brain stem system and the serotonin cell groups into the mechanisms underlying pain perception (Basbaum *et al.*, 1976; Nathan, 1977).

This raises an important point: the functions ascribed to the now more specified parts of the reticular formation have tended to proliferate over the last few years. In addition to the properties sketched out above, these pathways have been implicated in learning (but see Mason and Iversen, 1977; and Crow *et al.*, 1977), in responses of the autonomic nervous system, and in the control of movement (Fuxe *et al.*, 1970). The locus caeruleus has even been identified with the midbrain motor centre (Steeves *et al.*, 1975), and has been shown to be involved with motor activity in a general way (Donaldson *et al.*, 1976). (And this in spite of the massive known projections to the spinal cord from non-aminergic cells in the pons and medulla.)

In fact, there has been a remarkable tendency to ascribe to these pathways functions as multifarious as those originally applied to the classical reticular formation. Almost certainly, some of these results will eventually be revealed as different facets of a common phenomenon. For example, if various aminergic cell groups are involved in the control of the sleep/waking cycle, and if the laying down of effective memory traces is interlocked with the occurrence of a normal sleep pattern (Drucker-Colin and McGaugh, 1977), it is hardly to be wondered at that damage to these amine cell groups would interfere with at least some types of learning.

It must also be pointed out that in their dendritic and axonal configurations these 'systems' pose exactly the same problems as does the rest of reticular formation, and additional problems loom large. For example, the relationships of the monoamine pathways to the remainder of the reticular formation are not understood. Indeed, the sources of their afferents are unknown – a singularly striking omission in our knowledge, for if these pathways are capable of exerting influences as widespread as is supposed, to understand the factors to which they respond must be of paramount importance. The concentration of effort on unravelling their significance has, moreover, led to an ignoring of the other massive components of the central tegmental fasciculus and the 'classical', 'non-specific' input to the cerebral cortex through the 'non-specific' thalamus, not to mention that from the substantia nigra (possibly its non-aminergic part) via the ventromedial thalamus (Herkenham, 1976). The recent successes must not blind us to this any more than to the even more striking advances made in our knowledge of the organization of specific pathways. Science, as much as any other human activity, is subject to changes of fashion – brought about, one hopes, as much by the vicissitudes of technique as by the capriciousness of human nature – but a return to the 'reticular euphoria' of 20 years ago is surely undesirable.

REFERENCES

Basbaum, A. I., Clanton, C. H. and Fields, H. L. (1976). Opiate and stimulus-produced analgesia: functional anatomy of a medullo-spinal pathway. *Proc. Nat. Acad. Sci. USA*, **73,** 4685

Beckstead, R. M. (1976). Convergent thalamic and mesencephalic projections to anterior medial cortex in the rat. *J. Comp. Neurol.*, **166,** 403

Berger, B., Thierry, A. M., Tassin, J. P. and Moyne, M. A. (1976). Dopaminergic innervation of rat prefrontal cortex: a fluorescence histochemical study. *Brain Res.*, **196,** 133

Bonvallet, M. and Newman-Taylor, A. (1967). Neurophysiological evidence for a differential organization of the mesencephalic reticular formation. *Electroenceph. Clin. Neurophysiol.*, **22,** 54

Brodal, A. (1957). The reticular formation of the brain stem; anatomical aspects and functional correlations. (Edinburgh and London: Oliver & Boyd)

Burns, B. Delisle (1968). *The Uncertain Nervous System.* (London: Edward Arnold)

Carter, D. A. and Fibiger, H. C. (1977). Ascending projections of presumed dopamine-containing neurons in the ventral tegmentum of the rat as demonstrated by horseradish peroxidase. *Neuroscience*, **2,** 569

Chan-Palay, V. (1975). Serotonin axons in the supra- and sub-ependymal plexuses and in the leptomeninges. Their roles in local alterations of cerebrospinal fluid and vasomotor activity. *Brain Res.*, **102,** 103

Corvaja, N., Crofova, I., Pompeiana, O. and Walberg, F. (1977). The lateral reticular nucleus in the cat – I. An experimental anatomical study of its spinal and supraspinal afferent connections. *Neuroscience*, **2,** 537

Crow, T. J. (1972). A map of the rat mesencephalon for electrical self-stimulation. *Brain Res.*, **36,** 265

Crow, T. J., Longden, A., Smith, A. and Wendlandt, S. (1977). Pontine tegmental lesions, monoamine neurons, and varieties of learning. *Behav. Biol.*, **20,** 184

Dahlström, A. and Fuxe, K. (1964). Evidence for the existence of monoamine-containing neurons in the central nervous system. I. Demonstration of monoamines in the cell bodies of brainstem neurons. *Acta Physiol. Scand.*, **62,** Suppl. 232, 55

Demetrescu, M., Demetrescu, M. and Iosif, G. (1965). The tonic control of cortical responsiveness by inhibitory and facilitatory diffuse influences. *Electroenceph. Clin. Neurophysiol.*, **18,** 1

Descarries, L., Beaudet, A. and Watkins, K. (1975). Serotonin nerve terminals in adult rat neocortex. *Brain Res.*, **100,** 563

Descarries, L., and Lapierre, Y. (1973). Noradrenergic axon terminals in the cerebral cortex of rat. I. Radioautographic visualization after topical application of DL-[^{3}H]norepinephrine. *Brain Res.*, **51,** 141

Donaldson, I. MacG., Dolphin, A., Jenner, P., Marsden, C. D. and Pycock, C. (1976). The involvement of noradrenaline in motor activity as shown by rotational behaviour after unilateral lesions of the locus coeruleus. *Brain*, **99,** 427

Drucker-Colin, R. R. and McGaugh, J. L. (eds.) (1977). *Neurobiology of Sleep and Memory.* (New York: Academic Press)

Ellison, G. D. (1975). Behaviour and the balance between norepinephrine and serotonin. *Acta Neurobiol. Exp.*, **35,** 499

Emson, P. C., Björklund, A. and Stenevi, U. (1977). Evaluation of the regenerative capacity of central dopaminergic noradrenergic and cholinergic neurons using iris implants as targets. *Brain Res.,* **135,** 87

Emson, P. C. and Lindvall, O. (1976). Distribution of neurotransmitter candidates in the rat neo-cortex – a brief review. In O. Creutzfield, (ed.) *Exp. Brain. Res., Suppl. 1 – Afferent and Intrinsic Organization of Laminated Structures in the Brain.* pp. 329–336. (Berlin: Springer--Verlag)

Felton, D. L., Laties, A. M. and Carpenter, M. B. (1974). Monoamine-containing cell bodies in the squirrel monkey brain. *Am. J. Anat.,* **139,** 153

Fishbein, W. and Gutwein, B. M. (1977). Paradoxical sleep and memory storage process. *Behav. Biol.,* **19,** 425

Freedman, R., Foote, S. L. and Bloom, F. E. (1975). Histochemical characterization of a neocortical projection of the locus coeruleus in the squirrel monkey. *J. Comp. Neurol.,* **164,** 209

Fuxe, K., Hökfelt, T., Johansson, O., Jonsson, G., Lidbrink, P. and Ljungdahl, A. (1974). The origin of the dopamine nerve terminals in limbic and frontal cortex. Evidence for mesocortical dopamine neurons. *Brain Res.,* **82,** 349

Fuxe, K., Hökfelt, T. and Ungerstedt, U. (1970). Morphological and functional aspects of central monoamine neurons. *Int. Rev. Neurobiol.,* **13,** 93

Gatter, K. C. and Powell, T. P. S. (1977). The projection of the locus coeruleus upon the neocortex in the macaque monkey. *Neuroscience,* **2,** 441

Grillner, S. and Shik, M. L. (1973). On the descending control of the lumbosacral spinal cord from the 'mesemcephalic motor region'. *Acta Physiol. Scand.,* **87,** 320

Herkenham, M. (1976). The nigro-thalamic-cortical connection mediated by the nucleus ventralis medialis thalami: evidence for a widespread cortical distribution in the rat. *Anat. Rec.,* **184,** 462 (Abs.)

Hernández-Péon, R. (1955). Central mechanisms controlling conduction along central pathways. *Acta Neurol. Latinoam.,* **1,** 256

Hökfelt, T. (1968). *In vitro* studies on central and peripheral monoamine neurons at the ultrastructural level. *Z. Zellforsch.,* **91,** 1

Hökfelt, T., Ljungdahl, A., Terenius, L., Elde, R. and Nilsson, G. (1977). Immunohistochemical analysis of peptide pathways possibly related to pain and analgesia: enkephalin and substance P. *Proc. Nat. Acad. Sci. USA.,* **74,** 3081

Hughes, J. and Kosterlitz, H. W. (1977). Opoid peptides. *Br. Med. Bull.,* **33,** 157

Iversen, L. L. (1975). Dopamine receptors in the brain. *Science,* **188,** 1084

Jacobowitz, D. M. and Palkovits, M. (1974). Topographic atlas of catecholamine and acetylcholinesterase-containing neurons in the rat brain. I. Forebrain. *J. Comp. Neurol.,* **157,** 13

Jones, B. E. and Moore, R. Y. (1977). Ascending projections of the locus coeruleus in the rat. II. Autoradiographic study. *Brain Res.,* **127,** 23

Jones, E. G. and Leavitt, R. Y. (1974). Retrograde axonal transport and the demonstration of non-specific projections to the cerebral cortex and striatum from thalamic intralaminar nuclei in the rat, cat and monkey. *J. Comp. Neurol.,* **154,** 349

Jouvet, M. (1967). Neurophysiology of the states of sleep. *Physiol. Rev.,* **47,** 117

Jouvet, M. (1972). The role of monoamines and acetylcholine in the regulation of the sleep-waking cycle. *Ergebrisse. Physiol.,* **64,** 166

Jouvet, M. (1974). Monoaminergic regulation of the sleep-waking cycle in the cat. In F. O. Schmitt and F. G. Worden (eds.). *The Third Neurosciences Study Program,* pp. 499–508. (M.I.T. Press)

Kelly, P. H. (1975). Unilateral 6-hydroxydopamine lesions of nigro-striatal or mesolimbic dopamine-containing terminals and the drug-induced rotation in rats. *Brain Res.,* **100,** 163

Kievit, J. and Kuypers, H. G. J. M. (1975). Basal forebrain and hypothalamic connections to frontal and parietal cortex in the rhesus monkey. *Science,* **187,** 660

Kohnstamm, O. and Quensel, F. (1908). Das centrum receptorium (sensorium) der Formatio reticularis. *Neurol. Centralblatt,* **27,** 1046

Kuypers, H. G. J. M. (1973). The anatomical organization of the descending pathways and their contributions to motor control especially in primates. In J. E. Desmedt (ed.) *New Developments in Electromyography and Clinical Neurophysiology,* Vol. 3, pp. 36–38. (Basel: Karger)

Kuypers, H. G. J. M. and Maisky, V. A. (1975). Retrograde axonal transport of horseradish peroxidase from spinal cord to brainstem cell groups in the cat. *Neurosci. Lett.,* **1,** 9

Lapierre, Y., Beaudet, A., Demianczuk, N. and Escarries, L. (1973). Noradrenergic axon terminals in the cerebral cortex of rat. II. Quantitative data revealed by light and electron microscope radioautography of the frontal. *Brain Res.*, **63**, 175

Leontovich, T. A. and Zhukova, G. P. (1963). The specificity of neuronal structure and topography of the reticular formation in the brain and spinal cord of carnivora. *J. Comp. Neurol.*, **121**, 347

Lewis, P. R. and Schon, F. E. G. (1975). The localization of acetylcholinesterase in the locus coeruleus of the normal rat and after 6-hydroxydopamine treatment. *J. Anat. (London)*, **120**, 373

Lindsley, D. B. (1961). The reticular activating system and perceptual integration. In D. E. Sheer (ed.) *Electrical Stimulation of the Brain.* pp. 331–349. (Austin: University of Texas Press)

Lindsley, D. B., Bowden, J. W. and Magoun, H. W. (1949). Effect upon the EEG of acute injury to the brain stem activating systems. *Electroenceph. Clin. Neurophysiol.*, **1**, 475

Lindsley, D. B., Schreiner, L. H. and Magoun, H. W. (1949). Role of brainstem facilitatory systems in maintenance of spasticity. *J. Neurophysiol.*, **12**, 207

Lindvall, O. and Björklund, A. (1974). The organization of the ascending catecholamine neuron systems in the rat brain as revealed by the glyoxylic acid fluorescence method. *Acta Physiol. Scand. Suppl.*, **412**, 48

Lindvall, O., Björklund, A. Moore, R. Y. and Stenevi, U. (1974). Mesencephalic dopamine neurons projecting to neocortex. *Brain Res.*, **81**, 325

Lindvall, O., Björklund, A., Nobin, A. and Stenevi, U. (1974). The adrenergic innervation of the rat thalamus as revealed by the glyoxylic acid fluorescence method. *J. Comp. Neurol.*, **154**, 317

Lorez, H. P. and Richards, J. G. (1975). 5HT nerve terminals in the fourth ventricle of the rat brain: their identification and distribution studied by fluorescence histochemistry and electronmicroscopy. *Cell Tiss. Res.*, **165**, 37

Maeda, T., Pin, C., Salvert, D., Ligier, M. and Jouvet, M. (1973). Les neurons contenant des catécholamines du tegmentum pontique et leurs voies de projection chez le chat. *Brain Res.*, **57**, 119

Mannen, H. (1960). 'Noyau fermé' et 'noyau ouvert'. Contribution à l'étude cytoarchitectonique du tronc cérébrale envisagée du point de vue du mode d'arborisation dendritique. *Arch. Ital. Biol.*, **98**, 330

Mason, S. T. and Iversen, S. D. (1977). Effects of selective forebrain noradrenaline loss on behavioural inhibition in the rat. *J. Comp. Physiol. Psychol.*, **91**, 165

Moore, R. Y. (1970). Brain lesions and amine metabolism. *Int. Rev. Neurobiol.*, **13**, 67

Moore, R. Y., Bhatnagar, R. K. and Heller, A. (1971). Anatomical and chemical studies of a nigro-neostriatal projection in the cat. *Brain Res.*, **30**, 119

Moore, R. Y., Björklund, A. and Stenevi, U. (1971). Plastic changes in the adrenergic innervation of the rat septal area in response to denervation. *Brain Res.*, **33**, 13

Moruzzi, G. (1972). The sleep–waking cycle. *Ergeb. Physiol.*, **64**, 1

Moruzzi, G. and Magoun, H. W. (1949). Brain stem reticular formation and activation of the EEG. *Electroenceph. Clin. Neurophysiol*, **1**, 455

Nathan, P. W. (1977). Pain. *Br. Med. Bull.*, **33**, 149

Nauta, W. J. H. and Haymaker, W. (1969). Hypothalamic nuclei and fibre connections. In W. Haymaker *et al.* (eds.) *The Hypothalamus.* pp. 136–209. (Springfield: C. C. Thomas)

Nauta, W. J. H. and Kuypers, H. G. J. M. (1958). Some ascending pathways in the brainstem reticular formation. In H. H. Jasper *et al.*, (eds.) *Reticular Formation of the Brain.* pp. 3–30. (Boston: Little, Brown)

Nobin, A. and Björklund, A. (1973). Topography of the monoamine neuron systems in the human brain as revealed in fetuses. *Acta Physiol. Scand.*, Suppl. 388, 40

Olson, L., Borens, L. O. and Seiger, A. (1973a). Histochemical demonstration and mapping of 5-hydroxytryptamine- and catecholamine-containing neuron systems in the human foetal brain. *Z. Anat. Entwickl. Gesch.*, **139**, 259

Olson, L., Nyström, B. and Seiger, A. (1973b). Monoamine fluorescence histochemistry of human postmortem brain. *Brain Res.*, **63**, 231

Olszewski, J. and Baxter, D. (1954). *Cytoarchitecture of the Human Brain Stem.* (Basle: Karger)

Palkovits, M. and Jacobowitz, D. M. (1974). Topographic atlas of catecholamine- and acetylcholinesterase-containing neurons in the rat brain. II. Mesencephalon and rhomoncephalon. *J. Comp. Neurol.*, **157**, 29

Palkovits, M., Richardson, J. S. and Jacobowitz, D. M. (1974). A histochemical study of ventral tegmental acetylcholinesterase-containing pathway following destructive lesions. *Brain Res.*, **81**, 183

Pin, C., Jones, B. and Jouvet, M. (1968). Topographie des neurones monoaminergiques du tronc cérébral du chat: étude par histofluorescence. *C. R. Soc. Biol. (Paris)*,, **162,** 2136
Powell, T. P. S. (1973). Sensory convergence in the cerebral cortex. In L. V. Laitinen and K. E. Livingston (eds.) *Surgical Approaches in Psychiatry*. pp. 266–281. Lancaster: Medical and Technical Publishing Co.)
Ramón-Moliner, E. and Nauta, W. J. H. (1966). The isodendritic core of the brainstem. *J. Comp. Neurol.*, **126,** 311
Rittar, S. and Stein, L. (1974). Self-stimulation in the mesencephalic trajectory of the ventral noradrenergic bundle. *Brain Res.*, **81,** 145
Scheibel, M. E. and Scheibel, A. B. (1967). Anatomical basis of attention mechanisms in vertebrate brains. In G. C. Quarton, T. Melnechuk, and F. O. Schmitt (eds.) *The Neurosciences: A Study Programme*. pp. 577–602. (New York: Rockefeller University Press)
Shellenberger, M. K. and Gordon, J. H. (1975). Regional role of catecholamines and α-methyl-*m*-tyrosine-induced electroencephalographic arousal. *Exp. Neurol.*, **49,** 370
Sholl, D. A. (1953). Dendritic organization in the neurons of the visual and motor cortices of the cat. *J. Anat. (London)*, **87,** 387
Shute, C. C. D. and Lewis, P. R. (1967). The ascending cholinergic reticular system: neocortical, olfactory and subcortical projections. *Brain*, **90,** 497
Simantov, R., Kuhar, M. J., Uhl, G. R. and Snyder, S. H. (1977). Opioid peptide enkephalin: immuno-histochemical mapping in rat central nervous system. *Proc. Nat. Acad. Sci. USA*, **74,** 2167
Sladek,. J. R. (Jr.) and Bowman, J. P. (1975). The distribution of catecholamines within the inferior olivary complex of the cat and Rhesus monkey. *J. Comp. Neurol.*, **163,** 203
Sladek, J. R. (Jr.) and Parnavelas, J. G. (975). Catecholamine-containing dendrites in primate brain. *Brain Res.*, **100,** 657
Steeves, J. D., Jordan, L. M. and Lake, N. (1975). The close proximity of catecholamine-containing cells to the 'mesencephalic locomotor region' (MLR). *Brain Res.*, **100,** 663
Tennyson, V. M., Heikkila, R., Mytilineon, C., Côté, L. and Cohen, G. (1974). 5-Hydroxy-dopamine 'tagged' neuronal boutons in rabbit neostriatum: inter-relationship between vesicles and axonal membrane. *Brain Res.*, **82,** 341
Ungerstedt, U. (1971). Stereotaxic mapping of the monoamine pathways in the rat brain. *Acta Physiol. Scand. Suppl.*, **367,** 48
Ungerstedt, U. (1974). Brain dopamine neurons and behaviour. In F. O. Schmitt and F. G. Worden (eds.) *The Third Neurosciences Study Program*, pp. 695–703. (Cambridge: M.I.T. Press)
Valverde, F. (1962). Reticular formation of the albino rat's brainstem. Cytoarchitecture and corticofugal connections. *J. Comp. Neurol.*, **119,** 25
Webster, K. E. (1975). Structure and function of the basal ganglia – a non-clinical view. *Proc. R. Soc. Med.*, **68,** 203
Yahr, M. D. (ed.) (1977). The basal ganglia. *Assoc. Res. Neurol. Ment. Dis. Research Publication*, Vol. 55 (New York: Raven Press)
Zanchetti, A. (1967). Subcortical and cortical mechanisms in arousal and emotional behaviour. In O. G. C. Quarton, T. Melnechuk, and F. O. Schmitt (eds.) *The Neurosciences: A Study Programme*. pp. 602–614. (New York: Rockefeller University Press)

Since this essay was written, Sakai *et al. (Brain Res.* (1977). **119,** 21, and Cederbaum and Aghajanian *(J. Comp. Neurol.* (1978). **178,** 1) have described afferents to the locus caeruleus arising from numerous sources, including the hypothalamus, amygdala, septum, peri-aqueductal grey, cell groups A1–5, and the substantia nigra. Perhaps it should also be pointed out that there is evidence that the central aminergic systems control the blood vascular system of the brain, including perhaps the permeability of capillaries. The potential importance of this is considerable (see Ràichle *et al.* (1975). *Proc. Nat. Acad. Sci.*, **72,** 3726. Finally, although it appears likely that the aminergic endings lying in the cerebrospinal fluid of the brain ventricles are efferent, the possibility that they are afferent cannot be rigorously excluded.

SECTION 2:
Genetics

2

Clinical and biochemical manifestations of acute intermittent porphyria: A working model for schizophrenia as an inborn error of metabolism

L. WETTERBERG

INTRODUCTION

I want to consider schizophrenia as an inborn error of metabolism by comparing it with a disease in which the inborn error is already known. The disease chosen as a model for comparison is acute intermittent porphyria. Features of this disease include the presence of psychiatric symptoms, the onset of manifest disease symptoms post puberty, either an acute or chronic course, and the presence of hereditary factors and precipitating factors. The clinical material which has formed the basis for the comparison consists of two pedigrees, one of which has suffered from schizophrenia and the other from acute intermittent porphyria. Both families were from isolated geographical areas in Sweden, and both pedigrees have been traced back more than ten generations to the early 17th century.

Consideration will be given to the hypothesis that schizophrenia might be caused by enzyme deficiencies under genetic control. A preliminary study of 35 related persons, 8 schizophrenics and 27 non-schizophrenics, showed that dopamine-β-hydroxylase (DBH) in plasma and monoamine oxidase (MAO) in platelets were both at the lower end of the scale in the patients. By comparing schizophrenics in these families with their non-schizophrenic relatives it is easier to control both genetic and environmental factors and so avoid the diagnostic difficulties which arise when using a hospital population containing possibly heterogeneous types of schizophrenia.

Inborn errors of metabolism

Early in the century Garrod (1909) described alkaptonuria, cystinuria, pentosuria and albinism as diseases inherited according to Mendelian laws. Later Følling in 1934 described the genetic basis for phenylketonuria. There are now more than 250 well-defined inborn errors of metabolism and more than 2000 diseases of genetic origin. According to McKusick (1975) there are 2336 genetic diseases described. Possibly schizophrenia may provide a further instance. If this were found to be the case, then we should consider the aetiology, symptomatology, pathogenesis and precipitating factors of the schizophrenias, and also the mechanism of action of the therapeutically effective drugs in current use. Any model of schizophrenia as an inborn error has to take these

Table 1 General working model for the study of inborn errors of metabolism

	Acute intermittent porphyria	*Schizophrenia*
1. *Clinical characteristics*	1.	1.
(a) Symptoms I Latent	(a) I Latent UIS ↓ PBG ↑	(a) I Latent: MAO↓? DBH↓?
II Manifest	II Manifest: abdominal pain, neuropsychiatric symptoms	II Manifest: association and affect, disturbances, ambivalence and autism
(b) Age of onset	(b) Post puberty	(b) Post puberty
(c) Course of disease	(c) Acute attacks with spontaneous remissions or chronic course	(c) Acute attacks with spontaneous remissions or chronic course
(d) Hereditary factors	(d) Autosomal dominant gene	(d) Autosomal, one major gene? If close relative has manifest schizophrenia, 10 times greater risk
2. *Aetiological factors* Enzyme defect	2. Decrease of enzyme UIS activity 50% lower in patients	2. Enzyme or isoenzyme defect or defect in enzyme regulation
3. *Pathogenesis*	3. Neurotoxic products (?)	3. Neurotoxic products (?)
(a) Acute course	(a) Monopyrroles–development of tolerance	(a) Development of tolerance to the toxic product, e.g. bufotenine and others
(b) Chronic course	(b) Secondary factors	(b) No development of tolerance to the toxic product, e.g. *N,N*-dimethyltryptamine and others
4. *Precipitating factors*	4.	4.
(a) Permissive	(a) Altered steroid metabolism due to hormonal setting at puberty?	(a) Altered steroid metabolism due to hormonal setting at puberty?
(b) Direct precipitating	(b) Drugs and stressors	(b) Drugs and stressors influencing enzyme activity?
5. *Mechanism of therapeutic agents*	5. Glucose inhibition of overactive enzyme (ALAS)	5. Interference with faulty neurotransmission by drugs; removal of neurotoxic substance by haemodialysis (?)

UIS = Uroporphyrinogen-I-synthetase MAO = Monoamine oxidase

PBG = Porphobilinogen DBH = Dopamine-β-hydroxylase

factors into account and should also offer testable hypotheses for all the gaps in the model.

A working model for schizophrenia

On the bases of present knowledge I will present a general working model for the study of schizophrenia as an inborn error of metabolism (Table 1). Such a model is useful when trying to specify the priorities for necessary biochemical investigations. In studies together with Böök, Moderewska and Unge in Sweden,, presented in part at the World Congress of Psychiatry 1977, we have focused on a large sample of schizophrenic patients who, it is highly probable, represent one genetic entity. This provides us with a unique opportunity to study a homogeneous sample of schizophrenia.

ACUTE INTERMITTENT PORPHYRIA (AIP)

In the general working model (presented in Table 1) we decided to compare schizophrenia with a disease caused by a known inborn error of metabolism which, at least in some respects, shows similar features to schizophrenia. These include psychiatric symptoms, an acute attack or chronic course and clinical onset after puberty. We have for this reason chosen to compare schizophrenia with acute intermittent porphyria, sometimes named 'the royal disease' since it possibly affected George III (Macalpine and Hunter, 1969).

Let us first take a closer look at acute intermittent porphyria as it is seen in Sweden and then compare this disease with the disorder found in Swedish pedigrees with schizophrenia and finally compare the two diseases in different respects. Acute intermittent porphria (AIP) is characterized by neurological and psychiatric symptoms and by abdominal pain. The disease could until a couple of years ago be diagnosed only by its symptoms in the manifest form or by increased urinary excretion of porphobilinogen in the latent form. The increased excretion occurred only after puberty and rarely before the age of 15.

Like schizophrenia, AIP usually becomes clinically manifest – if at all – between the ages of 20 and 40. About 25% of the patients with manifest AIP have a mental syndrome with the following signs and symptoms: slight to moderate depression, transitional confusion, visual hallucinations and neurological signs.

Precipitating factors in AIP

It is well known that some drugs may precipitate acute attacks of AIP, including barbiturates, sulphonamides and general anaesthetics. Heavy metals such as lead, cadmium and mercury, alcohol and a low-calorie diet and malnourishment may also provoke acute attacks or make ongoing attacks worse. In a recent international survey of safe and unsafe drugs in AIP, several compounds with different chemical structures were reported to be dangerous (Wetterberg, 1976). Let us for a moment compare AIP with schizophrenia and consider the possibility that in schizophrenia certain drugs or other provoking factors could act upon the genetic predisposition to produce the disease. If such a factor were common, it would be difficult to detect since even the controls would have experienced the same agent although without deleterious effect. It may also be of some interest that in acute porphyria there is no clear dose–effect relationship between the adverse effect of barbiturates and symtomatology, e.g. even a small dose of a drug dangerous to an AIP patient may cause a metabolic catastrophy with pareses and respiratory trouble, psychiatric symptoms, hallucinations, paralyses and even fatal outcome.

Porphyrin biosyntheses

To understand the nature of the genetic lesion in AIP it is helpful to review the normal porphyrin synthesis which uses glycine and succinyl co-enzyme A to make δ-aminolevulinic acid (ALA) of which two molecules make porphobilinogen (PBG). Four molecules of PBG form tetrapyrroles which are precursors to haem which is incorporated into haemoglobin. AIP is characterized by a metabolic block between PBG and uroporphyrinogen. Due to this block PBG is not metabolized in a normal manner and PBG as well as ALA are excreted in the urine in increased amounts. The decreased haem formation results in a feed-back stimulation of the enzyme required for ALA formation, the ALA-synthetase activity. Furthermore the increase in PBG production may lead to formation of neurotoxic monopyrroles, one of which may be kryptopyrrole which has been used as a model substance in animal studies of AIP (Wetterberg and Formgren, 1976). The genetic lesion in AIP is thus characterized by a localized defect in the haem metabolism, more specifically a 50% decrease of the enzyme uroporphyrinogen-I-synthetase. This can be measured in the red blood cells. The 50% enzyme deficit is found both in males and females although females have clinical manifest disease symptoms twice as often as males.

Porphyric families

In Sweden there is a large family with AIP which we have been able to follow through 12 generations to an ancestor born in 1615. This pedigree consists of more than 5000 members. A small part of this pedigree has so far been examined by Formgren and Wetterberg (1978). All patients who had manifest symptoms showed a 50% decrease in uroporphyrinogen-I-synthetase activity in red blood cells (RBC) when compared with their non-porphyric siblings and the parent who did not have the AIP trait (Figure 1).

Some siblings, apparently healthy but with increased excretion of PBG in their urine, also showed a 50% decrease in RBC enzyme activity. There were further cases free of symptoms, especially among the children, with decreased enzyme activity. We assume that these family members have inherited the trait for AIP and we classify these as latent cases or carriers of AIP. The disease is inherited in a classical, autosomal, dominant manner.

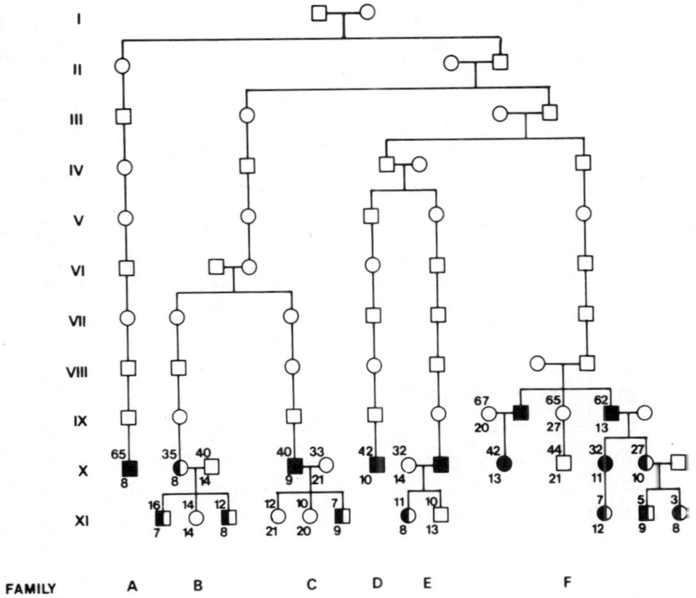

Figure 1 Pedigree of a minor part of a family from the north of Sweden with acute intermittent porphyria. The ancestor in the first generation was born in 1615. ○ = female; □ = male. The figures above the symbols indicate the age at the time of the test and the figures below the uroporphyrinogen-I-synthetase activity in the erythrocytes (nkatal per l). All individuals in generation XI were below 17 years of age and had normal excretion of porphobilinogen in the urine

The fact that females are more clinically affected than males may be due to endocrinological differences.

SCHIZOPHRENIC FAMILIES

A pedigree from the North of Sweden containing more than 50 cases of schizophrenia has been followed 12 generations back. The mode of inheritance has been studied by Böök (1953) and is now being re-investigated by Böök *et al.* (1977). It is possible that the underlying genetic defect could be an autosomal, dominant trait with about 20% penetrance expressed as clinical manifest schizophrenia. This hypothesis is now being tested on a larger scale. In Table 1 we have scheduled the previously mentioned general working model for the study of acute porphyria and schizophrenia as inborn errors of metabolism. When we compare the two diseases we can see that much more is known about porphyria than schizophrenia. Our present knowledge of porphyria is greater than it was 10 years ago, although the pathogenesis is still unclear and remains to be elucidated. When we consider schizophrenia in the model we can see that the lack of knowledge is profound and many points in the scheme remain to be determined.

Another hypothesis we have considered is that schizophrenia in the particular family we are studying might be caused by a gene-controlled enzyme deficiency (Böök *et al.,* 1977). This theory is neither new nor original. The situation today, however, is different from that of only a few years ago when the search for a specific factor in schizophrenia was paralleled with the proverbial 'looking for a needle in a haystack'. Increased knowledge about pathways in the nervous system has given us the opportunity to ask more precise questions and new methods of analysis have given us new tools, such as computerized two-dimensional chromatography, gas chromatography–mass spectometry and electron spin resonance combined with laser techniques. All these methods may help to answer some of the questions.

Haemodialysis in schizophrenia

In addition, new approaches in the treatment of schizophrenia have allowed us to study body fluids and metabolism in a new fashion for example: the dialysate from schizophrenic patients undergoing haemodialysis is being investigated by Wagemaker and Cade (1977).

Enzyme defects in schizophrenia

We have started the metabolic study of a section of a large pedigree in Sweden with a history of schizophrenia (Figure 2). The monoamineoxidases (MAO) and their metabolic pathways provide an interesting subject for research. We have just finished an interlaboratory study of the MAO enzyme in platelets (Ask *et al.*, 1978) and, in common with many previous reports in this field, we have found that the MAO activity in platelets is lower in schizophrenics. This only occurs when certain enzyme substrates are used

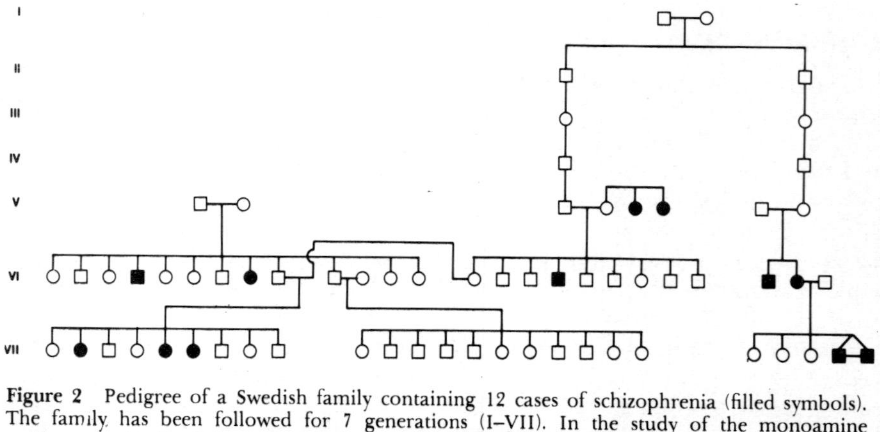

Figure 2 Pedigree of a Swedish family containing 12 cases of schizophrenia (filled symbols). The family has been followed for 7 generations (I–VII). In the study of the monoamine oxidase activity in platelets 8 patients with schizophrenia and 27 of their non-schizophrenic relatives have been examined. (Ask *et al.,* 1978). ○=females; □=males

but not with others. It is interesting that so far no one has reported higher MAO activities in platelets from schizophrenics when they have been compared with controls.

An advantage of using a family study is the possibility of comparing schizophrenics with their non-schizophrenic siblings. This gives a better opportunity of controlling both genetic and environmental factors than would be possible using a hospital population of schizophrenic patients which may have heterogeneous aetiology and differing control populations. Another approach we are trying is to use trace-metal analysis by the neutron activation technique. We assay the trace metals in blood and let the results serve as 'a metabolic probe' in the further explanation of the alleged error of metabolism in schizophrenia. In an attempt in this direction we have examined 22 trace metals in plasma from six schizophrenics and six of their non-schizophrenic siblings. No increase in the metals in the schizophrenic patients was found. Instead rather lower levels of some elements like phosphorus, antimony and arsenic were found in their plasma. Interestingly all these elements belong to group Vb of the Periodic Table. This group also contains nitrogen. We do not know the red blood cell content of these elements at the moment. Unfortunately the work along these lines tends to be slow since the cost of analyses of several trace metals simultaneously using neutron activation is very high at present.

Many more studies are under way; among other things we are examining the psychoendocrine profile as well as genetic linkage using serum and blood-cell markers. It is likely that the results will be inconsistent and confusing over a period, but eventually, if a metabolic correlate with schizophrenic behaviour exists, it will be elucidated.

REFERENCES

Ask, A-L., Böök, J. A., Heyden, T., Ross, S. B., Unge, C., Wetterberg, L., Eiduson, S. and Kobayashi, K. (1978). Platelet monoamine oxidase in a pedigree with schizophrenia: an interlaboratory comparison. *Clin. Genet.* (In press)

Böök, J. A. (1953). A genetical and neuropsychiatric investigation of a North Swedish population. *Acta Genet.*, **IV**, 1

Böök, J. A., Modrzewska, K., Unge, C. and Wetterberg, L. (1977). Schizophrenia in a North Swedish population 1900–75. Abstract from *VI World Congress of Psychiatry*. Honolulu, Hawaii, USA, August 28–September 3, 1977

Formgren, B. and Wetterberg, L. (1978). Uroporfyrinogen-I-Syntetasakti-vitet i röda blodkroppar som diagnostiskt index vid akut intermittent porfyri. *Läkartidningen*, **75**, 1921

Følling, A. (1934). Über Ausscheidung von Phenylbernztraubensäure in den Harn als stoffwechselanomalie in Verbindung mit Imbezzillität. *Z. Physiol. Chem.*, **227**, 169

Garrod, A. E. (1925). *Inborn Errors of Metabolism.* 2nd ed. (London: Henry Frowda)

Macalpine, I. and Hunter, R. (1969). *George III and the Mad-Business,* (Harmandsworth: Allen Lane) *Press)*

McKusick, V. A. (1975). The growth and development of human genetics as a clinical discipline. *Am. J. Hum. Genet.*, **27**, 261

Strauss, J. S. and Gift, T. E. (1977). Choosing an approach for diagnosing schizophrenia. *Arch. Gen. Psychiatry*, **34**, 1248

Wagemaker, J. R. and Cade, R. (1977). The use of hemodialysis in chronic schizophrenia. *Am. J. Psychiatry*, **134**, 6

Wetterberg, L. (1967). A neuropsychiatric and genetical investigation of acute intermittent porphyria. (Norstedts, Stockholm: Scandinavian University Books)

Wetterberg, L. (1976). Report on an international survey of safe and unsafe drugs in acute intermittent porphyria. Supplement to the Proceedings of the I International Porphyrin Meeting on *Porphyrins in Human Diseases* Freiburg, May 1–4, 1975. M. Doss and P. Nawrocki, (eds.). Univ. of Marburg, pp. 191–202

Wetterberg, L. and Formgren, B. (1976). Pharmacological and biochemical properties of kryptopyrrole and its oxidation products possibly related to acute intermittent porphyria. *Ann. Clin. Res.,* **8,** (suppl.) **17,** 162

SECTION 3:
Pathogenesis

3
Psychoses from digestive origins

H. BARUK

INTRODUCTION

Modern psychiatry has evolved in several phases. The first phase, illustrated in France by Pinel and Esquirol, in England by Tuke and in Italy by Chiarugi (preceded by Daquin at Chambéry), was characterized by a great philanthropic and moral movement followed by clinical observation and a meticulous description of the various mental syndromes: manic-depression by Pinel-Falret-Baillarger, mental confusion by Delasiauve, systemic delirium by Esquirol, the monomanias by Lasègue, Falret. Arnault. Sérieux and Capgras, hallucinations and hallucinatory delirium (Baillarger, Lasègue, Falret, Magnan, De Clérambault), development problems (Pinel, Esquirol, Bourneville, Voisin, Ferré, Wallon) and dementia praecox by Morel. An enormous amount of work followed in the description of the neuroses and the development of psychopathology with Charcot, the school of Nancy, Bernhein and Babinski and in the field of obsessions by Pierre Janet, etc.

The second phase was marked by an attempt to identify true autonomous mental illness with an organic and anatomical cerebral basis. This second phase was begun by Bayle (Antoine, Laurent, Jessé) who, in his thesis in 1822 at Charenton, discovered general paralysis, a true illness with a physical basis, the chronic arachnoiditis of Bayle, (diffuse meningoencephalitis), and its own special development. This discovery by Bayle was to become, according to his own expression in his treatise on the diseases of the brain and its membranes, the origin of a 'new doctrine of mental diseases'. Bayle's new doctrine was distinguished by the unitary theory, as opposed to Baillarger's dualism, that is to say by the idea that mental illnesses were entirely explicable by changes in the brain. These cerebral changes could not only throw light on dementia – that is to say the weakening of the intellectual faculties – but also on delirium, confusion of ideas, affective disorders and behaviour which until then had been considered as being of purely a 'mental' nature.

This new doctrine of the organic nature of mental illnesses which was subsequently taken up by Griesinger at Zurich and in Germany by Kahlbaum in his discovery of catatonia, which in some ways resembled the general paralysis of Bayle, was to result in the great synthesis of Kraepelin in Germany (Heidelberg–Munich) dividing mental illnesses into two large groups: dementia praecox, an illness presumed to be linked with incurable cerebral attacks, and the manic-depressive psychosis taken up by Baillarger and thought to be curable. Later on a study of a different kind into psychological factors, already stressed by Bernheim and the school of Nancy but systematized in a completely different way by Freud, led Bleuler to make a psychological interpretation of the dementia praecox of Kraepelin but without modifying its organic conception and its evolution towards incurability. This was the schizophrenia of Bleuler.

This systematization and simplification of mental illnesses had, by its very schematic form, considerable success throughout the world and tended to be substituted for the tentative discoveries of the older French psychiatry In particular the spread of Kraepelin's doctrine led to a break in the previously close relationship between French psychiatry and English and American psychiatry, a break that Professor Aubrey Lewis deplored and which has been partly corrected by a recent work (Hirsch and Shepherd, 1974) and by a new treatise of psychology (Krauss, 1960).

However neither physical research nor statistics have confirmed Kraepelin's ideas (Baruk, 1959). The notion in Germany of separating the curable and the incurable became the object of sharp criticism from Parchappe and has now been discredited. This is why since the congress at Zurich we have led a campaign for the revision of schizophrenia. We believe that schizophrenia is not a true illness with its own specific development but a simple reaction of the personality to various biological or psychological causes and its development depends on the causes and on the way in which they are resolved. Thus, an unthinking diagnosis of schizophrenia can do the greatest harm to the patient. The diagnosis of incurability, which such a diagnosis includes, may compromise the recovery of the patient, lead him to despair, discredit him and discourage his family. This is what we have called destructive prognosis and what Menninger and Ellenberger in the United States have also called diagnostic destruction. Furthermore, this idea of schizophrenia as a disease compromises the progress of psychiatry, prevents scientific research, reduces psychiatry to a simple stereotyped diagnosis and, finally, encourages 'blocking' therapies which hold the patient in a state of chronic infirmity and ensures the growth in numbers of the mentally sick.

The work of Kraepelin and Bleuler has even been surpassed by their followers and by their clumsy imitators. The schizophrenia of Bleuler comprised a psychic dissociation incoherence, confusion in the association of ideas, indifference in affect, autism, stereotyped behaviour and psychomotor disorders. Their imitators no longer even conform to this symptomatology. They see schizophrenia everywhere, confuse depression with periodic melancholia and in so doing they return to the pre-Pinel and, pre-Tuke fatalism, return to the obscurantism of the Middle Ages and subsequently advocate the therapeutics of despair 'blocking and mutilating the patient'. Kraepelin had at least distinguished dementia praecox from manic-depressive psychosis. Their imitators go further and reduce psychiatry to one single malady: schizophrenia. This is the position adopted in the treatise by Eliot Slater and Martin Roth (1969). According to this treatise, mania and depression which together contribute the most common and important mental illness, as Seglas and Delmas had so clearly shown and as we have insisted, are relegated to the vague category of 'affective disorders'.

This preamble has been necessary in order to make it quite clear that this trend must be overthrown. It is erroneous, despairing and sterilizing. It discredits psychiatry and has favoured the birth of anti-psychiatry. The only real mental illness is manic-depressive psychosis, a hereditary disease, which responds now to effective treatments such as lithium, depamide, etc. but an illness which also is affected by psychological and biochemical factors. Most of the mental symptoms of the psychoses and neuroses are in effect, apart from a predisposition in temperament, a reaction to moral or biological factors. The reactive character of such disorders has developed from Moreau de Tours up until our own time.

The third phase of psychiatry then is that of the reactive toxic psychosis. In fact the misconception that schizophrenia is an illness which develops to become an incurable disease derives from the general application to all psychiatry of Bayle's doctrine: that is to say the belief that a cerebral lesion is the origin of all the mental illnesses. This generalization now is shown to be arbitary. We have shown for example the catatonia, which up until now has been placed in the schizophrenia category and considered to be a definite organic illness Like GPI, has a toxic nature which has been demonstrated by the induction of experimental catatonia which we produced first with de Jong using bulbocapnine (de Jong and Baruk, 1930). This was verified throughout the world particularly in England by Richter and Paterson (1931). It was the ratification of this renowned conception of Moreau de Tours, the result of his famous work on hashish, which likened the dream to madness and delirium to a toxic dream. This is why we have founded the society and the Annals of Moreau de Tours.

The focus of psychiatry has also shifted from the concept of an incurable physical deterioration of the brain to that of a reaction to toxic factors which are more or less fleeting and produce a state of dream and delirium. This is the phase of reactive toxic psychosis. Amongst these toxic causes, digestive causes hold a principal place.

MENTAL DISORDERS OF DIGESTIVE ORIGIN

Colibacillary origin

It is again through the study of catatonia that our attention has been drawn to digestive causes and in particular by the observation of a catatonic state in the course of colibacillary pyelonephritis which had already been stressed by a urologist, M. Lepoutre of Lille. We have published with Devaux (Baruk and Devaux, 1933) the well known case of a woman patient as follows. In the course of a colibacillary pyelonephritis, followed by colibacillary septicaemia, she presented a severe state of catatonia with catatonic stupor, negativism and mutism interrupted by seemingly incoherent speech. She was completely cured after anti-colibacillus serotherapy (Vincent's serum) and, after her recovery explained her attitude during the catatonia and explained her utterances by a terrifying oneiroid dream of toxic origin. Following our observations of this patient and analogous cases, we have been able, using the neurotropic toxin of the colibacillus taken from our patients, to produce in animals, notably the cat, a typical colibacillary experimental catatonia (Baruk, 1933). As a result we have developed an effective therapeutic method, through the identification of syndromes hitherto classified as schizophrenic, and in fact curable through treatment of the collibacillary toxic infection when it is present.

Analogous cases have been published by Tomesco, Badenski, and Cosumilesco and have recently been the subject of a full bacteriological, immunological and clinical study by Lydia Mesrobéanu and I. Mesrobéanu (1971). Elsewhere numerous mental or nervous disorders have been found to be connected with the bacterium coli by Ferraro and Kilman, Fisch, Poppi (Umberto) Nieuwenhuyzen, Poppi, Bracaloni, Sicard and Buscaino. The action of the neurotropic toxin of the bacterium coli exerts itself not only on the nervous system in acute colibacillary infections such as pyelonephritis or septicaemia, for in these the toxicity produces a pathological sleep with an oneiroid state, dream and delirium thus producing the aspects of psychoses like mental confusion or schizophrenia, but also, when the neurotropic toxin exerts itself at a reduced or attenuated intensity on the nervous system, it can result in states of depression, characterized by insomnia, asthenia phenomena, of neurovegetative abnormal excitement, erethism with palpitations, depression, constipation, a saboural state of the digestive tract and black thoughts. These states of mind have been the object of the first study of this matter on colibacillary infection – that of Desgeorges (of Vichy) (1923), an excellent clinician who had already affirmed that the collibacillus can give rise to a true illness.

We have, with Claude and our pupil Forestier, who under our direction has written a thesis on this subject, made a study on the colibacillary nervous disorders (Claude *et al.,* 1952). Professor Vincent in his turn emphasized these facts at the Academy of Science (1933). We have returned to these problems many times with the same results (Baruk, 1939). We have accumulated many conclusive observations proving that the neurotropic toxin isolated by Vincent could cause not only attacks of oneiric delirium but also the manic depressive states like that of the woman whose case we have published with Trubert (Baruk and Trubert, 1933). Whilst pregnant this woman suffered a feverish pyelonephritic attack during which she suddenly threw herself out of the window under the influence of a toxic dream and landed on electric railway lines thus burning her back. After this a severe manic condition developed with loss of ideas, euphoria and raving. Afterwards colibacilli found in the patient's urine gave rise, in a group of mice, to a pathological sleep followed by catalepsy, which was in turn followed by terrifying hyperkinesia (leaping, jumping and throwing themselves violently against the glass walls of the tank resulting in their deaths). The subcutaneous injection of this same toxin in cats (5 cc) and guinea pigs (2 cc) and a pigeon gave the same results. Another case concerned a young man who presented with a typical catatonia and schizophrenic state of mind, and who had been considered incurable, who also showed a colibacillary toxic infection in his urine and after anticolibacillary treatment regained contact with reality. He then fell victim to a transitory manic attack, and then recovered completely – a recovery that has been totally maintained for 30 years.

From this we can see how useless it is to give a prognosis of schizophrenia and to talk of the concept of schizophrenia as an illness. Schizophrenia is the reaction of the personality to varying causes and it can be cured, when the cause is found and cured, as can be seen, in the cases of toxic colibacillary schizophrenia. We have shown moreover *a propos* our neurophysiological research into catatonia that catatonia is only a type of pathological sleep with oneiroid symptoms, curable but induced by a variety of causes. On this subject our research with our student Cornu has shown that the neurotropic toxin of colibacillus (Vincent's toxin) has a drowsy effect so that one could pass from sleep to catalepsy and to catatonia (Cornu, 1937).

We have also studied the role of associated infections, in particular the relationship between colibacillary and typhoid infections and the role played by the increase of the virulence of the colibacillus in typhoid nervous disorders and in typhoid encephalitis (Baruk *et al.,* 1933). Elsewhere we have studied at length on the psychological level the passage from dream to delirium (Baruk, 1934) whether the disorder lasts for a long time; and the passage of schizophrenic dissociation as the result of colibacillary poisoning. From these we studied the steps in the reconstitution of the personality and its recovery in getting in touch with reality as the result of the ethological treatment (Baruk, 1938) in the case that we published with Devaux (Baruk and Devaux, 1933). Colibacillary mental disorders have given rise to a large number of publications such as those of Laignel. Lavastine and their colleagues (1934), Cossa (1934), Hoven (1935) in Belgium, Mestrallet and Larrive (1934), Martimoore (1932), Warembourg (1936), Fisch, and a certain number of monographs (Des Georges: the colibacillus of Maloine (1935); Strominger).

Mental disorders of hepatic or biliary origin

The facts we have quoted above concerning colibacillary infections also explain the oft-stressed connection between appendicitis and mental disorders, notably concerning depression immediately following appendicectomy or appendicular peritonitis. It must not be forgotten in this respect that appendicitis is an infection linked with the colibacillus and that surgical intervention often has to include a specific general anti-infection treatment in order to neutralize toxic absorption.

The same considerations apply to the gall bladder which is often infected and secondly to the intestine by the action of the colibacilli. These facts explain attacks of depression which frequently follow the removal of the gall bladder or the removal of gall stones. A disinfecting treatment must always accompany the ablation of the gall bladder. Together with Briand, Camus and Cornu, (Baruk *et al.,* 1935) we have drawn attention to biliary anxiety and have recalled the experimental work of L. Crandall and Arthur Wed (1933) in America. Their experiments were carried out at the Institute of Neurology in Chicago on dogs and rats. Following biliary intoxication by ligature of the bile duct these animals developed lesions at the level of the ganglia at the base of the corpus striatum and the ventricles. The main cause of this biliary intoxication is to be found in the bile salts, the effects of which have been studied in France by Bariety. His injection into a rabbit's marginal vein has shown secondary neurovegetative disorders in the animal, notably bradycardia. Following this we undertook with Dr Camus (Baruk and Camus, 1934) a series of researches into the toxicity of the bile in mental patients. This toxicity was demonstrated by the injection of 2 cc of bile from the duodenal tubes in a pigeon. The toxic biles caused catalepsy in the pigeon. From this we concluded that these toxic biles contained a special toxic substance which we have named 'biliary catatonia'.

This biliary catatonia has been rediscovered in France in a study of migraine by Caroli, Paraf and Allot (1949), in asthma by Hesse (1950), in Germany by von Mall (1958), who found it not only in schizophrenics but also in epileptics during the prodromal stage of the attack, and in Belgium by P. Guilmot (1956) who, with his experiments on cats and mice, stressed the toxicity of bile produced by schizophrenics. In Switzerland Géorgi (from Basle) and his collaborators have also emphasized hepatic-psychic relationships (1950). Next the question was to identify biliary catatonia. The research that we did with Camus (Baruk and Camus, 1934) enabled us to show that biliary catatonia does not belong to the normal constituents of bile and cholesterol salts and that it does not dialyse but belongs to or is linked to the molecules expected in the duodenal bile (Launay *et al.*, 1961). Furthermore the catatonic property of duodenal bile is fragile; it is thermolabile and does not tolerate lyophilization (Baruk *et al.*, 1963).

As early as 1931 with Mlle Halina Jankovska (Baruk and Jankovska, 1931) we discovered alterations in the metabolism of nitrogen in certain schizophrenics, with Fabiani (Baruk and Fabiani, 1962) alterations of ammonia levels, which Gjessing (1936) had already identified in periodic catatonia and with Claude and Oliver (Claude *et al.*, 1932) we showed the marked increase of polypeptides in the cerebrospinal fluid. We took up this problem again in a series of researches with Olivier and Liteanu (1967). Together we applied to the study of biles electrophoretic analysis using the properties of molecular filtration with Sephadex resins and following the technique of Ambert and Hartman.

The conclusions resulting from this research, the details of which can be found in our paper at the Academy of Medicine, are as follows: (1) the lipids of the duodenal lumen are toxic whether they contain bile or not. Consequently the toxicity is not connected with the constituents of hepatic bile. (2) Atoxic biles contain a relatively high concentration of fast-moving protein fractions on the electrophoretic columns. The B biles rich in heavy fractions have been shown to be particularly toxic. (3) With regard to the lipids from the duodenum (duodenal biles A) the average of relative concentrations in fast-moving electrophoresis protein fractions is higher in atoxic fluids. To conclude the toxicity of fluids in the duodenal tube is linked to the proteins formed or modified in the gall bladder or the second part of the duodenum, the pancreatic part. The absence of toxicity of the bile in the duodenal fluid coincides with the raising of the ratio of the rapid fractions to the slow fractions calculated on paper electrophoresis.

Thus, if the identification of the toxic psychotropic substance found in the bile of certain mental, hepatic or allergic patients is not yet completely resolved, we are approaching this goal. This modern biological research conforms with previous work by Klippel in France and Jelgersma in Holland and other authors. These facts conform with Buscaino's theory of amine abnormalities being the origin of schizophrenic disorders, and with Hoffer's and the role of the indoles (1957). We have ourselves done experimental work with indoles and tryptamine (Baruk *et al.*, 1958). All must be continued and developed.

CONCLUSION

As we have insisted in a work published in the Journal of Medicine (Baruk, 1953), instead of considering illnesses whose progress is hopeless it is altogether preferable to consider the majority of psychoses or neuroses as reactions either to biological factors or to nervous psychological or moral factors (Krauss, 1960). These biological factors are very often digestive in origin and psychiatry must acknowledge them. These toxic causes are disregarded far too often as are also the moral factors which are often linked with them and to which we have also called attention in psychiatry and in psychology.

REFERENCES

Baruk, H. (1933). Catatonie sommeil pathol et onirisme par intoxication colibacillaire. La catatonie expérimentale et les psychoses colibacillaires. La catatonie colibacillaire expérimentale et clinique. *Ann. Méd. Psychol.*, **4 Nov**

Baruk, H. (1934). L'état mental au cours de l'accès catatonique. Rôle de l'onirisme et des idées fixés postoniriques dans le négativisme les délires et les hallucinations des catatoniques. Faux aspects de simulation étiologique toxique. *Ann. Méd. Psychol.* **3 Mar**

Baruk, H. (1938). Etude psychologique de la catatonie. In *Psychiatrie Médicale Physiologique Expérimentale*. Vol. 1, p. 143 (Paris: Masson)

Baruk, H. (1939). Apropos des psychoses colibacillaires. *Rev. Méd.*, **56,** 367

Baruk, H. (1953). Origine digestive et hepato-intestinale de certaine maladies mentales. *Suisse J. Méd.* (suppl.) **38,** 1517

Baruk, H. (1959). *Traité de Psychiatrie*, Vol. 1. pp. 54–84 (Paris: Masson)

Baruk, H. and Janovska, H. (1931). *Encephall.*, **4,** 315

Baruk, H. and Devaux. (1933). Catatonie grave colibacillaire. Délire onirique intiqué avec la catatonie. Guérison après sérotherapie

Baruk, H. Poumeau, Delille and Sicard, M. (1933). Accès catatonique avec état onirique transitoire a décours d'une typhoide, rôle respectif de la toxi-infection typhique et colibacillaire. *Rev. Neurol.*, **5 Nov** and Sicard (th) (Paris)

Baruk, H. and Trubert, E. (1933). Psychose colibacillaire à forme onirique puis maniaque au cours d'une pyélonéphrite post puerpérale tardive. *Ann. Méd. Psychol.* **4 Nov**

Baruk, H. and Camus, L. (1934). Sur un principe toxique cataleptisant décilé dans la bile de tubage duovénal de 5 malades atteintes d'icter. *C.R. Soc. Biol.*, **115,** 403, et la catalepsie bilaire expérimentale. *Ann. Méd. Psychol.*, **5 Nov**

Baruk, H., Briand, Camus and Cornu. (1935). L'anxiété bilaire. Données cliniques et expériments sur l'action de la bile et des sels bilaires sur les centres neuro-vegetatifs. *Ann. Méd. Psychol.*, **Jan**

Baruk, H. and Launay, B. (1958). Effects neuropsychiques de quelques derives indoliques. *Ann. Méd. Psychol.*, **1**

Baruk, H. and Fabiani, P. (1962). *Ann. Méd. Psychol.*, **5,** 971 and (1963), **2,** 257

Baruk, H. and Launay, J. (1962). Du hachisch et de l'aliénation mentale. Moreau de Tours, 1845. See *Annale Moreau de Tours P.U.F.*

Baruk, H., Asfar, M. and Vittoz, A. (1963). Etude des effets de la liophilisation sur la catatonie billaire. *C.R. Soc. Biol. Paris,* **157,** No. 1, 110

Baruk, H., Olivier, E. and Liteanu, D. (1967). Recherches de relations entre les toxicités des lipides dans le tubage duodénal et leurs protéinogrames au cours des syndromes depressifs avec ou sans réaction psychophréniques. *Acad. Méd. Paris,* **6 July**

Caroli, Paraf and Allot. (1949). *Semaine des hôpitaux de Paris.*, **41,** 1743

Claude, M., Baruk, H. and Olivier, H. R. (1932). *C. R. Soc. Biol.*, **60,** 1275

Claude, Baruk and Forestier. (1952). Éncephalites colibacillaires de type schizophréniques. *Ann. Méd. Psychol.*, **5 Dec**

Cornu, R. (1937). *Sur une forme léthargique et onirique d'encéphalite toxique colibacillaire.* (Paris: Jouve)

Cossa. (1934). De quelques psychoses toxi-infectiaux d'onirique intestinale. *Soc. Méd. Psychol,* **June**

Crandall, L. and Wed, A. (1933). Pathology of central nervous system of diseases of the liver. *Arch. Neurol. Psychol.,* **29,** 1066

De Jong and Baruk, H. (1930). *La Catatonie Expérimentale par la Bulbocapine.* Vol. 1 (Paris: Masson)

Des Georges. (1923). La colibacillose. *Soc. Méd. Gannat.*

Fisch. (1930). L'évolution du colibacille intestinal et ses conséquences. *Rev. Méd.,* **June**

Géorgi, Fischer *et al.* (1950). *Sweez. Méd. Wichr.,* **80,** 129

Gjessing. (1936). Bertage zur Menntnis der pathophysiologie du katatomen erregung. *Arch. Psychiatr. Nervenkr.,* **104,** 355

Guilmot. (1956). *Acta. Neurol. Psychol. Belgica.* **2,** 81

Hesse. (1950). *Bull. Acad. Nat. Méd,* No. 15, 16, 136 fol. 310

Hirsch, S. and Shepherd, M. (1974). *Themes and Variations in European Psychiatry* (Bristol: Wright)

Hoffer, A. (1957). Second International Congress of Psychiatry at Zurich. Congress Report, 1–7 Sept., Zurich. Vol. 1

Hoven. (1935). Apropos des psychoses colibacillaires. *J. Belge Neurol. Psychiatr.,* **March**

Krauss, S. (1960). In *Encyclopaedic Handbook of Medical Psychology.* (London: Butterworth)

Launay, Peters and Cornut. (1961). *Ann. Méd Psychol.,* **II,** No. 1, 99

Laignél, Lavastine d'Hencqueville and Guilly. (1934). Evolution schizophrénique et colibacillon puerpériale. *Soc. Méd Psychol.* **8 Feb**

Martimoore. (1932). *Soc. Méd Psychol.,* **Nov**

Mesrobeanu, L. and Mesobeanu, I. (1971). Salmonella typhimuruimand Eschérica coli. neurotoxins. In *Microbial Toxins.* Vol. 2A pp. 301–336. (New York and London: Academic Press)

Mestrallet and Larrive. (1934). Psychose colibacillaire avec pyelonéphrite évoluant depuis plusieurs semaines. Guérison par sérothérapie. *Congrès des Aliénistes et Neurol, Lyon*

Richter, D. and Paterson. (1931). Catalepsy induced by bulbocapine and the grasp reflex. *J. Pharmacol. Exp. Ther.,* **43,** 677

Slater and Roth. (1969). *Clinical Psychiatry.* (London: Balliére, Tindal and Cassell)

Tomesco, Badenski and Cosmulesco. *Soc. Psych.* **2,** 175

Vincent, H. (1933). Rôle de l'intoxication colibacillaire dans la genes de certaines troubles mentaux. *Acad. Sci.,* **28 Aug**

Von Mall. (1958). (b) *Confin. Neurol.,* **18,** 263

Warembourg and Bédunes. (1936). Accidents nerveaux au cours de la colibacillose. *Paris Méd.,* 121

4

The amino-hepato-entero-toxic theory of schizophrenia: an historical evaluation

G. A. BUSCAINO

INTRODUCTION

On the 17th February, 1921, Vito Maria Buscaino, while boiling for a few minutes 5 ml of urine from an acute schizophrenic together with 25 ml of 5% silver nitrate, observed the immediate formation of a black precipitate. A second test soon after with the urine from a normal subject formed a white precipitate. It was in that moment that a new path was opened in his research on the biology of schizophrenia.

Already in 1922 it was possible with this reaction, later called 'black reaction', to identify in schizophrenics a particular type of dismetabolism characterized by the quantitative and qualitative abnormal elimination of basic organic substances (deriving from ammonia). In fact, the formation of a black precipitate with the above-mentioned test was due to the presence of substances of the *amine* type (Buscaino V. M., 1922).

In the winter of 1921, the knowledge gained on the pathology of schizophrenia gave the go-ahead to studies on the reaction of heated silver nitrate. Out of about 650 autopsies carried out up to that time by at least 120 different people, besides the usual non-specific findings of neuronal damage both in the cortex and in the basal ganglia and brainstem, and of involvement of the glia, there were also reports of *focal* cellular damage and considerable alterations *spread* through the nerve fibres: metachromatic formations of myelin of various sizes, areas of hypo and demyelinization, and, above all, the so-called 'clods of disintegration in clusters' as reported by V. M. Buscaino (1921).

These appeared as limited ovoidal or bullet-shaped swellings with a granular or amorphous content often grouped in clusters, and differentiated from the surrounding tissue also by their metachromasia and birefringence through the polarizing microscope. Pecchiai (1964) reported their prevailing glyco-lipidic character with protidic, glycidic and glycoprotidic fragments.

The 'clods' do not appear to be specific but there is a vast quantitative difference depending on whether one is dealing with the brain of schizophrenics or non-schizophrenic psychotics. They form mainly in the cerebral white matter, but are also found in the basal ganglia with, in the case of catatonic schizophrenia, emphasized participation of the corpus striatum. The existence of these 'clods' has been confirmed, among others, by Del Rio Hortega; Ferraro; Nagasaka; Freeman; Roussy; Lhermitte and Oberling;

Guiraud and Ey; Snessarew; and Grynfelt (who preferred to call them 'foci of mucocitic degeneration') (cf. Buscaino V. M., 1939).

In the winter of 1921, in order to rule out the possibility that the 'clods' in schizophrenics could be a consequence of intoxication similar to that from e.g. formic acid it was already known that after intravenous injections with formic acid, formations very similar to the above-mentioned 'clods' appeared in the brain of dogs), V. M. Buscaino applied the reaction of hot silver nitrate to the urine of a schizophrenic – that being the method used to trace the presence of formic acid in fluids – and as mentioned in the opening paragraph, a black precipitate immediately appeared.

Further detailed and complex controls showed that it was not a question of formic acid but of basic substances deriving in particular from ammonia, amines and, above all, histamine. (Already in 1917, Holmes mentioned the presence of "toxic amine" in 2 cases of schizophrenia and reported on the "intestinal stasis" as possible histamine poisoning in dementia praecox). In fact, histamine, when injected into rabbits, provokes the appearance of 'clods of disintegration in clusters' in the brain and a black reaction in the urine, besides serious degenerative changes in the liver and in the gastro-intestinal tract. When dogs are injected intracisternally, it gives rise to catatonia. Moreover, hyperhistaminaemia has been noted in schizophrenics together with a rise of the imidazolic derivatives, the presence of histamine breakdown products and an increase of serum histaminolitic activity.

Also, inoculation with serum from schizophrenics provokes an increase of histamine in the CNS of experimental animals.

There then followed a series of researches on 'Buscaino's black reaction' (known as Kimbarowski's reaction in Poland and as Rosa's reaction in Austria). The positivity of the reaction, more frequent in acutely ill patients and in the worsening phases of the disease, soon made certain the existence of changes in the biochemistry of schizophrenics. In England, Namm and Slipp, Bayard-Holmes, and Katzenelbogen worked at that time on this topic.

A series of reports followed on the presence of indole compounds in the urine and serum from chronic schizophrenics: Gullotta in 1929, Noto in 1930, Longo in 1937 and Sano in 1954, followed by many other researchers who were stimulated by the knowledge gained on the psychotomimetic effects, sometimes schizophrenic-like, of mescaline, and in minimal doses, of LSD, a derivative of diethylamine, and by the presence in their chemical structure of the indole nucleus. This is a chemical grouping also present in the human body.

It was logical to question whether particular substances of an indole derivation formed from a metabolic abnormality in the human body could be implicated in mental illness (V. M. Buscaino *et al.*, 1955; McGeer *et al.*, 1956). Kemali *et al.*, of V. M. Buscaino's group, in 1956 reported the presence of methylated tryptamines in the black precipitates and of 5-methoxytryptamine 6-methoxytryptamine, 5-methoxyindoleacetic acid in the serum and urine of schizophrenics; it was thus that for the first time the presence of tryptamine (also psychoactive) and especially methylated tryptamines was signalled in schizophrenics. In 1957, I carried out similar experiments on urine as, in 1958, did Leyton, Riegelhaupt, Rodnight and Aves, and Feldstein *et al.*

It should be mentioned that Smythies, Osmond and Harley-Mason in 1952, perhaps on the grounds of the work of Hoffer on adrenochrome and the chemical similarity between norepinephrine and mescaline, suspected the importance of the endogenous synthesis of unspecified 'methylated abnormal derivatives' which could function as hallucinogens.

Also Woolley and Shaw in 1954 suggested that upsets of serotonin metabolism caused alterations of the human mental equilibrium, while in 1959 Erspamer considered the possibility that it was the formation of methylated compounds of serotonin that caused mental disturbances.

These authors, who can be considered as the pioneers of such experiments, were followed by many others, and a vast range of substances were reported, out of which bufotenine (Fischer *et al.*, 1961; Brune *et al.*, 1963), 3,4-dimethoxyphenylethylamine (Friedhoff and van Winkle, 1962), 4-methoxyphenylethylamine (Sen and McGeer, 1964), 3-methyldopamine (Gjessing, R.) and 6-hydroxydopamine (Stein and Wise, 1971), many of which experimentally proved to be psychotomimetic and with potent behavioural effects (e.g. catatonia, hallucinations).

The history of the pathology of the liver of schizophrenics is a long one, as far back as 1904 Dide demonstrated the complete steathosis of the liver in some of these patients. It should be said that up to 1952 the liver of schizophrenics was reported examined in at least 207 cases; there were histological findings of the acute type in 172 cases, of the chronic type (fibrosis) in 25; alterations, that is, in about 83% of the cases examined (Buscaino, V. M., 1953). Some of the more common pathological data are: fat infiltration, torbid swelling, vacuolar degeneration, focal spread disintegration of the parenchyme; these were often found in the centre of the hepatic lobule (the area of afflux to the liver of substances coming from the gut).

I would also like to recall the work of H. Baruk who in 1933 reported the existence of the 'colibacillaire catatonia' of intestinal origin. This research demonstrated the presence in 'human bile' from the duodenum of a substance different from those normally found in the bile and able, if taken from the duodenal content of catatonic schizophrenics, to experimentally provoke (by intramuscular injections, preferably in pigeons) characteristic cataleptic behaviour. It should be noted that this does not exclude the activity of non-biliary fractions present or formed in the gut especially following the report of Stano (1969) on the existence of a bacterial flora also in the duodenum and the jejunum. Summerfield *et al.* (1976) showed evidence of 6-α-hydroxylation of bile acids in man.

But investigations carried out with the most varied techniques reported both in the Italian and International literature (and I mention only at random: deamination capacity of the liver, hippuric acid synthesis, bilirubinaemia, disprotidaemia, cupraemia, procaino-esterasic activity, serum test of retention of coloured substances, Bengal pink, Congo red, etc.) have all proved, sometimes with very high percentages, that the liver really functions abnormally in these patients. One could therefore conclude that there are no doubts regarding the existence of hepatic metabolic changes in the biological manifestations of schizophrenia.

The early research of V. M. Buscaino on the pathology of the gastro-intestinal tract of the patients with dementia praecox dates back to 1923: in five cases congestion of the mucosa in spots and also haemorrhaging was noted in the small intestine and, in one case, even diffused patchy areas of atrophy.

Up until 1933 there were 82 schizophrenic patients autopsied (Buscaino, V. M., 1953) with reports of gastritis in 50%, of enteritis in 88% and colitis in 92% of the cases (signs of catarrhal and haemorrhagic inflammation of the intestinal mucosa, patchy areas of sclerosis and also of atrophy). Manic-depressive patients did not show these changes (Meyer, 1935).

There was furthermore a wide documentation on the abnormality of the intestinal flora of schizophrenics; beginning in 1921 with Ford Robertson and followed by Stewart in 1928, on the increased number of cases with coliform and anaerobe germs in the faeces and the marked frequency of particular types of pneumococci, streptococci, coli-like or diphtheroid germs, etc. A bacterial pathology in about half of the 99 schizophrenics examined was reported by Kanig and Kludas in 1958. But Platania's data (1940) are more precise; out of 193 acute schizophrenics, he obtained a positive serum-agglutination test for entero-tropic germs (typhus, paratyphoid A and B, brucella, Bang, *coli,* Flexner, Shiga) in 61.6%; out of 82 chronic schizophrenics, a positivity of 58.5%; out of 100 non-schizophrenic psychotics a positivity of 6.8% and out of 41 non-psychotic controls, a positivity of 4.8%.

More recently Malis (1959) reported the presence of *Escherichia coli* in the blood of schizophrenics. He even arrived at the conclusion that schizophrenic psychosis is fundamentally an infectious disease.

The role played by the intestinal pathology regarding schizophrenia is underlined by: (1) the observation that the intestinal content, and especially the duodenal one, is in itself toxic, as is shown by several cases of porta-cava anastomosis in patients with hepatic cirrhosis. In these conditions, due to the impairment of the liver function, substances coming from the intestinal lumen cause simple mind obnubilation, mental confusion with time-space disorientation, apathy or excitement, verbal and gesticulatory perseveration, incoherence when replying and also serious hallucinatory phenomena and disturbances of the body scheme, similar to those seen during intoxication from mescaline and LSD.

(2) Chromaffin cells of the gastro-intestinal mucosa secrete serotonin, a 5-hydroxytryptamine. But if it is bimethylated it turns into bufotenin which is a well-known psychotomimetic compound.

(3) Serotonin can form in the gut also under the influence of *E. coli* through the enzyme apotryptophanase that catalyses the breakdown of tryptophan in indole + pyruvate + ammonia. Also other germs act similarly synthesizing the indole nucleus.

The interest, therefore, that the gastro-intestinal tract has for those studying schizophrenia is due to the fact that histamine and serotonin, among other substances, originate in the gut from the chemical activity of the intestinal contents and the intestinal mucosa; histamine and serotonin being two substances with quantitative variations (hyperhistaminaemia) and qualitative variations (appearance of methylated tryptamines) that came to light some years ago in the field of schizophrenia.

To this can be added the recent reports by Dohan (1976) on the possible schizogenous effect of some types of cereal grains in the diet, and the relation between mental illness, changes in the intestine, coeliac disease and schizophrenia. In 1977 Dr Dohan, during a meeting of 'The Schizophrenia Association of Great Britain', held an interesting conference on the subject, underlined the fact that schizophrenics in a phase of reactivation improve more rapidly when fed on a diet without milk or grains than if fed on a diet rich in cereals. Gluten in the diet annuls such beneficial effects.

We now come to the role of methylations in schizophrenia research; this has developed into a theory, the so-called 'transmethylation hypothesis of schizophrenia'. Much research has been carried out on this subject, after having known of the hallucinogenic action of methyl- and dimethyltryptamines on man (Szara, 1956) – that is the psychotoxic effect of many methylated tryptamines – and after having learnt that in our organism there is an enzyme capable of forming *N,N*-dimethyl-tryptamine from non-methylated tryptamine usually present in the body (Axelrod, 1961).

There then followed (and I mention only a few positive results) Losowski's data (1962) on the increase of methylnicotinamide (64.4% in normal subjects and 109.8% in schizophrenics) after tryptophan administration; the results of Pollin *et al.*, Brune and Himwich (1961–1962) and many others on the worsening of schizophrenic symptoms after the administration of methyl-donors; the report of Berlet *et al.* (1964) on the worsening of clinical conditions in schizophrenics after loading with tryptophan + a methyl donor; the observations of Heyman and Merlis (1962) and myself (1965) on the increase of the methylating activity in the blood and urine of schizophrenics; Friedhoff and van Winkle's data (1963) on the ability of the schizophrenic body to methylate dopamine; the results of Narasimhachari *et al.* (1970) on the appearance in schizophrenics and not in normal subjects of three different *N*-dimethyl-tryptamine urinary compounds after loading with cysteine and tranylcypromine, before and during the exacerbations of behaviour observed with the test, and finally the fact that an injection of a methylating enzyme (COMT) worsens the schizophrenia.

All these reports seem to lead to the conclusion that the organism of a schizophrenic is a kind of mini laboratory able to produce psychotomimetic (schizophrenic-like) substances. To sum up, keeping to the basic data of the amino-entero-hepatic-toxic doctrine, we can above all underline:

(1) The 'non-specific' structural brain pathology especially characterized by diffused damage ('clods of disintegration in clusters', foci of alterations or disappearance of the neurons and glia). (Up to 1970 almost 1,200 schizophrenic brains were autopsied (Buscaino, V. M., 1970)). It was this very evident spreading that over half a century ago led V. M. Buscaino to the interpretation of the *dissociative* manifestations that characterize the disease. This 'dissociation' could be due to the disruption of the activity of the nervous pathways, which in normal conditions, together with the sensorial

periphery and language, make up the so-called mental activity: indeed without 'neuronal activity' mental activity is impossible.

(2) Alterations of the liver.

(3) A pathology of the gastro-intestinal tract, sometimes even evident prior to the appearance of mental disturbances.

(4) The presence in the body of toxic substances. I could name more than 120 authors from more than 50 institutes worldwide who have studied the toxicity of the urine, the plasma, the serum, the cerebrospinal fluid, the bile and the intestinal content of schizophrenics in the mouse, the hamster, the pigeon, the cat, the dog, the monkey and man with the production of catatonic conditions, irregular behaviour or schizophrenic-like phenomenology. Also the fighting fish of Siam, spiders, pine processionaries, tadpoles, and parameci have all served to show the toxicity, often deadly, of the body fluids of schizophrenics and, likewise, also chicken embryos, yeast cells, the spore of some fungi, germination of the lupin and other cellular groupings in culture have been used. Among the first toxic components to be noted were oxyproteic acids, imidazolic derivatives, xantinic bases, histamine, various globulins (α_1, α_2, β) among which Heath's taraxein, and then many other compounds with an indole nucleus: adrenochrome, adrenolutin, the 'mauve factor', bufotenin, DMPEA, methoxyphenylethylamine, 3-methyl-dopamine, almost all being methylated tryptamines, psychotoxic, as are the methylated tryptamines (hallucinogen) studied by Szara (1956). The importance of methylation is, moreover, enhanced by the increase of methylating ability of the blood of schizophrenics observed by me almost 10 years ago.

At the beginning of 1961 I wrote '. . . among the amine derivatives the methylated and ethylated ones are the most active and it is known that the introduction of a methyl group in the side chain in the alpha position renders many amines completely immune from attack by aminoxidases; the lack of enzymatic action could allow the methylated metabolites to exercise their abnormal action longer'.

This lengthy and perhaps boring statement shows, according to me, that schizophrenia in its biological characteristics is, in fact, a somatic disease; everything, in these patients, functions abnormally; not only in the brain, but also in the liver and gut. The biochemical aetiopathogenesis is, however, very complicated.

In 1964 I attempted to give an over-all interpretation by grouping the more significant biological aspects in a series of factors: (1) predisposing, (2) preparatory, (3) facilitating and (4) triggering.

(1) Among the first, apart from genetic faults with the relevant hereditary metabolic changes (supposed for schizophrenia), I emphasized the functional state of the liver (hepatic meiopragia) and an eventual excessive blood–brain permeability (Bogoch, 1958).

(2) Among the second I mainly included the gastro-intestinal disturbances and the abnormal virulence of the intestinal flora (dysbatteria with an over-production of the usual indole components or even neoformation of abnormal indole molecules) which made the absorption and the transport

by the walls of the gut to the liver of products (mainly indoleamines) of a simple structure possible.

(3) As far as the facilitating factors are concerned, a non-efficient liver enhances the activity of any type of psychotomimetic and the binding of the harmful molecule to carrier proteins is one of the protective mechanisms the liver uses to neutralize toxic substances of an aminic structure (Waelsch, 1961). If the detoxicant capacity of the liver (constitutionally meiopragic, or insufficient due to a disease, or impaired due to the noxious action of the indoleamines coming, maybe continuously, from the gut) is disturbed, some of the (psycho-) toxic molecules can break through the defensive barrier even though attached to a carrier protein. Hence the almost constant increase of the serum globulins and the reports of many 'toxic factors', mostly globulins, in the body fluids of schizophrenics.

Once the harmful molecules free themselves at the blood–brain barrier, they penetrate the cerebral parenchyme and act on the nervous cells *per se* or after having undergone biochemical modifications, among others methylation or transmethylation as well as hydroxylation in particular sites of the molecule all being very important for the acquisition of psychotoxic capacity. Another quota of noxious molecules could be metabolized by aminoxidases – the second protective mechanism against the harmful NH_2 group – and the last catabolites eliminated with the urine (aromatic and diazo reacting compounds likewise found in the urine of schizophrenics). And it is the activity of the intestinal mucosa (especially the small intestine) that through enzymatic mechanisms of bacterial origin is thought to play a fundamental role in the formation of not only histamine and serotonin, but also other eventual indole tryptamines. Even today this is a sufficient argument in favour of the hypothesis that an intestinal abnormality (also bacterial) may play a role in the pathogenesis of schizophrenia.

On this subject I would like to point out that such an intestinal impairment with complications of a bacterial origin was demonstrated over 50 years ago, before tryptamines and especially methylated indole-tryptamines were known.

(4) These metabolites, once in the nervous tissue, could act as 'triggers' of development of schizophrenic symptoms, probably by means of different metabolic changes at a neuronal level perhaps in various specific areas. These changes while compromising the energy and the functioning of some nerve cells, or glia cells (oligodendroglia?) initiate the mental disturbances. And here, one of the most valuable mechanisms could well be the effect on the neurotransmitters either as specific impairment of the 'turnover' of one of them, or as a disturbance of the biohumoral synaptic equilibrium, or for the chain-alterations of the physiological balance between acetylcholine, dopamine, serotonin, adrenaline, noradrenaline, etc. Even histamine seems to have a certain role just as a mediator in certain hypothalamic structures.

This is not the place to go into this much more modern aspect: that will certainly be treated with more competence by someone else in this volume. I only wish to put forward my point of view that it is not necessary to discover a specific and characteristic compound to which to attribute the origin of the schizophrenia.

It could also be that some mediators (or their derivatives, qualitatively or quantitatively aberrating) act as endogenous psychotoxins determining a kind of chemical block of synaptic receptors. But such an active participation could be neither indispensible nor necessarily primitive.

Anyway, my father's conviction that true schizophrenia (and not only some schizophrenic syndromes) appears to be the result of chronic intoxication from indoleamines, especially from methylated tryptamines, is still, today, valid. This doesn't rule out that other psychotoxic factors *similar* to those mentioned may be found, or proved to be the only ones pathogenetically responsible for certain forms of schizophrenia.

REFERENCES

Axelrod, J. (1961). Enzymatic formation of psychotomimetic metabolites from normally occurring compounds. *Science*, **134**, 343

Baruk, H. (1933). La catatonie experimentale et les psychoses coli-bacillaires. *Ann. Med. Psychol.*, **4**

Bayard-Holmes. Cited by Buscaino, V. M. (1970)

Berlet, H. H., Matsumoto, K., Pscheidt, G. R., Spaide, J., Bull, C. and Himwich, H. E. (1965). Biochemical correlates of behaviour in schizophrenic patients. *Arch. Gen. Psychiatry.*, **13**, 521

Bogoch, S. (1958). Cerebrospinal fluid neuraminic acid deficiency in schizophrenia. *Arch. Neurol. Psychol.*, **80**, 221

Brune, G. G. and Himwich, H. E. (1962). Effects of methionine loading on the behaviour of schizophrenic patients. *J. Nerv. Ment. Dis.*, **134**, 447

Brune, G. G., Hohl, H. H. and Himwich, H. E. (1963). Urinary excretion of bufotenin-like substance in psychotic patients. *J. Neuro psychiatr.*, **5**, 14

Buscaino, G. A. (1961). Serotonina e psichiatria. *Acta Neurol.*, **16**, 93

Buscaino, G. A. (1964). Il fattore tossico nella schizofrenia. *Acta Neurol.*, **19**, 1

Buscaino, G. A., Spadetta, V. and Carella, D. (1965). Metilazione della nicotinamide negli schizofrenici. *Acta Neurol.*, **20**, 453

Buscaino, G. A. and Stefanachi, L. (1957). Contributo allo studio del metabolimo delle sostanze indoliche nelle malattie del S. N. III). Ricerche cromatografiche sulle urine di schizofrenici (e di altri malati del sistema nervoso). *Acta Neurol.*, **12**, 1188

Buscaino, V. M. (1920). Le cause anatomo patologiche delle manifestazioni schizofreniche nella demenza precoce. *Riv. Pat. Nerv. Ment.*, **25**, 197

Buscaino, V. M. (1921). I dati attuali sull'anatomia patologica del sistema nervoso dei dementi precoci. *Riv. Pat. Nerv. Ment.*, **26**, 87

Buscaino, V. M. (1922). Sostanze basiche tossiche-amine a nucleo imidazolico – presenti nelle orine di neuro- e psicopatici. *Riv. Pat. Nerv. Ment.*, **27**, 178

Buscaino, V. M. (1923). Alterazioni del fegato e dell'intestino tenue in malati (amenti, dementi precoci encefalitici con amine abnormi nelle orine. *Riv. Pat. Nerv. Ment.*, **28**, 437

Buscaino, V. M. (1924). I dati più recenti (1920–1923) d'istologia patologica del sistema nervoso dei dementi precoci. *Rass. St. Psichiatr.*, **13**, 274

Buscaino, V. M. (1932). Componenti enterogene della demenza precoce. II. Dati clinici e batteriologici. *Schizofrenie*, **2**, fasc. 3

Buscaino, V. M. (1939). Tossicosi aminiche e demenza precoce. *Rass. St. Psichiatr.*, **28**, 792

Buscaino, V. M. (1952). Extraneural pathology of schizophrenia. *Proc. First Int. Congr. of Neuropathol., Roma, 8–13 September, 1952. Acta Neurol.*, **8**, 1

Buscaino, V. M. (1953). Patologia extraneurale della schizofrenia. *Acta Neurol.*, **8**, 1

Buscaino, V. M. (1970). Biologia e terapia della schizofrenia. *Acta Neurol.*, **25**, 1

Buscaino, V. M., Kemali, D. and Bagnulo, R. (1955). Nuove indagini in tema di tossicosi aminiche in schizofrenici. I. Dati orientativi. *Acta Neurol.*, **10**, 547

Dide, M. (1904). Stéathose hépatique chez les aliénés. *Rev. Neurol.*, **12**, 516
Dohan, F. C. (1976). The possible pathogenic effect of cereal grains in schizophrenia. Celiac disease as a model. *Acta Neurol.*, **31**, 195
Feldstein, A., Hoagland, H. and Freeman, H. (1958). On the relationship of serotonin to schizophrenia. *Science*, **128**, 358
Fischer, E., Fernandez la Gravere, T. A., Vazquez, A. J. and di Stefano, A. O. (1961). A bufotenin-like substance in the urine of schizophrenics. *J. Nerv. Ment. Dis.*, **133**, 441
Ford Robertson (1921). Cited by Buscaino, V. M. (1932)
Friedhoff, A. J. and van Winkle, E. (1962). The characteristics of an amine found in the urine of schizophrenic patients. *J. Nerv. Ment. Dis.*, **135**, 550
Friedhoff, A. J. and van Winkle, E. (1963). Conversion of dopamine to 3,4-dimethoxyphenyl-ethylacetic acid in schizophrenic patients. *Nature*, **199**, 1271
Giessing, R. (1974). A review of periodic catatonia. *Biol. Psychiatr.*, **8**, 23
Gullotta, S. (1929). Esplorazione della funzionalità epatica in casi di amenza e di demenza precoce. *Riv. Pat. Nerv. Ment.*, **34**, 852
Heyman, J. J. and Merlis, S. (1962). Paper given at the Proceedings of the 17th, Ann. Meeting of Soc. Biol. Psychiatr., Toronto (Canada), May 4–6, 1962. Transmethylation of nicotinamide in schizophrenics and normals. *Rec. Adv. Biol. Psychiatr.*, **5**, 211 (New York: Plenum Press)
Kanig, K. and Kludas, M. (1958). Indikanurie und Darm-flora bei psychiatrisch-neurologischen Erkrankungen. *Psichiatr. Neurol.*, **136**, 408
Katzenelbogen. Cited by Buscaino, V. M. (1970)
Kemali, D., Buscaino, V. M. and Balbi, R. (1956). Nuove indagini in tema di tossicosi aminiche in schizofrenici II. Dati sul siero di sangue. *Acta Neurol.*, **11**, 209
Kemali, D. and Romano, G. (1956). Ulteriori dati cromatografici sul dismetabolismo indolico in schizofrenici. *Acta Neurol.*, **11**, 959
Leyton, G. B. (1958). Indolic compounds in the urine of schizophrenics. *Br Med. J.*, **5105**, 1136
Longo, V. (1937). Nuovi reperti di insufficienza epatica in malati nervosi e mentali. *Riv. Sperim. Freniatr.*, **61**, 3
Losovskii, D. V. (1962). Triptofan u boglnich scizofreniei. *Vopz. Mediz. Kim.*, **8**, 6 6
Malis, G. Y. (1959). *Research on the Etiology of Schizophrenia.* (New York: Consultants Bureau Enterprises, Inc.)
McGeer, P. L., McGeer, E. G. and Boulding, Y. E. (1956). Relation of aromatic amino acids to excretory patterns of schizophrenics. *Science*, **123**, 1076
McGeer, P. L., McGeer, E. G. and Gibson, W. (1956). Aromatic excretory pattern of schizophrenics. *Science*, **123**, 1029
Meyer, F. R. (1935). Anatomisch-histologische Untersuchungen an Manisch-Depressiven. *Monatschr. Psychiatr. Neurol.*, **91**, 137
Namm e Slipp. (1970). Cited by Buscaino, V. M.
Narasimhachari, N., Heller, B., Spaide, J., Harkovec, L., Fujimori, M., Tabushi, K. and Himwich, H. E. (1970). Comparative behavioural and biochemical effects of tranylcypromine and cysteine on normal controls and schizophrenic patients. *Life Sci.*, **9**, 1021
Noto, G. (1930). Aromatemia ed aromaturia da tirosina nei dementi precoci. *Riv. Pat. Nerv. Ment.*, **36**, 2
Pecchiai, L. (1964). Ricerche istochimiche sulle zolle di disintegrazione a grappolo del sistema nervoso centrale e considerazioni sulla loro genesi. *Biol. Lat.*, **7**, 30
Platania, S. and Pappalardo, P. (1940). Etiologia dell'amenza e della demenza precoce. Ricerche sierodiagnostiche di agglutinazione. *Riv. Neurol.*, **13**, 3
Pollin, W., Cardon, P. V. Jnr. and Kety, S. S. (1961). Effects of amino acid feedings in schizophrenic patients treated with iproniazid. *Science*, **133**, 104
Riegelhaupt, L. M. (1956). Investigations on the glyoxylic acid reactions on urines from schizophrenics and other psychotic patients. *J. Nerv. Ment. Dis.*, **123**, 383
Riegelhaupt, L. M. (1958). *J. Nerv. Ment. Dis.*, **127**, 128
Rodnight, R., Aves, E. K. (1958). Body fluid indoles of normal and mentally-ill subjects. I. Preliminary survey of the occurrence of some urinary indoles. *J. Ment. Sci.*, **104**, 1 49
Sano, I. (1954). Uber di kalte Millon-Reaktion beim schizophrenen Formenkreis und den Träger derselben. *Folia Psychiatr. Neurol Jpn.*, **8**, 218
Sen, N. P. and McGeer, P. L. (1964). 4-methoxyphenylethylamine and 3-4-dimethoxyphenyl-ethylamine in human urine. *Biochem. Biophys. Res. Commun. (Canada)*, **14**, 227
Smythies, Osmond and Harley-Mason (1952). Schizophrenia: a new approach. *J. Ment. Sci.* **98**, 309

Stano, G. (1969). Studio della flora del tenue. I. Ricerche preliminari sulla flora prelevata in corso di laparatomia. *Q. Sclavo Diagnost.*, **5,** 169
Stein, L. and Wise, C. D. (1071). Possible etiology of schizophrenia. *Science*. **171,** 1032
Stewart, (1928). Cited by Buscaino, V. M. (1932)
Summerfield, J. A., Billing, B. H. and Shackleton, H. L. (1976). Identification of bile acid in the serum and urine in cholestasis. *Biochem. J.*, **154,** 507
Szara, S. (1956). Dimethyltryptamine: its metabolism in man; the relation of its psychotic effect to the serotonin metabolism. *Experientia*, **12,** 441
Waelsch, H. (1961) In Jordy Folch-Pi (ed.) *Chemical Pathology of the Nervous System*. (Oxford: Pergamon Press)
Woolley, D. W. and Shaw, E. (1954). Some neurophysiological aspects of serotonin. *Br. Med. J.*, **2,** 122

5
Clues to the causation of schizophrenia

D. RICHTER

INTRODUCTION

At the present time opinion is sharply divided on the factors mainly responsible for the causation of schizophrenia. At one extreme are those who believe that psychological and social factors are the most important, while at the other extreme are those who attribute greater significance to etiological factors of a genetic, physiological or organic kind (Kemali *et al.*, 1976). Research in various different fields has yielded several pieces of evidence which, although not in themselves conclusive, may serve as clues in trying to extend our understanding of the mechanisms concerned. In the present article it is proposed to consider the relation of such clues as are available to a model based on the hypothesis that environmental and genetic factors of a physiological or physical kind are operative in the causation of the commoner forms of schizophrenia.

DISORGANIZATION OF TRANSMITTER MECHANISMS

There is now considerable evidence for the postulate that the symptoms of schizophrenia are due to a disorganization of the transmitter mechanisms in subcortical regions of the brain. It could hardly be regarded as an accident that the phenothiazines, butyrophenones and other drugs of different chemical types which alleviate the symptoms of schizophrenia can all be shown to act as powerful inhibitors of dopaminergic transmission, whereas drugs like the amphetamines which induce the symptoms of schizophrenia potentiate the action of dopamine (DA) in the brain. Hence the 'dopamine hypothesis', which postulates that schizophrenics have an imbalance of transmitters and a relative over-activity of dopaminergic transmission at central synapses in the brain. The precise form of the imbalance may differ to some extent in different cases, and the relative over-activity of dopaminergic transmission could be due to under-activity of inhibitory cholinergic or GABA-liberating neurones. A disturbance of other metabolites which influence synaptic transmission, such as peptides, cations, prostaglandins and steroid hormones must also be considered (Richter, 1976). There is evidence in some cases of a disturbance of adrenergic as well of dopaminergic transmission: this is suggested by the apparent inability of some schizophrenics to experience any kind of pleasure (anhedonia), as if the adrenergic mechanisms of the 'pleasure centres' were impaired. It is unlikely that the dopamine hypothesis is the whole story: nevertheless it would appear that a partial disorganization of central synaptic transmitter mechanisms is one of the best authenticated features of the schizophrenic psychoses.

FAULTY PROCESSING OF SENSORY STIMULI

Patients are said to suffer from schizophrenia if they have certain combinations of mental and behavioural symptoms. The symptoms generally regarded as diagnostically important include certain forms of thought disorder such as thought insertion, faulty perception, inappropriate response, inappropriate affect, delusions of control and auditory hallucinations: but the symptoms vary considerably in different cases and leave room for differences of opinion as to what should be included under the heading of 'schizophrenia'. It is therefore helpful to use specific criteria such as the presence of Schneider's first-rank symptoms (delusions of control, thought insertion, etc.) to define more precisely the way in which we are using the term (Schneider, 1959). Besides the first-rank symptoms, there are many other symptoms that may be present in individual cases.

Careful studies by psychologists of the behaviour of schizophrenics have shown that they often give an abnormal response to sensory stimuli (Shakow, 1971). One characteristic is their failure to adapt in the normal way to a stimulus that is repeated many times by reducing the response (faulty habituation). Often they over-react or under-react, so that the response is inappropriate. Gruzelier and Venables (1973) concluded that there is a disturbance of transmitter mechanisms in the limbic system affecting especially the amygdala and hippocampus, which are believed to mediate the control of sensory input and habituation. Specially characteristic of schizophrenics is their apparent inability to exclude irrelevant stimuli from their attention and maintain a consistent train of thought. Their tendency to over-inclusive thinking suggests a defect in the filtering or gateing mechanism by which specific stimuli are selected for attention. It was shown many years ago by Pfister (1938) that the physiological responses of schizophrenics to stimuli are also frequently abnormal, suggesting a disorder of the basic neurological controlling systems operated by transmitter mechanisms in the hypothalamus. More recently it was reported that schizophrenics show a form of sleep disturbance in that they fail to react in the same way as normal control subjects to the loss of REM sleep (Zarcone *et al.*, 1975).

It may be seen that many of the signs and symptoms found in schizophrenics could result from defects in the processing of sensory data. The brain is constantly receiving stimuli, not only from the special senses, but also from the sensory nerve endings in the skin, joints and viscera. The tasks of sorting out the vast flow of sensory information, relating it to associations in the memory stores, assigning significance in relation to affective potentials, directing attention to the signals of highest priority and defining the autonomic and motor responses, are the function of the transmitter systems operating especially in certain brain-stem and central brain areas. Closely related mechanisms are concerned also in maintaining an appropriate state of arousal during the waking state and in controlling the working out of sensory data during times of paradoxical or REM sleep.

Any serious disorganization of the transmitter mechanisms in the brain-stem and central brain regions would be expected to affect the normal processing of sensory data. It is therefore not unreasonable to believe that

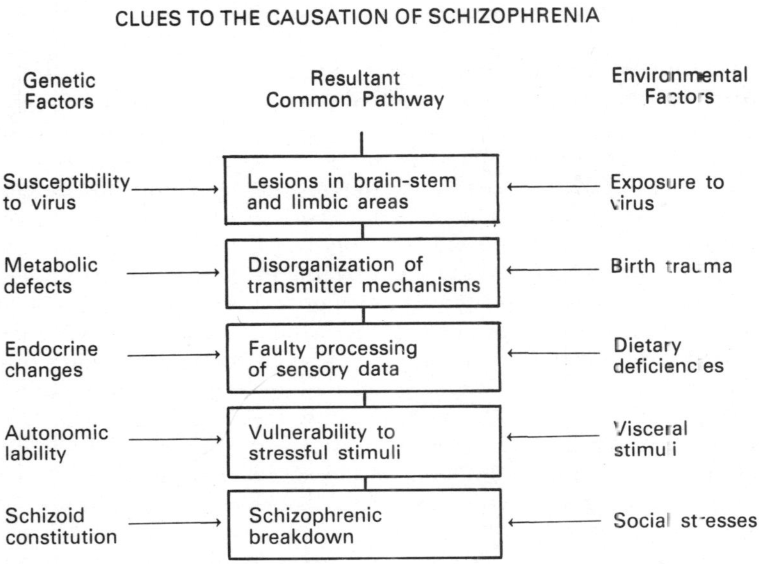

Figure 1 Contribution of genetic and environmental factors to the common pathway resulting in schizophrenic breakdown

the signs and symptoms of defective processing found in schizophrenics are attributable to the transmitter disturbance indicated by the actions of drugs (Figure 1). In agreement with this view is the observation that the physiological mechanisms concerned in the selection or 'gateing' of sensory stimuli and in habituation are closely associated with the mesolimbic dopaminergic system of Dahlström and Fuxe (1964), which is believed to be the main target of the antipsychotic drugs. Further evidence of the part of the brain which is mainly concerned in giving rise to the symptoms of schizophrenia was obtained by Davison and Bagley (1969), who made a computer analysis of the symptoms in 80 cases of brain injury with localized lesions. They found a strong association (1) between diencephalic (central brain) lesions and auditory hallucinations, and (2) between brain-stem lesions and thought disorder, including Schneider's symptoms of the first rank. There are therefore several independent observations indicating that the characteristic symptoms of schizophrenia can be related mainly to a disturbance focused on brain-stem and central areas of the brain (Stevens, 1973).

REACTION TO STRESSFUL STIMULI

A defect in the processing of sensory data can affect behaviour in a number of different ways. Defective habituation implies an inability to adapt in the normal way by reducing the response to a stimulus that is repeated many times. It may mean that a person is unable to develop tolerance and to ignore the many minor sources of friction that commonly occur in contacts with others in everyday life. Such an individual is therefore specially vulnerable to stressful stimuli and liable to break down under their influence

Some indication of this happening in schizophrenics is given by the clinical observation that the onset of a schizophrenic psychosis commonly coincides with a situation of special stress, such as an unhappy love affair. It may be noted that the age of onset of schizophrenia rises to a peak at about the age of 20, an age when sexual arousal tends to reach a maximum. The associated endocrine changes could be relevant in view of the presence of specific receptors for steroid hormones in the brain and their action in altering the firing pattern and habituation properties of neurones in the hypothalamus, septum, amygdala and hippocampus (Stevens, 1973).

At a physiological level the defective gateing of afferent stimuli would be expected to interfere with the operation of the homeostatic controlling mechanisms of the hypothalamus, leading to maladjustment of the body functions. Defective habituation could also result in an abnormal reaction to prolonged stimulation coming from an internal organ such as an inflamed intestine, and this might account for the special sensitivity of some schizophrenics to allergens such as wheat gluten which can set up a chronic inflamation of the gut.

It is evident that the perceptual distortion caused by the faulty processing of sensory data could readily give rise to a subjective sense of unreality and to delusions, while the tendency to over-inclusive thinking must be detrimental to a rational approach in dealing with the practical problems of everyday life. Broadly it can be said that the subject would suffer from a general inability to cope with stressful stimuli, and the natural result would therefore be withdrawal from situations in which stressful stimulation might arise. Of interest in this connection is the secondary system of 'neophobia', or aversion to the unknown, which was found by Shakow (1971) to characterize the behaviour of the schizophrenics he examined.

Under conditions when withdrawal is impossible and there is no escape from exposure to stressful stimuli, the outcome could be a general breakdown of the kind seen in the fully developed schizophrenic psychoses.

CAUSES OF DISORGANIZATION OF SYNAPTIC TRANSMISSION

A disorganization of synaptic transmission such as is postulated in the 'dopamine hypothesis' offers a reasonable explanation for the primary symptoms of schizophrenia, but we still need to know how the disorganization arises. It is evident that some of the characteristics of different individuals are genetically determined; and those with experience of post mortem examinations can testify that there are surprisingly large individual variations in the form and structure of the brain. It appears likely that genetic factors contribute to some extent to the general qualities that go to make up a schizoid personality. They may also operate in individual cases in which a condition such as autonomic lability contributes to the difficulty of coping with a stressful situation. Of interest in this connection is the considerable range of individual variation in the activity of enzymes concerned in the synthesis and breakdown of the various transmitter amines. A genetically determined abnormality in the metabolism of a metabolite such as phenylethylamine or tryptophan is therefore the kind of variation that might play a part in some cases (Sandler and Reynolds, 1976; Huszak *et al.*, 1972).

It is unlikely that a disorganization of synaptic transmission as severe as that which apparently occurs in schizophrenics could be inherited directly by the operation of genetic factors alone. Among the environmental factors that could be held responsible for a disturbance of synaptic organization are birth injuries, including prolonged anoxia, which is known to be capable of causing damage to the brain. There may be individual cases in which birth injuries are a contributing factor, but they can hardly account for the many cases of schizophrenia in subjects who suffered no known birth injury of any kind.

Evidence of synaptic disorganization in the brains of schizophrenics could not easily be obtained by the traditional methods of neuropathology, which are able to show gross changes in the neurones but which were not designed to show changes of a more subtle kind such as those affecting the delicate membranes of the synaptic junctions. Most of the earlier neuropathological studies related in any case mainly to the cerebral cortex which, in the light of more recent work, is probably not the region mainly concerned. More recent investigations by Nieto and Escobar (1972) showed no abnormality in the cerebral cortex of schizophrenics, but gave consistent evidence in every case of a patchy glial proliferation in the region of the hypothalamus, hippocampus and other diencephalic structures. They concluded that the lesions would be consistent with a virus infection or anoxic brain damage at an earlier age. Fisman (1975) has recently reported the presence in the brain-stem region of seven out of eight schizophrenics, but not in the brains of normal controls, of glial nodules that could be attributed to a virus infection. It is known that viruses such as the common herpes simplex virus from time to time invade the brains of individuals who are susceptible to them, and cases of herpes encephalitis have sometimes been diagnosed at first as suffering from schizophrenia (Raskin and Frank, 1974), or have later developed a schizophrenic psychosis (Misra and Hay, 1971). It has long been known that a proportion of schizophrenics have abnormally high levels of proteins in the cerebrospinal fluid, a finding that would agree with a subacute or recurrent virus infection. More recently it has been found that some schizophrenics have raised levels of IgG immunoglobulins in the CSF and high serum antibody levels to herpes simplex virus (Torrey and Peterson, 1976).

There are also some observations that would be consistent with a virus infection of the brain at a very much earlier age. An older report that schizophrenic women produce an abnormally high proportion of infants that are stillborn or malformed has recently been confirmed, and an increased frequency of stillbirths has been reported in the mothers of schizophrenics (Reider *et al.*, 1975; MacSweeney *et al.*, 1976). These findings could well be due to an inherited susceptibility to a neurotropic virus which kills some of the foetuses and leaves others with residual brain damage. In this connection it is of interest that schizophrenics have been found to differ from the general population in the antigens they carry: the frequency level of HLA-A9 is relatively high whereas that of some other antigens may be decreased (Eberhard *et al.,* 1975). The view that genes conferring a predisposition to schizophrenia operate at an early foetal or paranatal stage is supported by the work of Mednick *et al.* (1971) who studied the high-risk children of schizophrenic mothers and found that early birth complications associated with low birth weight and retarded development were often present in those who had a psychiatric illness later in life: nearly 50 per cent showed neurophysiological deviations which included poor habituation, verbal irrelevance and defective autonomic control, as well as deviations at a behavioural level.

Several investigations in different countries of the northern and southern hemisphere have shown that the birthdays of schizophrenics are not randomly distributed, but show an excess in the winter months ranging from about 3 to 13% above the level for the general population (Torrey *et al.,* 1977). It appears unlikely that this finding can be attributed to a difference in the seasonality of conception of schizophrenics (Hare, 1976), but a number of virus infections show a seasonal variation with a higher morbidity rate during the winter months. That might therefore offer an alternative explanation for the higher proportion of schizophrenics born in the winter season.

SUMMARY

It is now well established that genetic and environmental factors both play a part in the causation of schizophrenia. There is no reason to believe that the causes are the same in every case and it appears likely that in individual cases a number of different factors contribute to the common pathway leading up to a schizophrenic psychosis. Consideration has been given to the view that the symptoms most characteristic of schizophrenia are attributable to a partial disorganization of the synaptic transmitter mechanisms involved in the processing of sensory data. It is concluded that this constitutes a special vulnerability to stressful stimuli which can lead to withdrawal and ultimately to schizophrenic breakdown under the influence of social and other stresses. It is suggested that genetic and environmental factors are both relevant at every stage and that in some cases infection by a neurotropic virus is the main cause of the dysfunction which results in the later development of a schizophrenic psychosis.

REFERENCES

Dahlström, A. and Fuxe, K. (1964). Evidence for the existence of monoamine-containing neurones in the CNS. *Acta Physiol. Scand.,* **62,** (Suppl. 232), 1

Davison, K. and Bagley, C. R. (1969). Schizophrenia-like psychoses associated with organic disorders of the CNS. In *Current Problems in Neuropsychiatry.* (R. N. Herrington, ed.) pp. 113–184. (Ashford: Headley Bros.)

Eberhard, G. Franzen, G. and Low, B. (1975). Schizophrenia susceptibility and HLA–A antigen. In *Neuropsychobiology.* (J. Mendelwicz, ed.) pp. 211–217. (Basel: S. Karger

Fisman, M. (1975). The brain-stem in psychoses. *Br. J. Psychiatry,* **126,** 414

Gruzelier, J. and Venables, P. (1974). Bimodality and lateral assymmetry of skin conductance orientating activity in schizophrenics. *Biol. Psychiatry,* **8,** 55

Hare, E. H. (1976). The season of birth of siblings of psychiatric patients. *Br. J. Psychiatry,* **129,** 49

Huszak, I., Durko, I. and Karsai, K. (1972). Experimental data to the pathogenesis of cryptopyrrole excretion in schizophrenia. *Acta Physiol. Acad. Sci. Hungariene,* **42,** 79

Kemali, D., Bartholini, G. and Richter, D. (1976). *Schizophrenia Today.* (Oxford: Pergamon Press)

MacSweeney, D. A., Johnson, A. L. and Timms, P. E. S. (1978). Thyro-endocrine pathology, obstetric morbidity and schizophrenia: Survey of a hundred families with a schizophrenic proband. *Psychol. Med.,* **8,** 151

Mednick, S. A., Mura, E., Schulsinger, F. and Mednick, B. (1971). Perinatal conditions and infant development in children with schizophrenic parents. *Soc. Biol.,* **18,** Suppl. S.103–S.113

Misra, P. C. and Hay, G. G. (1971). Encephalitis presenting as acute schizophrenia *Br. Med. J.,* **5748,** 532

Nieto, D. and Escobar, A. (1972). Major psychoses. In *Pathology of the Nervous System.* Vol. III, (J. Minckler, ed.) pp. 2654–2670. (New York: McGraw-Hill Inc.)

Raskin, D. E. and Frank, S. W. (1974). Herpes encephalitis with catatonic stupor. *Arch. Gen. Psychiatry,* **31,** 544

Rieder, R. O., Rosenthal, D., Wender, P. and Blumenthal, H. (1975). The offspring of schizophrenics. *Arch. Gen. Psychiatry,* **32,** 200

Richter, D. (1976). The impact of biochemistry on the problem of schizophrenia. In *Schizophrenia Today.* (D. Kemali, G. Bartholini and D. Richter, eds.) pp. 71–83 (Oxford: Pergamon Press)

Sandler, M. and Reynolds, G. P. (1976). Does phenylethylamine cause schizophrenia? *Lancet,* **i,** 70

Schneider, K. (1959). *Clinical psychopathology.* (London: Grune and Stratton)

Shakow, D. (1971). Some observations on the psychology (and some fewer on the biology) of schizophrenia. *J. Nerv. Ment. Dis.,* **153,** 300

Stevens, J. R. (1973). An anatomy of schizophrenia? *Arch. Gen. Psychiatry,* **29,** 177

Torrey, E. F. and Peterson, M. R. (1976). The viral hypothesis of schizophrenia. *Schizophrenia Bull.,* **2,** 136

Torrey, E. F., Torrey, B. B. and Peterson, M. R. (1977). Seasonality of schizophrenic births in the US. *Arch. Gen. Psychiatry,* **34,** 1065

Zarcone, V., Azumi, K., Dement, W., Gulevich, G., Kraemer, H. and Pivik, T. (1975). REM phase deprivation and schizophrenia II *Arch. Gen. Psychiatry,* **32,** 1431

6

An evaluation of the dopamine hypothesis of schizophrenia

T. J. CROW

INTRODUCTION

In recent years no hypothesis of the chemical basis of schizophrenia has proved more productive than the conjecture that dopaminergic mechanisms are hyperactive and that the pathological effects of this hyperactivity are reduced by adminstration of neuroleptic drugs. Some neurohumoural theories (e.g. the serotonin deficiency hypothesis, (Gaddum, 1954; Woolley and Shaw, 1954) have, like the dopamine hypothesis been founded upon observations on certain hallucinogenic drugs. Others such as the noradrenaline neurone degeneration hypothesis of Stein and Wise (1971) have been more sophisticated in attempting a psychological as well as a chemical explanation of some features of the disease. The dopamine hypothesis, perhaps because it was formulated partly to explain the well established therapeutic effects of the neuroleptic drugs, has proved highly fertile. It continues to stimulate much basic and some clinical research.

THE ORIGINS OF THE DOPAMINE HYPOTHESIS

The hypothesis had two major origins: the observation that the psychosis which is sometimes seen after amphetamine abuse closely resembles acute paranoid schizophrenia, and the finding that many of the drugs which had been found to be effective in schizophrenia have actions on central dopaminergic mechanisms. The recognition of the significance of amphetamine psychosis owes much to Connell's monograph (Connell, 1958), and to accounts of the psychiatric sequelae of the epidemics of amphetamine abuse which affected various countries in the 1950s and 1960s (Ellinwood, 1967; Jönsson and Gunne, 1970; Rylander, 1972). The efficacy of the neuroleptic drugs in acute schizophrenia was by this time well-established, and the observation that they frequently induced extra-pyramidal parkinsonian) side effects had stimulated discussion concerning their possible mechanisms of action (Flügel, 1953; Deniker, 1960). The description of the distribution of dopamine in the brain (Bertler and Rosengren, 1959; Carlsson, 1959) and the discovery that this substance was reduced in the brains of patients dying from Parkinson's disease (Ehringer and Hornykiewicz, 1960) were the findings that led to the concept of a specific interaction between neuroleptic drugs and dopaminergic mechanisms (Carlsson and Lindqvist, 1963; van Rossum, 1966).

Randrup and Munkvad (1966) and their colleagues appear to have been the first to associate the behavioural actions of the amphetamines specifically with central dopaminergic transmission. In a series of studies (Randrup and Munkvad, 1967) they demonstrated that the central actions of the amphetamines consisted not, as had previously been thought, of a general increase of motor activity, but of a complex change in the pattern of behaviour (the development of stereotyped behaviours) and the appearance of certain situationally inappropriate behaviours (e.g. sniffing, licking and gnawing behaviours, in the rat). These amphetamine-induced changes were selectively anatagonised by neuroleptic drugs (Randrup and Munkvad, 1965). From these animal experiments has been developed much later theorising about the nature of the abnormalities observed in schizophrenia and their reversal by drugs.

THE AMPHETAMINE PSYCHOSIS

The similarities of the phenomena of amphetamine psychosis to those seen in acute schizophrenic illnesses have been stressed by Connell (1958) and by other authors (Ellinwood, 1967; Jönsson and Gunne, 1970; Rylander, 1972; Angrist, Sathananthan, Wilk and Gershon, 1974a). Whether or not the amphetamine psychosis lacks certain features (e.g. flattening of affect) of acute schizophrenic psychoses has been debated (Angrist *et al.*, 1974a), but it is clear that the amphetamine psychosis more closely resembles the idiopathic illness than do the psychoses induced, for example, by lysergic acid diethylamide and mescaline. However the relevance for understanding the pathogenesis of schizophrenia would be diminished if, as has been suggested.

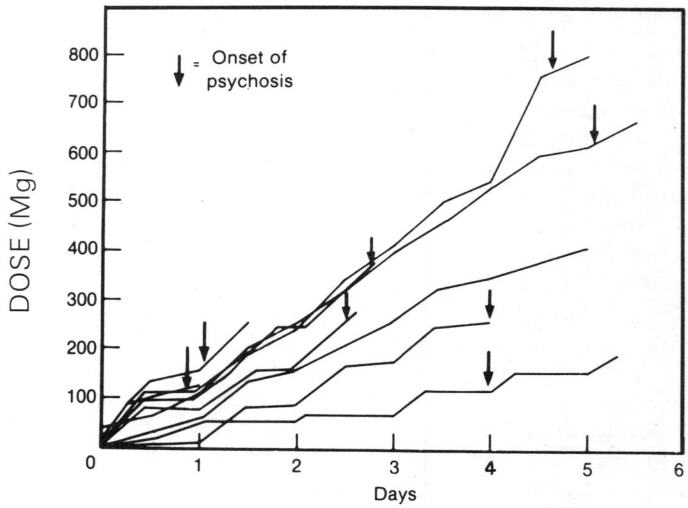

Figure 1 The cumulative dose of amphetamine administered to eight volunteer subjects over a 5-day experiment. Arrows indicate the point at which psychotic changes were seen (from Griffith, *et al.*, 1972)

psychotic symptoms occured following amphetamine only in subjects predisposed to a schizophrenic illness, or were a secondary consequence of the sleep deprivation induced by the drug. However Griffith, Cavanagh, Held and Oates (1972) were able to show that psychotic symptoms occur in most if not all volunteer subjects (Figure 1) if sufficient doses are given, and also that such symptoms can occur before the extent of the sleep deprivation approaches the duration (generally in excess of 72 hours) at which psychotic changes have been observed. Such findings establish the psychotic changes as a direct pharmacological action. Therefore interest in the chemical mechanism is increased.

Randrup and Munkvad (1966) found that the syndrome of amphetamine stereotypies in rodents is abolished by administration of the compound α-methyl-*p*-tyrosine, which inhibits the enzyme tyrosine hydroxylase and depletes the brain of the two catecholamines dopamine and noradrenaline. Pre-treatment with drugs which block the enzyme dopamine-β-hydroxylase, and therefore inhibit the synthesis of noradrenaline alone, does not diminish the syndrome. Similar findings are obtained in other species (Randrup and Munkvad, 1967). The dependence of amphetamine-induced changes in behaviour upon the integrity of central dopaminergic transmission is further substantiated by a series of studies using the neurotoxic agent 6-OH-dopamine which can induce a relatively selective degeneration of catecholamine neurones. Stereotaxically placed injections into the region of the substantia nigra, where the cell-bodies of the dopaminergic nigro-striatal system are located, or into the corpus striatum, the region of the terminals, substantially diminish the ability of the amphetamines to elicit stereotypies (Creese and Iversen, 1975). Similar lesions of the nucleus accumbens, a nucleus innervated by dopamine-containing terminals which arise from cell bodies in the mid-line area, over the interpeduncular nucleus, and between the two substantiae nigrae, diminish the locomotor increases induced by amphetamine (Kelly *et al.*, 1975). Both major components of the amphetamine syndrome therefore appear to depend on amine release from central dopamine-containing neurones.

Although the psychological changes observed in the amphetamine psychosis in man are not closely related to the behaviours elicited by amphetamine in lower mammals there are similarities, particularly in the incidence of repetitive and stereotyped activities, and it is argued that the neurochemical basis may be the same. There is some evidence that this may be the case. The amphetamine psychosis can be blocked by administration of neuroleptic drugs such as haloperidol (Angrist *et al.*, 1974b) and amphetamine euphoria by the tyrosine hydroxylase inhibitor α-methyl-*p*-tyrosine (Gunne *et al.*, 1972). It has been argued that since the psychosis is easily provoked by the (+) as by the (–) isomer of amphetamine it is more likely to be related to dopamine than noradrenaline release (Angrist, Shopsin and Gershon, 1971) on the basis that the amphetamine isomers show a degree of selectivity in their actions on the two catecholamines. However the precise neurochemical effects of the two isomers are uncertain (Matthysse, 1974) and the significance of these observations in man is still equivocal.

Direct evidence for increased dopamine release following amphetamine administration in man has been sought in c.s.f. studies following probenecid. This substance blocks the egress of acidic monoamine metabolites from c.s.f. and the increase in the levels of the dopamine metabolite homo-vanillic acid can therefore be taken as an index of dopamine release in the brain. Angrist *et al.* (1974a) have found that HVA levels in c.s.f. are increased following amphetamine and this suggests rather strongly that dopamine release is increased by amphetamine, and also that the changes in monoamine function which accompany the psychosis can be reliably assessed by the probenecid technique (Figure 2).

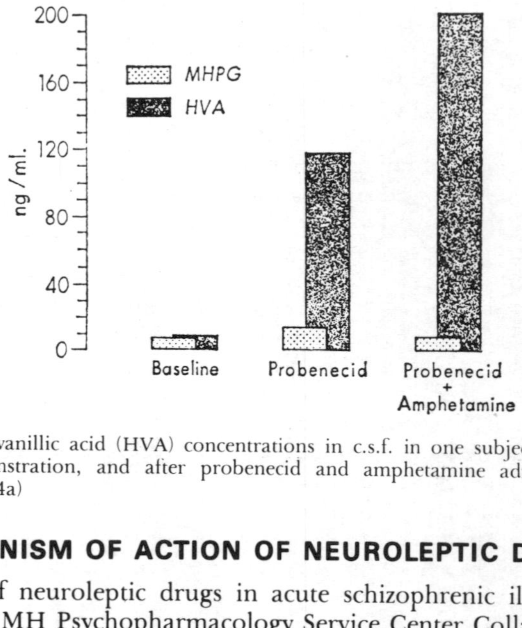

Figure 2 Homovanillic acid (HVA) concentrations in c.s.f. in one subject before and after probenecid adminstration, and after probenecid and amphetamine administration (from Angrist *et al.*, 1974a)

THE MECHANISM OF ACTION OF NEUROLEPTIC DRUGS

The efficacy of neuroleptic drugs in acute schizophrenic illnesses is well-established (NIMH Psychopharmacology Service Center Collaborative Study Group, 1964). An analysis of the placebo–drug differences for a range of symptoms in the NIMH 1964 study (Goldberg *et al.*, 1965) has shown that the beneficial effects of these drugs, at least in the short term, are rather widely distributed across the various manifestations of the disease. Thus these drugs may interact in some way with the basic disease process rather than merely suppress the more florid symptoms. There is also substantial evidence (Leff and Wing, 1971; Hirsch *et al.*, 1973; Hogarty and Goldberg, 1974) that these drugs are effective in some patients in preventing relapse. It is reasonable to suppose that an understanding of these pharmacological effects might tell us something about the pathological process.

Three major groups of compounds – phenothiazines, butyrophenones and thiaxanthenes – are known to include members which have anti-psychotic activity. It is a striking fact that most if not all of the compounds which are active are also able to induce extrapyramidal side effects if given in sufficient doses. Since the structures of some of these drugs are quite dissimilar this provides some support for the view (Flügel, 1953; Deniker, 1960) that these properties are related.

Carlsson and Lindqvist (1963) observed that certain neuroleptic drugs increase the levels of the dopamine metabolites homo-vanillic acid (HVA) and dihydroxy-phenylacetic acid (DOPAC) in brain. They suggested that this might be due to increased activity in the presynaptic neurone induced by a feedback mechanism from the blocked post-synaptic dopamine receptor. Other observers (e.g. van Rossum, 1966; Randrup and Munkvad, 1967; Ernst, 1967) had concluded on the basis of pharmacological and behavioural experiments that neuroleptic drugs have powerful dopamine blocking activity. The demonstration that dopamine is depleted in the brain in Parkinson's disease (Ehringer and Hornykiewicz, 1960) suggested that the extrapyramidal side effects of the neuroleptic drugs might well be due to impaired dopaminergic transmission, resulting not from depletion of dopamine stores, but from blockade of the post-synaptic receptor site. Later studies (Laverty and Sharman, 1965; O'Keefe, Sharman and Vogt, 1970) established that the increase in dopamine turnover occurs with a variety of neuroleptic drugs, and behavioural experiments demonstrated that ability to block the syndrome induced by amphetamine, or the closely similar behaviour induced by administration of apomorphine, a drug which acts as an agonist at the dopamine receptor, is a good predictor of antipsychotic potency (Janssen *et al.*, 1965).

A more direct approach to the dopamine receptor was opened up by the discovery of a dopamine-sensitive adenylate cyclase in the corpus striatum (Kebabian *et al.*, 1972). The concept that some post-synaptic actions of neurohumours are mediated by cyclic nucleotide formation in the post-synaptic cell is now well accepted, and it appears that the adenylate cyclase enzyme in the striatum may be closely related to the dopamine receptor itself. A series of studies (Miller *et al.*, 1974; Clement-Cormier *et al.*, 1974) have established that the sensitivity of the enzyme to dopamine is inhibited by low concentrations of various neuroleptic drugs, and that there is a good correlation between antipsychotic potency and ability to block the dopamine-sensitive adenylate cyclase. Phenothiazines such as promazine with low anti-psychotic potency are relatively poor blockers of adenylate cyclase stimulation. Drugs with high potency such as fluphenazine are more effective than standard compounds such as chlorpromazine and trifluoperazine which themselves are probably as effective clinically, but only when given in higher doses (Figure 3).

In general the correlation between *in vitro* activity in this system and therapeutic activity in schizophrenia holds well over a wide range of pheno-thiazine and thiaxanthene compounds. There are, however, two difficulties. Firstly that the incidence of extrapyramidal side effects, which are also due to these drugs' ability to block dopamine receptors, is not perfectly correlated with therapeutic potency. Secondly, the activity of the butyrophenones in the adenylate cyclase preparation is much less (perhaps by a factor of 60 in the case of haloperidol) than would be expected on the basis of the anti-

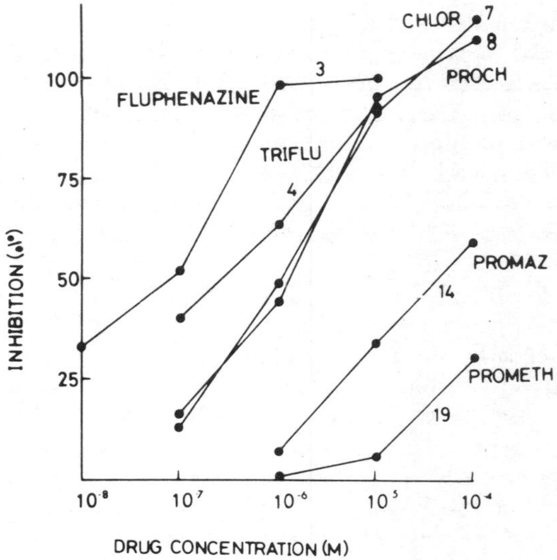

Figure 3 Inhibition of adenylate cyclase stimulation by dopamine as a function of increasing concentrations of various neuroleptic drugs (from Miller *et al.*, 1974)

psychotic doses used in practice. The former difficulty can now be satisfactorily resolved and two possible explanations for the latter have recently been advanced.

The less than perfect correlation between extrapyramidal side effects and clinical potency has been explained by reference to the anticholinergic blocking actions of certain neuroleptic drugs. It has long been recognised that drugs such as chlorpromazine have peripheral anticholinergic actions, and techniques have recently been developed for studying their central antimuscarinic effects. Two groups (Miller and Hiley, 1974; Snyder *et al.*, 1974) have examined the relationship between these actions and the abilities of various neuroleptic drugs to induce parkinsonian side effects. The two actions are strongly negatively correlated. Thus drugs such as thioridazine with few extrapyramidal side effects are potent blockers of the central muscarinic cholinergic receptor. Drugs with a high incidence of side effects, like fluphenazine, have little anticholinergic activity. Therefore it appears that the explanation for the limited correlation between side effects and therapeutic effects is that some drugs possess their own 'in-built' anti-parkinsonian actions.

The two explanations that are offered for the apparent ineffectiveness of the butyrophenones in the adenylate cyclase test are: (1) that these compounds may block release from the presynaptic dopamine terminal Seeman and Lee (1975) have demonstrated in striatal tissue slices that there is a surprisingly high correlation between therapeutic potency (assessed mainly from data on daily dosage as recommended by the pharmaceutical houses) and ability to inhibit dopamine release induced by electrical stimulation. (2) That neuroleptics may interact with a dopamine receptor site distinct from that associated with the dopamine-sensitive adenylate cyclase. For example a 'haloperidol binding site' has been studied by isotope labelling techniques as a possible model for the dopamine receptor, and an interaction between haloperidol and dopamine at this site has been demonstrated. Various neuroleptics interfere with haloperidol binding in direct relation to their antipsychotic effects and in this situation the potency of the butyrophenones falls into line with the clinically effective doses (Creese *et al.*, 1976; Seeman *et al.*, 1976).

With the removal of these apparent anomalies the dopamine blockade hypothesis of neuroleptic action is able to accommodate most, if not all, of our present knowledge of the pharmacology of the antipsychotic effect. Lately, on the basis of some findings in the adenylate cyclase preparation, it has been possible to devise a rather stringent clinical test of the hypothesis. Previous studies in the preparation *in vitro* (Miller *et al.*, 1974) had shown that some thiaxanthene compounds which exhibit isomerism have a stereo-specific ability to block the dopamine-induced increase. For example flu-penthixol has a *cis*-(α), and a *trans*-(β) isomerism determined by the deviation of the side chain with respect to the CF_3 substituent, and only the α-isomer possesses significant dopamine-blocking activity. Since the standard oral preparation includes both isomers it was of particular interest to determine whether all of the therapeutic activity was due to the α-isomer or whether the β-form also contributed. If, for example, it could be shown that the two isomers were equally active this finding would effectively eliminate the dopamine blockade hypothesis. If the β-isomer possessed no activity the hypothesis would survive unscathed, but if the α-isomer were more effective than the β- but the β-itself were more effective than placebo this would suggest that although dopamine blockade is a significant component other pharmacological actions are also important.

To test these possibilites a trial was designed to compare the antipsychotic activities of α- and β-flupenthixol with placebo in patients suffering from acute schizophrenic illnesses (Crow *et al.*, 1977, submitted for publication). Since patients on placebo, at least, might require further medication chlor-promazine adminstration was allowed in addition to the trial medication. Thus two dependent variables were assessed: weekly symptom ratings, and amount of additional medication received. By both criteria the results were clear-cut; α-flupenthixol was superior to β-flupenthixol, and the latter was not significantly different from placebo. On the rating scales the differ-ences between α-flupenthixol and the other two treatments were significant at the third and fourth weeks of the 4-week trial.

The dopamine blockade hypothesis has therefore survived a rather exacting experimental test and the results suggest that the entire antipsychotic effect must be associated with a pharmacological action, such as dopamine blockade, possessed by the α- but not the β-isomer of flupenthixol. Phar-macological actions on which the two isomers do not differ can be ruled out. This has now been demonstrated for the acetylcholine, opiate (Enna *et al.*, 1976) and the noradrenergic receptors (Horn and Phillipson, 1975).

Thiothixene has an isomerism similar to that of flupenthixol, and it has been shown that the two thiothixene isomers do not differ from each other in their abilities to block the glycine and GABA receptors (Enna *et al.*, 1976). It seems likely that the flupenthixol isomers will show a similar lack of selectivity, and therefore that ability to block the glycine and GABA receptors as well as the cholinergic, noradrenergic, and opiate receptors can be ruled out as the basis of the antipsychotic effect.

There is however one action besides dopamine receptor blockade in which the isomers of flupenthixol are known to differ, and that is with respect to their ability to block the 5-hydroxytryptamine receptor (Enna *et al.*, 1976). Therefore on the basis of the trial result 5-HT blockade cannot be ruled out. However there is other evidence (Bennett and Snyder, 1975) that the 5-HT blocking activity of various centrally-acting drugs show a poor correlation with antipsychotic potency. For example drugs such as promazine and amitriptyline which are known to have little or no antipsychotic activity are almost as potent blockers of the 5-HT receptor as chlorpromazine and fluphenazine. On these grounds it appears unlikely that 5-HT blockade is related to therapeutic effectiveness.

In summary the hypothesis that ability to block the central dopamine receptor is necessary for the antipsychotic effect has survived a number of critical tests. No other pharmacological action approaches dopamine blockade as a predictor of clinical potency.

THE SITE OF ANTIPSYCHOTIC ACTION

There is an important corollary of the assumption that both the antipsychotic and the extrapyramidal effects are due to dopamine blockade and the observation that the two can vary independently. This is that these actions cannot be occuring at the same site in the brain. It is widely assumed that the extrapyramidal effects are due to dopamine receptor blockade in the striatum and are to a certain extent antagonised by cholinergic blockade in the same structure. If the antipsychotic effects were also due to dopamine blockade in the striatum it would be expected that, in the case of a drug like thioridazine with a high anticholinergic potency, the therapeutic effects would be antagonised by the blockade of the acetylcholine receptor. However this is not the case. Thioridazine and chlorpromazine are approximately equally effective dose for dose clinically (NIMH–PSC Collaborative Study Group, 1964) and inhibit the dopamine-sensitive adenylate cyclase at similar concentrations (Miller and Hiley, 1974), but thiorizadine has fewer extrapyramidal effects. The conclusion appears to be inescapable that if the antipsychotic effects are due to dopamine blockade they do not occur in the striatum.

One is led to ask what other dopaminergic receptor sites in the brain there may be at which neuroleptic drugs could be exerting their antipsychotic action. With the fluorescence histochemical technique of Flack and Hillarp, Ungerstedt (1971a) described two major ascending dopamine-containing pathways: (1) the weil-known nigro-striatal pathway arising from cell-bodies in the pars compacta (the A9 area- of the substantia nigra innervate the corpus striatum, and

(2) the 'mesolimbic' dopamine system which arises from a group of cell-bodies (the A10 area) situated in the mid-line over the interpeduncular nucleus to terminate in the nucleus accumbens, olfactory tubercle and some related nuclei. More recently a small dopaminergically-innervated area of the frontal cortex has been described (Berger *et al.,* 1976) and this system may also arise from the A10 cell body group.

In order to test the hypothesis that neuroleptic drugs might be exerting their antipsychotic effects within the mesolimbic system we compared three neuroleptic drugs, differing in their incidence of extrapyramidal side effects, in their actions on dopamine turnover in the striatum and nucleus accumbens, using dose ratios approximating to therapeutically equivalent levels in man. The index of action on dopaminergic mechanisms is the extent to which these drugs are able to increase the accumulation of the dopamine metabolite homovanillic acid (HVA), an effect which is interpreted as a secondary consequence of receptor blockade (Carlsson and Lindqvist, 1963).

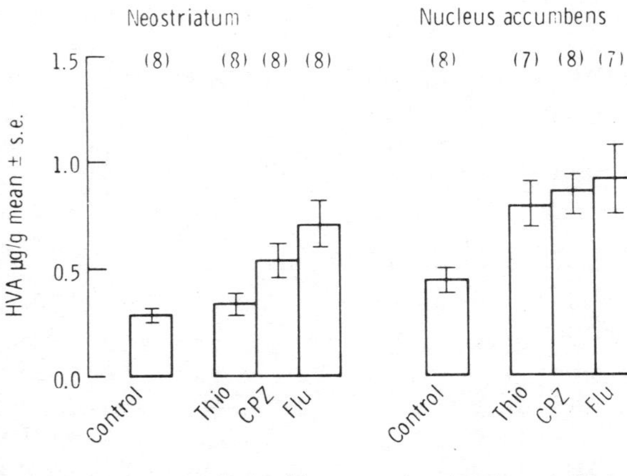

Figure 4 Effects of thioridazine (Thio), chlorpromazine (CPZ), and fluphenazine (Flu), on dopamine turnover (assessed by the accumulation of the metabolite HVA) in the neostriatum and nucleus accumbens. The dose ratios (1:1:0·05) were selected to correspond to therapeutically equivalent daily dosages. Figures in parentheses represent nos. of animals studied (adapted from Crow *et al.*, 1977)

The results show quite clearly that there are differences between various neuroleptic drugs in their actions on the two areas. In the striatum, fluphenazine, a drug with a high incidence of extrapyramidal side effects, has the largest effect, while thioridazine, with relatively few side effects at this dose level, has little effect, and chlorpromazine is intermediate. The effects on HVA are therefore in direct proportion to the extrapyramidal effects. By contrast in the nucleus accumbens each of the three drugs causes a similar increase in HVA. Since the dose ratio has been selected to correspond as closely as possible to equivalent antipsychotic potencies in man the effects in the accumbens are closely related to the antipsychotic effects.

These results are therefore entirely consistent with the suggestion (Andén, 1972; Stevens, 1973) that the antipsychotic effects of neuroleptic drugs may be due to their ability to block dopamine receptors in the nucleus accumbens. They do not rule out the possibility that the therapeutic effects may be due to an action elsewhere within the mesolimbic dopamine system, for example in the frontal cortex, and this alternative hypothesis remains to be tested. The relationship between the nucleus accumbens and the hippocampus and amygdala (Swanson and Cowan, 1975) is of some interest in view of the evidence (Slater *et al.*, 1963; Flor-Henry, 1969) that there may be a particular association between temporal lobe epilepsy and schizophrenia-like states. It appears that there is a reciprocal relationship between the nucleus accumbens and these limbic structures which is analagous to that which exists between the corpus striatum and the neocortex. It appears possible that the nucleus accumbens processes descending information from the hippocampus and amygdala in the way in which the corpus striatum processes that from the cerebral cortex.

THE DOPAMINE OVER-ACTIVITY HYPOTHESIS OF SCHIZOPHRENIA

With the survival of the dopamine blockade hypothesis of neuroleptic action it is natural to ask whether the findings of these various investigations tell us anything about the nature of the disease itself. Why should it be, as now appears likely, that blockade of dopamine receptors reverses some of the manifestations of the disease? The simplest current explanation – the dopamine over-activity hypothesis of schizophrenia – is that excess transmitter release from dopaminergic neurones occurs in schizophrenia and forms the basis of at least some of the psychiatric symptoms. There have now been a number of tests of this hypothesis. In general the results do not appear favourable to the hypothesis as originally stated (Randrup and Munkvad, 1972; Klawans *et al.*, 1972; Metthysse, 1973; Snyder, 1973; Stevens, 1973), and it is instructive to ask whether our present techniques are able to give information of a decisive nature, and if so whether alternative hypotheses can be formulated to account for the apparent relationship between the therapeutic effects of the neuroleptics and their actions on dopamine receptors.

There have been three major types of investigation of dopaminergic processes in schizophrenia – (1) studies of dopamine metabolites in c.s.f., (2) studies of the coincidence of schizophrenia with Parkinsonism, a disease in which dopamine metabolism is known to be disturbed and (3) studies of prolactin secretion in acute and chronic schizophrenic illnesses.

The most direct approach to c.n.s. dopamine turnover currently available appears to be the technique of combining measurements of the concentration of the dopamine metabolite (HVA) with probenecid administration. This technique depends upon the fact that probenecid blocks the mechanism which removes the acid metabolites of the monoamines (such as HVA) from c.s.f. The rise in concentration of HVA in c.s.f. after probenecid may therefore be taken as an index of the rate at which this metabolite is leaving the brain and spinal cord, and therefore of the rate of turnover of the parent amine dopamine. This strategy has been tested in Parkinson's disease (Korf and van Praag, 1971), where it is possible to detect the decrease in dopamine turnover, and it is of particular interest that in amphetamine psychosis increased concentrations of HVA have been detected after probenecid (Angrist *et al.*, 1974a). There seems no reason therefore why increased dopamine turnover if it occurs in schizophrenia should not be demonstrated by the probenecid technique. However Bowers (1974), in a study of 17 acute schizophrenics, found HVA concentrations after probenecid to be significantly lower than in a group of 11 patients with depressive illnesses, and there is other evidence (Sjöström and Roos, 1972) that such patients with affective illness may have lower concentrations than neurological and normal controls. In patients judged to have a worse prognosis Bowers found HVA levels after probenecid to be less than those in patients with a better prognosis. A similar study by Post *et al.*, (1975) yielded no evidence of decreased dopamine turnover by comparison with controls but within the patient group revealed an inverse relationship between HVA accumulation and severity of illness, assessed by number of Schniederian first-rank symptoms. Both studies have therefore given results precisely the opposite of those found in amphetamine intoxication by Angrist *et al.* (1974a), and the reverse of the prediction of the dopamine over-activity hypothesis. **

A further prediction appears to be that schizophrenia, in which dopamine release is held to be increased, should exhibit a relationship of mutual antagonism with Parkinson's disease, where it is highly likely that degeneration of dopamine neurones accounts for the major symptoms of the disease (Hornykiewicz, 1973). One might predict either that the two diseases would not occur together, or that if they did, they might interact in such a way that, for example, the onset of Parkinson's disease was associated with an amelioration of the symptoms of schizophrenia or vice versa. There is little evidence that this is the case. Schizophrenic symptoms were recognised as a possible sequel of the epidemic encephalitis which swept the world in the 1920s, and was a frequent precursor of a parkinsonian syndrome, and it appears that schizophrenic and extrapyramidal symptoms could co-exist (see e.g. McCowan and Cook, 1928). In a recent study (Crow *et al.*, 1976) we were able to identify four patients with long-standing parkinsonian symptoms, in two cases of the post-encephalitic, and in two of the idiopathic types, who subsequently developed psychotic illnesses which in each case included schizophrenic features which were not explicable on the basis of changes in medication or affect. While these illnesses did not clearly belong to the category of nuclear schizophrenia it appeared that they had to be classified within the 'schizophrenia spectrum'. Such cases therefore establish the point that increased dopamine release is not necessary for the emergence of schizophrenia-like symptoms.

Against this conclusion it may be objected that the increased dopamine release takes place not from the terminals of the nigro-striatal dopamine pathway which presumably has degenerated in Parkinson's disease, but from the terminals of the mesolimbic dopamine pathway, e.g. in the nucleus accumbens and related nuclei. However it has recently been demonstrated (Farley *et al.,* 1977) that in the brains of patients dying with Parkinson's disease dopamine is as depleted in mesolimbic structures as it is in the corpus striatum. The disease process appears to affect at least all those dopamine systems which arise from the ventral mesencephalon, and observations that schizophrenic symptoms can arise in the context of an otherwise typical parkinsonian syndrome are perhaps therefore of more critical significance for the dopamine over-activity hypothesis that might otherwise have been the case.

A further approach to the hypothesis has been through investigations of prolactin secretion, following the discovery that the small tubero-infundibular dopamine system in the median eminence of the hypothalamus exerts an inhibitory influence on prolactin secretion (Fuxe *et al.,* 1969). It is well-established that neuroleptic drugs increase prolactin secretion. For example serum prolactin concentrations in patients on chlorpromazine are related both to extrapyramidal side effects and to serum levels of chlorpromazine (Kolakowska *et al.,* 1975), and it is particularly interesting that thioridazine which, as previously mentioned, has a low incidence of side effects but possesses undoubted dopamine receptor blocking activity, is a potent releaser of prolactin secretion (Wilson *et al.,* 1975). These findings, and the prediction that increased dopamine release, if it includes the tubero-infundibular system, should lower prolactin, make observations of prolactin secretion in unmedicated schizophrenic patients of particular interest. Meltzer, Sachar and Frantz (1974) studied a group of 22 patients with acute schizophrenia and found that the serum concentrations of prolactin were not significantly different from those of a group of 13 normal subjects, and that within the patient group those with paranoid symptoms, whose illnesses might be thought to resemble the amphetamine psychosis more closely, did not differ from those without such symptoms. In a group of hospitalized patients with chronic schizophrenic illnesses who had for many years been free of medication Johnstone, Crow and Mashiter (1977) also found no evidence that prolactin secretion was low by comparison with the normal range, and in a few patients the serum concentrations appeared abnormally high. However in this population there was an interesting relationship between symptom change and serum prolactin. When clinical state and serum prolactin were each assessed on two occasions a significant inverse relationship was observed between positive schizophrenic symptoms and prolactin secretion, i.e. increasing severity of symptoms was associated with decreased prolactin secretion. This relationship can be explained if increased symptom severity results in increased activity of the tubero-infundibular system. However the investigations of prolactin secretion in general give little support for the hypothesis that there is a widespread over-activity of dopaminergic systems in either acute or chronic schizophrenic illnesses.

Thus all three lines of investigation have failed to provide definite evidence that dopamine release is increased in schizophrenic illnesses. In view of the findings with the probenecid test in amphetamine psychosis the c.s.f. studies are perhaps the most cogent and in this case the results are the opposite of those predicted by the hypothesis.

SOME ALTERNATIVE HYPOTHESES

The site of action of an effective drug does not necessarily correspond to the site of the primary pathological process. Diuretic drugs are effective in heart failure and anticholinergic drugs in Parkinson's disease. If the effectiveness of these drugs were the only clues to the site of the primary abnormality it might well be suggested that this was in the kidney and the cholinergic neurone respectively. In both cases the suggestion would be mistaken. So it may be that in schizophrenia the primary disturbance is not in the dopamine neurone which appears to be so closely related to the site of action of the antipsychotic drugs.

Nevertheless the apparent necessity of dopamine receptor blockade for neuroleptic effectiveness requires explanation. Two possibilities deserve consideration – (1) that the defect lies not in the dopamine neurone, but in some closely related and reciprocally balanced system. If the activity of this system were reduced, dopaminergic transmission, although in absolute terms within normal limits, might be in relative excess, and neuroleptics would restore the balance. (2) That the defect lies, not in the presynaptic dopamine neurone, but in the post-synaptic receptor. 'Denervation supersensitivity' is a well-known phenomenon and can probably affect central dopaminergic mechanisms (Ungerstedt, 1971b). The mechanism of the change in post-synaptic response is unclear, but the fact that such changes can occur suggests the possibility that increased responsiveness might be the basis of a pathological change. An increased response at the post-synaptic level in schizophrenia might explain not only the absence of evidence for increased dopamine release but even the apparent decreases observed in the c.s.f. studies (Bowers, 1974). For it would be expected that the feed-back mechanism from the post-synaptic site would come into effect and decrease activity in the presynaptic neurone, and thus the turnover of dopamine itself.

SUMMARY

The phenomena of the amphetamine psychosis and observations on the effectiveness of neuroleptic drugs have stimulated much research on dopaminergic mechanisms in schizophrenia, and have given rise to two separate, although potentially related, hypotheses – (1) that neuroleptic drugs act by blocking dopamine receptors and (2) that dopaminergic mechanisms are over-active in schizophrenia. The dopamine blockade hypothesis has survived a number of critical tests, and it is now established that antipsychotic potency of the thiaxenthene flupenthixol is associated only with the α-(dopamine receptor blocking) isomer of this compound. The dissociation between the therapeutic and extrapyramidal side effects of neuroleptic drugs can be explained on the basis that, while both are due to dopamine receptor blockade, they may be related to actions at different sites in the brain. In particular the hypothesis that the antipsychotic effects occur within the mesolimbic dopamine system explains the differing ratios of extrapyramidal and therapeutic effects in chlorpromazine, thioridazine and fluphenazine.

By contrast the dopamine over-activity hypothesis of schizophrenia has fared less well. Studies of dopamine metabolites in c.s.f. and of prolactin secretion have provided no evidence for increased dopaminergic activity, and the observation that schizophrenic symptoms can occur in patients with pre-existing Parkinson's disease suggests that increased dopamine release is not a necessary condition for a schizophrenia-like illness. Two hypotheses which would explain the viability of the dopamine blockade hypothesis of neuroleptic action but the failure of the dopamine over-activity hypothesis of schizophrenia are — (1) that there is a deficit of a system which normally acts in antagonism to the mesolimbic dopamine system, and (2) that supersensitivity develops to the effects of dopamine at the post-synaptic level.

REFERENCES

Andén, N.-E. (1972). Dopamine turnover in the corpus striatum and the limbic system after treatment with neuroleptic and anti-acetylcholine drugs. *J. Pharm. Pharmacol.*, **24**, 905

Angrist, B. M., Lee, H. K. and Gershon, S. (1974b). The antagonism of amphetamine-induced symptomatology by a neuroleptic. *Am. J. Psychiatry*, **131**, 817

Angrist, B., Sathananthan, G., Wilk, S. and Gershon, S. (1974a). Amphetamine psychosis: behavioural and biochemical aspects. *J. Psychiat. Res.*, **11**, 13

Angrist, B. M., Shopsin, B. and Gershon, S. (1971). Comparative psychotomimetic effects of stereoisomers of amphetamine. *Nature (London)*, **234**, 152

Bennett, J. P. and Snyder, S. H. (1975). Stereospecific binding of D-lysergic acid diethylamide (LSD) to brain membranes: relationship to serotonin receptors. *Brain Res.*, **94**, 523

Berger, R., Thierry, A. M., Tassin, J. P. and Moyne, M. A. (1976). Dopaminergic innervation of the rat prefrontal cortex: a fluorescence histochemical study. *Brain Res.*, **106**, 133

Bertler, A. and Rosengren, E. (1959). Occurrence and distribution of catecholamines in brain. *Acta Physiol. Scand.*, **47**, 350

Bowers, M. B. (1974). Central dopamine turnover in schizophrenic syndromes. *Arch. Gen. Psychiatry*, **31**, 50

Carlsson, A. (1959). The occurence, distribution and physiological role of catecholamines in the nervous system. *Pharmacol. Rev.*, **11**, 490

Carlsson, A. and Lindqvist, M. (1963). Effect of chlorpromazine and haloperidol on formation of 3-methoxytyramine and normetanephrine in mouse brain. *Acta Pharmacol. Toxicol.*, **20**, 140

Clement-Cormier, Y. C., Parrish, R. G., Petzold, G. L., Kebabian, J. W. and Greengard, P. (1975). Characterisation of a dopamine-sensitive adenylate cyclase in the rat caudate nucleus. *J. Neurochem.*, **25**, 143

Connell, P. H. (1958). *Amphetamine Psychosis*. Maudsley Monograph No. 5., (London: Chapman and Hall)

Creese, I., Burt, D. R. and Snyder, S. H. (1976). Dopamine receptor binding predicts clinical and pharmacological potencies of antischizophrenic drugs. *Science*, **192**, 481

Creese, I. and Iversen, S. D. (1975). The pharmacological and anatomical substrates of the amphetamine response in the rat. *Brain Res.*, **83**, 419

Crow, T. J., Johnstone, Eve, C. and McClelland, H. A. (1976). The coincidence of schizophrenia and Parkinsonism: some neurochemical implications. *Psychol. Med.*, **6**, 227

Deniker, P. (1960). Experimental neurological syndromes and the new drug therapies in psychiatry. *Comp. Psychiatry*, **1**, 92

Ehringer, H. and Hornykiewicz, O. (1960). Verteilung von Noradrenalin und Dopamin (3-Hydroxytyramin) im Gehirn des Menschen und ihr Verhalten bei Erkrankungen des Extrapyramidalen-Systems. *Klin. Wochenschr.*, **38**, 1236

Ellinwood, E. H. (1967). Amphetamine psychosis: I. Description of the individuals and process. *J. Nerv. Ment. Dis.*, **144**, 273

Enna, S. J., Bennett, J. P., Burt, D. R., Creese, I. and Snyder, S. H. (1976). Stereospecificity of interaction of neuroleptic drugs with neurotransmitters and correlation with clinical potency. *Nature (London)*, **263**, 338

Ernst, A. M. (1967). Mode of action of apomorphine and d-amphetamine for grawing compulsion in rats. *Psychophamacologia,* **10,** 316

Farley, I. J., Price, K. S. and Hornykiewicz, O. (1971). Dopamine in the limbic regions of the human brain: normal and abnormal. In *Non-Striatal Dopamine,* (E. Costa and G. L. Gessa eds.) (New York: Raven Press)

Flor-Henry, P. (1969). Psychosis and temporal lobe epilepsy, a controlled investigation. *Epilepsia,* **10,** 363

Flügel, F. (1953). Thérapeutique par médication neuroléptique obtenue en réalisant systématiquement des états Parkinsoniformes. *L'Encephale,* **45,** 1090

Fuxe, K., Hökfelt, T. and Nilsson, O. (1969). Factors involved in the control of the activity of the tubero-infundibular dopamine neurons during pregnancy and lactation. *Neuroendocrinology,* **5,** 257

Gaddum, J. H. (1954). Drug antagonistic to 5-hydroxytryptamine. In *Ciba Foundation Symposium on Hypertension.* (G. W. Wolstenholme, ed.). pp. 75–77

Goldberg, S. C., Klerman, G. L. and Cole, J. O. (1965). Changes in schizophrenic psychopathology and ward behaviour as a function of phenothiazine treatment. *Br. J. Psychiatry,* **111,** 120

Griffith, J. D., Cavanagh, J., Held, J. and Oates, J. A. (1972). Dextroamphetamine: evaluation of psychotomimetic properties in man. *Arch. Gen. Psychiatry,* **26,** 97

Gunne, L. M., Angåard, E. and Jönsson, L. E. (1972). Clinical trials with amphetamine blocking drugs. *Psychiat. Neurol. Neurochir. (Amsterdam),* **75,** 225

Hirsch, S. R., Gaind, R., Rohde, P. D., Stevens, B. C. and Wing, J. K. (1973). Out-patient maintenance of chronic schizophrenic patients with long-acting fluphenazine: double-blind placebo trial. *Br. Med. J.,* **1,** 633

Hogarty, G. E., Goldberg, S. C., Schooler, N. R. and Ulrich, R. F. (1974). Drug and sociotherapy in the after-care of schizophrenic patients. *Arch. Gen. Psychiatry,* **31,** 603

Horn, A. S. and Phillipson, O. T. (1975). Noradrenaline-sensitive adenylate cyclase in rat limbic forebrain homogenates: effects of agonists and antagonists. *Br. J. Pharmacol.,* **55,** 299

Hornykiewicz, O. (1973). Dopamine in the basal ganglia. Its role and therapeutic implications. *Br. Med. Bull.,* **29,** 172

Janssen, P. A. J., Niemegeers, C. J. E. and Schellekens, K. H. L. (1965). Is it possible to predict the clinical effects of neuroleptic drugs (major tranquillizers) from animal data? Part I. 'Neuroleptic activity spectra' for rats. *Arzneimittel-Forschung,* **15,** 104

Johnstone, E. C., Crow, T. J. and Mashiter, K. A. Anterior pituitary hormone secretion in chronic schizophrenia – an approach to neurohumoural mechanisms. *Psychol. Med.*

Jönssen, L.-E. and Gunne, L.-M. (1970). Clinical studies of amphetamine psychosis. In *Amphetamines and Related Compounds.* (E. Costa and S. Garrattini, eds.) pp. 929–936 (New York: Raven Press)

Kebabian, J. W., Petzold, G. L. and Greengard, P. (1972). Dopamine-sensitive adenylate cyclase in caudate nucleus of rat brain, and its similarity to the 'dopamine receptor'. *Proc. Nat. Acad. Sci. USA,* **69,** 2145

Kelly, P. H., Seviour, P. W. and Iversen, S. D. (1975). Amphetamine and apomorphine responses in the rat following 6-OHDA lesions in the nucleus accumbens septi and corpus striatum. *Brain Res.,* **94,** 507

Klawans, H. L., Goetz, C. and Westheimer, R. (1972). Pathophysiology of schizophrenia and the striatum. *Dis. Nerv. Syst.,* **33,** 711

Kolakowska, T., Wiles, D. H., McNeilly, A. S. and Gelder, M. G. (1975). Correlation between plasma levels of prolactin and chlorpromazine in psychiatric patients. *Psychol. Med.,* **5,** 214

Korf, J. and van Praag, H. M. (1971). Amine metabolism in the human brain: further evaluation of the probenecid test. *Brain Res.,* **35,** 221

Laverty, R. and Sharman, D. F. (1965). Modification by drugs of the metabolism of 3,4-dihydroxyphenylethylamine noradrenaline and 5-hydroxytryptamine in the brain. *Br. J. Pharmacol. Chemother.,* **24,** 759

Leff, J. P. and Wing, J. K. (1971). Trial of maintenance therapy in schizophrenia. *Br. Med J.,* **3,** 599

Matthysse, S. (1973). Antipsychotic drug actions, a clue to the neuropathology of schizophrenia? *Fed. Proc.,* **32,** 200

McCowan, P. K. and Cook, L. C. (1928). The mental aspect of chronic epidemic encephalitis. *Lancet,* **i,** 1316

Meltzer, H. Y., Sachar, E. J. and Frantz, A. G. (1974). Serum prolactin levels in unmedicated schizophrenic patients. *Arch. Gen. Psychiatry,* **31,** 564

Miller, R. J. and Hiley, C. R. (1974). Antimuscarinic properties of neuroleptics and drug-induced Parkinsonism. *Nature, (London)*, **248**, 596

Miller, R. J., Horn, A. S. and Iversen, L. L. (1974). The action of neuroleptic drugs on dopamine-stimulated adenosine-3,',5'-monophosphate production in the rat neostriatum and limbic forebrain. *Mol. Pharmacol.*, **10**, 759

National Institute of Mental Health, Psychopharmacology Service Center Collaborative Study Group. (1964). Phenothiazine treatment in acute schizophrenia. *Arch. Gen. Psychiatry*, **10**, 246

O'Keefe, R., Sharman, D. F. and Vogt, M. (1970). Effect of drugs used in pychoses on cerebral dopamine metabolism. *Br. J. Pharmacol.*, **38**, 287

Post, R. M., Fink, E., Carpenter, W. T. and Goodwin, F. K. (1975). Cerebrospinal fluid amine metabolites in acute schizophrenia. *Arch. Gen Psychiatry*, **32**, 1013

Randrup, A. and Munkvad, I. (1965). Special antagonism of amphetamine-induced abnormal behaviour. Inhibition of stereotyped activity with increase of some normal activities. *Psychopharmacologia*, **7**, 416

Randrup, A. and Munkvad, I. (1966). On the role of catecholamines in the amphetamine excitatory response. *Nature (London)*, **211**, 540

Randrup, A. and Munkvad, I. (1967). Stereotyped activities produced by amphetamine in several animal species and man. *Psychopharmacologia*, **11**, 300

Randrup, A. and Munkard, I. (1972). Evidence indicating an association between schizophrenia and dopaminergic hyperactivity in the brain. *Orthomolec. Psychiatry*, **1**, 2

Rylander, G. (1972). Pyschoses and the punding and choreiform syndromes in addiction to central stimulant drugs. *Psychiat. Neurol. Neurochir. (Amsterdam)*, **75**, 203

Seeman, P. and Lee, T. (1975). Antipsychotic drugs: direct correlation between clinical potency and presynaptic action on dopamine neurons. *Science*, **188**, 1217

Seeman, P., Lee, T., Chau-Wong, M. and Wong, K. (1976). Antipsychotic drug doses and neuroleptic/dopamine receptors. *Nature (London)*, **261**, 717

Sjöström, R. and Roos, B.-E. (1972). 5-Hydroxyindoleacetic acid and homovanillic acid in cerebrospinal fluid in manic-depressive psychosis. *Eur. J. Clin. Pharmacol.*, **4**, 170

Slater, E., Beard, A. W. and Glithero, E. (1963). The schizophrenia-like psychoses of epilepsy. *Br. J. Psychiatry*, **109**, 95

Snyder, S. H. (1973). Amphetamine psychosis: a model of schizophrenia mediated by catecholamines. *Am. J. Psychiatry*, **120**, 61

Snyder, S. H., Greenberg, D. and Yamamura, M. I. (1974). Anti-schizophrenic drugs and brain cholinergic receptors. *Arch. Gen. Psychiatry*, **31**, 58

Stein, L. and Wise, C. D. (1971). Possible etiology of schizophrenia: progressive damage to the noradrenergic reward system by 6-hydroxydopamine. *Science*, **171**, 1032

Stevens, J. R. (1973). An anatomy of schizophrenia. *Arch. Gen Psychiatry*, **29**, 177

Swanson, L. W. and Cowan, W. M. (1975). A note on the connections and development of the nucleus accumbens. *Brain Res.*, **92**, 324

Ungerstedt, U. (1971a). Stereotoxic mapping of the monoamine pathways in the rat brain. *Acta Physiol. Scand.*, **82**, (suppl.) 367, 1

Ungerstedt, U. (1971b). Post-synaptic supersensitivity after 6-hydroxydopamine induced degeneration of the nigro-striatal dopamine system. *Acta Physiol. Scand.*, (suppl.) **82**, 367, 69

van Rossum, J. M. (1966). The significance of dopamine-receptor blockade for the mechanism of action of neuroleptic drugs. *Arch. Int. Pharmacol. Ther.*, **160**, 492

Wilson, R. G., Hamilton, J. R., Boyd, W. D., Forrest, A. P. M., Cole, E. N., Boyns, A. R. and Griffiths, K. (1975). The effect of long-term phenothiazine therapy on plasma prolactin. *Br. J. Psychiatry*, **127**, 71

Woolley, D. W. and Shaw, E. (1954). A biochemical and pharmacological suggestion about certain mental disorders. *Proc. Nat. Acad. Sci. USA*, **40**, 228

POSTSCRIPT

The findings of the trial of the isomers of flupenthixol described in this paper have recently been published in full (Johnstone, E. C. *et al.* (1978). *Lancet*, **i, 848**). Recent post-mortem studies (Owen, F., Cross, A. J., Crow, T. J., Longden, A., Poulter, M. and Riley, G. J. *Lancet*. (In press)) have found no evidence of increased dopamine turnover in schizophrenia but have demonstrated increased post-synaptic receptor sensitivity.

7

The dopamine hypothesis revisited

M. SANDLER

A generation ago, it would have been unthinkable to attempt to define schizophrenia in terms of anything other than the somewhat mysterious psychological concepts of the time. This approach, which had little contact with everyday physical experience, produced theoretical constructs that were blinkered by their own limited set of assumptions. The major questions were pre-empted, the arguments circular and, scientifically, no progress was possible.

Although far from gaining universal acceptance, a revolution has taken place in our thinking over the past quarter of a century. Whilst, in the absence of an aetiological agent, definitions of schizophrenia remain phenomenological, the advent and remarkable therapeutic success of neuroleptic drugs in the 1950s made a connection between biochemical processes and the functioning of the mind inescapable. Such biochemical manipulations threw into bold relief lessons which might well have been learned many years earlier had we drawn the correct conclusions from the close interrelationship between certain forms of organic disease and disturbed mental function. But perhaps the pendulum has now swung too far. In our anxiety to define the physical foundations of schizophrenia, we espouse too readily certain hypotheses and explanations which attempt to provide a global explanation for the disease, despite insufficient information. The pieces of the jigsaw are all too few for the picture to be clearly visible: even if we can discern the beginnings of a pattern, we must not hesitate to rearrange these pieces to a different design when the gaps start to be filled.

Perhaps biological explanations of schizophrenia lean too heavily on data obtained from the observation of drug responses, whether therapeutic as with the neuroleptics or provocative, to instance the model psychoses produced by hallucinogens. The actual pinpointing of physicochemical deficits or aberrations in untreated patients has, despite careful search, proved disappointing and even the identification of such putative 'markers' as decreased platelet monoamine oxidase activity (Buchsbaum *et al.*, 1976), particularly in the paranoid variant of the disease (Schildkraut *et al*, 1976), has been disputed (Owen *et al.*, 1976). Even if the platelet deficit proves real, it has not been possible to identify a corresponding decrease of activity in the brains of schizophrenic subjects (Schwartz *et al.*, 1974). Indeed, until recently, had we used the biochemical lesion within the platelet as a pointer and tried to link it to schizophrenia within a unitarian framework – I refer particularly to the widely held dopamine hypothesis (Randrup and Munkvad, 1968) – we would have been hard pressed: platelet monoamine oxidase is of the B variety (Murphy and Donnelly, 1974), whereas dopamine oxidation in the brain, or so it seemed, is predominantly degraded by the A form of the enzyme (Waldmeier *et al.,* 1976). However, my colleagues and I have recently shown that in man (Glover *et al.,* 1977), in contradistinction to the rat, where all the earlier data were obtained (Waldmeier *et al.,* 1976), both platelet and brain monoamine oxidase B oxidise dopamine vigorously. Thus, from this viewpoint at least, the question of a contribution by dopamine to the biochemical sequence culminating in the florid disease is still an open one. Lest protagonists of the dopamine hypothesis clutch at this straw, however, it should be pointed out that monoamine oxidase B has other preferred substrates, the most important of which perhaps, in the present context, is phenylethylamine (Yang and Neff, 1973).

On balance, it now seems to me that the dopamine hypothesis of schizophrenia is untenable. One may try to prolong its life by invoking the existence of excitatory and inhibitory central dopamine receptors (Cools and Van Rossum, 1976), and indeed I do not doubt that they exist; but, as I shall explain shortly, I also have little doubt that there are many other receptors, uncharacterized and unsuspected, which have to be taken into consideration.

There seems to be general agreement that the closest human model of schizophrenia, at least of the paranoid variant, is amphetamine psychosis (Connell, 1958). Almost invariably, authors have attempted to explain this clinical entity by invoking dopamine release (Snyder *et al.,* 1974), perhaps throwing in a supersensitive dopamine receptor for good measure: certainly, smaller doses of amphetamine provoke schizophrenic relapse compared with the drug loading required for the model disease in otherwise normal subjects (Janowsky *et al.,* 1972). If this indirect mechanism of action of amphetamine were a true one, it would mean that a high doseage L-dopa regimen should produce a rather better model psychosis in normal subjects than amphetamine for, certainly, the brain is flooded with dopamine generated from the amino acid by the action of dopa decarboxylase at both regular and adventitious sites. However, no syndrome similar to the amphetamine psychosis has, to my knowledge, been reported in non-schizophrenics after L-dopa ingestion and although L-dopa has been reported by some (Yaryura-Tobias *et al.,* 1970) to cause a relapse in schizophrenia, this is by no means invariable and, indeed, some authors have claimed that L-dopa is beneficial in this disease (Inanaga *et al.,* 1975). It should be mentioned, however, that the situation is far from clear; published trials designed to test the beneficial effects of L-dopa in schizophrenia have been performed on subjects already under treatment with neuroleptic drugs.

If, in accordance with dopamine-hypothesis prediction, L-dopa turns out to have a deleterious effect in schizophrenia, one might expect that the putative dopamine receptor agonists, piribedil, apomorphine and bromocriptine, would similarly cause schizophrenics to deteriorate but, despite some preliminary observations (Angrist *et al.,* 1975), no very clear evidence of this has so far been obtained.

What seems to have been lost sight of is the possibility of amphetamine acting *directly* on a set of receptors, different from those specific for dopamine. Reynolds and I (Sandler and Reynolds, 1976) have suggested the possibility, based on a body of evidence assembled from the literature, of the existence of a phenylethylamine receptor and we envisage the likelihood of amphetamine, which only differs from phenylethylamine by the possession of an α-methyl group, producing its effect via that receptor. This view is supported by the observation that when one gives a monoamine oxidase inhibiting drug to an experimental animal and then administers phenylethylamine, the observed pharmacological effect is indistinguishable from that of amphetamine (Mantegazza and Riva, 1963).

Thus we proposed that endogenously produced phenylethylamine might give rise to the amphetamine-like psychosis we call schizophrenia, either by increased synthesis, decreased degradation or receptor hypersensitivity. Because of evidence, obtained in germ-free rats, that most of the phenylethylamine elaborated in the body derives from the action of gut flora (Goodwin *et al.*, in preparation), presumably on dietary phenylalanine residues, it seemed that the association claimed between coeliac disease and schizophrenia (Dohan *et al.*, 1969 and Singh and Kay, 1976) and described elsewhere in this volume, might have a basis in this finding. However, gut sterilization in a small group of chronic paranoid schizophrenics resulted in no benefit (Sandler *et al.*, in preparation (a)), whilst evidence of increased phenylethylamine production could not be found in patients with untreated coeliac disease (Sandler *et al.*, in preparation (b)). Whether the small decrease in monoamine oxidase B claimed by some in schizophrenia is sufficient to cause a build-up of phenylethylamine similarly seems doubtful. If the hypothesis is a viable one, it must probably be conceived in terms of some form of receptor hypersensitivity to phenylethylamine.

The main argument evinced by opponents of hypotheses invoking a direct action of amphetamine and thus, presumably, of an analogue such as phenylethylamine, at some post-synaptic receptor site is that the tyrosine-hydroxylase inhibiting drug, α-methyl-*p*-tyrosine, prevents the amphetamine response (Snyder *et al.*, 1974): thus, it is argued that dopamine or noradrenaline formation and release must play a role. However, α-methyl-*p*-tyrosine also inhibits the direct dopaminergic agonist effect of bromocryptine, in which tyrosine hydroxylase seems unlikely to be involved. It seems plausible to suggest that it does so by generating α-methyl-*p*-tyramine which competes for whatever receptor the drug acts on, whether membrane bound (Burt *et al.*, 1975) or dopamine-sensitive adenylcyclase (Kebabian *et al.*, 1972) (this conjecture has the merit of being testable!). In a similar manner, α-methyl-*p*-tyramine might compete for whatever receptor amphetamine acts upon. Surely there are lessons to be drawn from α-methyldopa which now seems likely to exert its hypotensive effect by direct central α-agonist stimulation by α-methylnoradrenaline (Henning, 1973). In this particular site at least, the α-methyl amine may have a more powerful and prolonged action than noradrenaline itself, a 'super transmitter' rather than a false transmitter (Baldessarini, 1975).

The strongest plank that supporters of the dopamine hypothesis of schizophrenia have in their platform is that central dopamine receptor blocking drugs, the neuroleptics, alleviate the illness. This argument is circular, however, for the drug is already defined in terms of one single observed action which is then, and by definition, used to explain the global effect. Since when has *any* drug had a *single* action? True, some drugs are 'dirtier' than others but one is hard put to think of a drug which possesses one pure effect. Let us consider haloperidol, for instance, a butyrophenone which has been widely used in the treatment of schizophrenia. There is evidence that this drug also blocks the opiate receptor (Clay and Brougham, 1975 and Creese *et al.,* 1976a). Although the opiate receptor has been recognized for some time (Snyder, 1975), a series of endogenous agonists, the endorphin group of compounds, has recently been identified (Hughes, 1975 and Bradbury *et al.,* 1976). The fact that haloperidol blocks this receptor may just as easily imply that schizophrenia stems from some distortion of endorphin activity rather than or as well as of dopamine activity. This possibility has, in fact, already been noted, suggested by the ability of the endorphins to produce a catatonic state when injected into animals (Bloom *et al.,* 1976 and Jacquet and Marks, 1976). This type of argument must be viewed with some caution: even apart from the fact that catatonia is an extremely non-specific phenomenon (De Jong, 1945), which can be produced by substances as disparate as the neuroleptics (Stille, 1971), and the prostaglandins (Feldberg, 1976), the catatonic state itself should not necessarily be equated with schizophrenic illness (Abrams and Taylor, 1976).

There are still further reasons why the dopamine hypothesis is suspect. If haloperidol binding represents the antagonist state of the dopamine receptor, as claimed by Snyder and his school (Creese *et al.,* 1975), one might have expected the binding of this drug and that of the receptor agonist, dopamine, to run in parallel. In fact, there does not appear to be full anatomical correspondence (Creese *et al.,* 1976b). To what extent Snyder's membrane dopamine binding sites (Burt *et al.,* 1975) represent the true dopamine receptor, as opposed to the dopamine-sensitive adenyl cyclase of Greengard and his colleagues (Kebabian *et al.,* 1975) is unresolved. Perhaps the specificity of the membrane receptor is to some extent suspect. Apomorphine for instance appears to bind to it twice as well as dopamine (Burt *et al.,* 1975); and it may be unwise to assume that apomorphine is neither more nor less than a dopamine receptor agonist. There are many ways in which apomorphine differs from dopamine; for instance, Cotzias and his colleagues have demonstrated that, in certain circumstances, apomorphine antagonises the effect of L-dopa. One might have predicted that, if it were acting on the identical receptor, the process would be additive. There are other points of difference. Apomorphine produces a qualitatively different growth hormone response compared with L-dopa (Rotrosen *et al.,* 1976). The anti-emetic drug, metoclopramide, blocks apomorphine-induced stereotypy, and also apomorphine reversal of reserpine locomotor suppression. It also blocks apomorphine (or amphetamine) turning behaviour. However, this drug has no effect in parkinsonism. It does not interfere with the therapeutic efficacy of L-dopa or prevent L-dopa dyskinesias. Apomorphine (Strian *et al.*, 1972) seems to be more helpful towards parkinsonian tremor than L-dopa. If the dopamine-sensitive adenyl cyclase be used as a receptor model, then apomorphine, as opposed to dopamine, is only a partial agonist, while the butyrophenones do not react as avidly with it as might have been predicted from their therapeutic efficacy (Miller *et al.*, 1974).

As the discovery of the opiate receptor eventually led to the identification of conformationally correct but non-opiate endogenous peptide agonists (Editorial, Lancet, 1976), I would put forward the thesis that the apomorphine receptor may similarly possess its own endogenous and as yet unidentified agonist. Even though it is tempting to suggest that this may be a derivative of a Pictet–Spengler condensation product (Whaley and Govindachari, 1951), it is just as likely to be an unrelated peptide, to judge from the endorphin precedent.

What I envisage is rather more than a single receptor in search of an agonist. As I see it, there may be overlapping banks of receptors with similar but not identical properties. There may be excitatory and inhibitory dopamine receptors and there may also be very similar but not identical apomorphine receptors, piribedil receptors, bromocryptine receptors and LSD receptors. All these agonists, together with L-dopa, have in common the property of stimulating the so-called supersensitive dopamine receptor animal model, the 'turning' rat or mouse preparation (Ungerstedt, 1968). They do more. They also share the ability to produce visual hallucinations. Some representatives of the group, such as LSD, are able to do this with greater facility than others which only give rise to hallucinations as an occasional adverse reaction. It is of interest, however, that if the ability to initiate hallucinations be considered as the link then another drug used in the treatment of Parkinson's disease, amantadine, the therapeutic ability of which has been difficult to classify in terms of orthodox dopamine receptor theory, also possesses the ability to give rise to this adverse reaction. Perhaps, then, there is an amantadine receptor too which acts against parkinsonian clinical signs in some subtler way than by mere dopamine replacement. The idiopathic human pathological entity, Parkinson's disease, seems likely to differ in many subtle ways from the animal models of it we have constructed. We have been prisoners of our animal models for too long and, to my mind, this is where much of the present confusion has arisen. Perhaps the greatest error of all has been to model our concept of the central receptor on what we know of peripheral receptors. We are in urgent need of some new concept, such as the one I have outlined here, in order to break out of the conceptual strait-jacket in which we find ourselves.

If we accept for the sake of argument that new and unsuspected types of receptors might exist in the central nervous system, it might be instructive to view an old situation in reverse and extrapolate from the brain to the periphery, scrutinising such adverse reactions as the red, swollen tender feet sometimes observed during the bromocriptine treatment of parkinsonism (Teychenne *et al.*, 1975), or the livedo reticularis which occasionally supervenes during amantadine therapy. As careful search revealed evidence of dopamine receptors in the periphery after a central role of this amine had been established, so the opiate receptor and the banks of receptors I have tried to delineate, possessing as yet uncharacterised endogenous agonists, may similarly have their peripheral counterpart. But that is another story!

REFERENCES

Abrams, S. R. and Taylor, M. A. (1976). Manic and schizo-affective disorder, manic type: a comparison. *Am. J. Psychiatry,* **33,** 579

Angrist, B., Thompson, H., Shopsin., B. and Gershon, S. (1975). Clinical studies with dopamine-receptor stimulants. *Psychopharmacologia,* **44,** 273

Baldessarini, R. J. (1975). In *Handbook of Neuropsychopharmacology,* (L. Iversen, S. Iversen and S. Snyder, eds.) p. 37 (New York: Plenum)

Bloom, F., Segal, D. and Guillemin, R. (1976). Endorphins: Profound behavioral effects in rats suggest new etiological factors in mental illness. *Science,* **194,** 630

Bradbury, A. F., Smyth, D. G., Snell, C. R., Birdsall, M. and Hulme, E. C. (1976). C fragment of lipoprotein has a high affinity for brain opiate receptors. *Nature (London),* **260,** 793

Buchsbaum, M. S., Cousey, R. D. and Murphy, D. L. (1976). The biochemical high-risk paradigm: Behavioral and familial correlates of low platelet monoamine oxidase activity. *Science,* **194,** 339

Burt, D. R., Enna, S., Creese, I. and Snyder, S. H. (1975). Dopamine receptor binding in the corpus striatum of mammalian brain. *Proc. Nat. Acad. Sci. US,* **72,** 4655

Clay, G. A. and Brougham, L. R. (1975). Haloperidol binding to an opiate receptor. *Biochem. Pharmac.,* **24,** 1363

Connell, P. H. (1958). *Amphetamine Psychosis.* (London: Chapman and Hall)

Cools, A. R. and van Rossum, J. M. (1976). Excitation-mediating and inhibition-mediating dopamine receptors: a new concept towards a better understanding of electrophysiological, biochemical, pharmacological, functional and clinical data. *Psychopharmacologia,* **45,** 243

Creese, I., Burt, D. R. and Snyder, S. H. (1975). Dopamine receptor bindings: differentiation of agonist and antagonist states with ^{3}H dopamine and ^{3}H haloperidol. *Life Sci., II,* **17,** 993

Creese, I., Feinberg, A. P. and Snyder, S. H. (1976a). Butyrophenone influences on the opiate receptor. *Eur. J. Pharmac.,* **36,** 231

Creese, I., Burt, D. R. and Snyder, S. H. (1976b). Dopamine receptor binding predicts clinical and pharmacological potencies of anti-schizophrenic drugs. *Science,* **192,** 481

De Jong, H. (1945). *Experimental Catatonia.* (Baltimore: Williams and Wilkins)

Dohan, F. C., Grasberger, J. C., Lowell, F. M., Johnston, H. I. Jr. and Arbergast, A. (1969). Relapsed schizophrenics: more rapid improvement on a milk and cereal-free diet. *Br. J. Psychiatry.,* **115,** 595

Feldberg, W. (1976). *Psychol. Med.,* **6,** 359

Glover, V., Sandler, M., Owen, F. and Riley, G. J. (1977). Dopamine is a monoamine oxidase B substrate in man. *Nature (London),* **265,** 80

Goodwin, B. L., Ruthven, C. R. J. and Sandler, M. (in preparation).

Henning, M. (1973). In *Frontiers in Catecholamine Research,* (E. Usdin and S. Snyder, eds.) p. 595 (New York: Pergamon)

Hughes, J. (1975). Isolation of an endogenous compound from the brain with pharmacological properties similar to morphine. *Brain Res.,* **88,** 295

Inanaga, K., Nakazawa, Y., Inoue, K., Tachibana, H., Oshima, M., Kotorii, T., Tanaka, M. and Ogawa, N. (1975). Double blind controlled study of L-dopa therapy in schizophrenia. *Fol. Psychiatr. Neurol. (Jpn.),* **29,** 123

Jacquet, Y. F. and Marks, N. (1976). The C-fragment of -lipoprotein: an endogenous neuroleptic or antipsychotogen? *Science,* **194,** 632

Janowsky, D. S., El-Yousef, M. K. and Davis, J. M. (1972). The elicitation of psychiatric symptomology by methylphenidate. *Compr. Psychiatry.,* **13,** 83

Kebabian, J. W., Petzold, G. I. and Greengard, P. (1972). *Proc. Nat. Acad. Sci. USA,* **69,** 2145

Mantegazza, P. and Riva, M. J. (1963). Amphetamine-like activity of β_I-phenylethylamine after a monoamine oxidase inhibitor *in vivo. J. Pharm. Pharmac.,* **15,** 472

Miller, R. J., Horn, A. S. and Iversen, L. L. (1974). The action of neuroleptic drugs on dopamine-stimulated adenosine—3′5′-monophosphate production in the rat neostriatum and limbic forebrain. *Mol. Pharmac.,* **10,** 759

Murphy, D. L. and Donnelly, C. H. (1974). In: *Neuro-psychopharmacology of Monoamines and their Regulatory Enzymes,* (E. Usdin, ed.) p. 71 (New York: Raven)
Owen, F., Bourne, R., Crow, T. J., Johnstone, E. C., Bailey, A. R. and Hershon, H. I. (1976). *Arch. Gen. Psychiat.,* **33,** 1370
Randrup, A. and Munkvad, I. (1968). Behavioural stereotypes induced by pharmacological agents. *Pharmakopsychiat. Neuro-Psychopharmak.,* **1,** 18
Rotrosen, J., Angrist, B. M., Gershon, S., Sachar, E. J. and Halpern, F. S. (1976). *Psychopharmacology,* **51,** 1
Sandler, M. and Reynolds, G. P. (1976). Does phenylethylamine cause schizophrenia? *Lancet,* **i,** 70
Sandler, M., Goodwin, B. L., Ruthven, C. R. J. and Coppen, A. (In preparation, a)
Sandler, M., Goodwin, B. L., Ruthven, C. R. J. and Kumar, P. (In preparation, b)
Schildkraut, J. J., Herzog, J. M., Orsulak, P. J., Edelman, S. E., Shein, H. M. and Frazier, S. H. (1976). Reduced platelet monoamine oxidase activity in a sub-group of schizophrenic patients. *Am. J. Psychiatry,* **133,** 438
Schwartz, M. A., Aikens, A. M. and Wyatt, R. J. (1974). Monoamine oxidase activity in brains from schizophrenic and mentally normal individuals. *Psychopharmacologia,* **38,** 319
Singh, M. M. and Kay, S. R. (1976). Wheat gluten as a pathogenic factor in schizophrenia. *Science,* **191,** 401
Snyder, S. H., Banerjee, S. P., Yamamura, H. I. and Greenberg, D. (1974). Drugs, neurotransmitters and schizophrenia. *Science,* **184,** 1234
Snyder, S. H. (1975). Opiate receptor in normal and drug altered brain function. *Nature (London),* **257,** 185
Stille, G. (1971). *Zur Pharmakologie katatonigener Stoffe.* (Aulendorf: Cantor)
Strian, F., Micheler, E. and Benkert, O. (1972). *Pharmakopsychiat. Neuro-Psychopharmak.,* **5,** 198
Taychenne, P. F., Calne, D. B., Leigh, P. N., Greenacre, J. K., Reid, J. L., Petrie, A. and Bamji, A. N. (1975). Idiopathic Parkinsonism treated with bromocriptine. *Lancet,* **ii,** 473
Ungerstedt, U. (1968). 6-Hydroxydopamine induced degeneration of central monoamine neurones. *Eur. J. Pharmac.,* **5,** 107
Waldmeier, P. C., Delini-Stula, A. and Maître, L. (1976). Preferential deamination of dopamine by an A type monoamine oxidase in rat brain. *Naunyn-Schmiedeberg's Arch. Pharmac.,* **292,** 9
Whaley, M. and Govindachar, T. R. (1951). In *Organic Reactions,* (R. Adams (ed.) vol. 6, p. 151, (New York: Wiley)
Yang, H. Y.-T. and Neff, N. H. (1973). Beta phenylethylamine: a specific substrate for type B monoamine oxidase of brain. *J. Pharmac. Exp. Ther.,* **187,** 365
Yaryura-Tobias, J. A., Diamond, B. and Merlis, S. (1970). The action of L-dopa on schizophrenic patients. *Curr. Ther. Res.,* **12,** 528

8

Tryptophan and serotonin in schizophrenia: a clue to biochemical defects?

D. A. BENDER

There have been many reports implicating abnormalities of tryptophan metabolism in the pathogenesis of schizophrenic diseases; Gilka (1975) has reviewed much of this evidence. Pollin, Cardon and Kety (1961) showed that administration of tryptophan and a monoamine oxidase inhibitor to chronic schizophrenics led to an exacerbation of symptoms in some cases. This was followed by an apparent 'rebound' period, during which the patients were somewhat better than prior to the trial. This finding was confirmed by Alexander and co-workers (1963). However, relatively less attention has been paid to the results of tryptophan administration observed by these two groups of workers than to their observation that administration of methionine under the same conditions had the same effect in some patients. This effect of methionine (and other methyl group donors such as betaine) was interpreted as suggesting that an abnormal methyl derivative of a normal brain metabolite might be an endogenous psychotogen, and hence a major biochemical factor in the pathogenesis of schizophrenia. One compound that has been proposed for such a role is dimethyltryptamine, which is known to induce hallucinations when administered to normal subjects. In view of the reports from Pollin and co-workers and from Alexander's group, cited above, dimethyltryptamine is an especially interesting compound, since it can be regarded as a derivative of both tryptophan and methionine.

A number of hallucinogenic drugs, such as lysergic acid diethylamide (LSD), mescaline, bufotenine and psilocybin, have been thought to act by way of a serotoninergic mechanism in the brain, because of the structural similarity between the hallucinogens and 5-hydroxytryptamine (5HT). Recent studies show that both 5HT and LSD can bind to brain membrane preparations which are assumed to be, or to contain, the physiological 5HT receptor sites. Both 5HT and LSD can be displaced from membrane binding by a variety of compounds, at broadly similar concentrations, and each inhibits the binding of the other (Bennett and Snyder, 1976). The interaction between hallucinogens and the 5HT receptor site raises the possibility that part of the symptomatology of schizophrenia could be due to interactions with, or abnormalities of, the 5HT receptor. However, although compounds such as LSD will induce hallucinations and even frank psychosis, these may be qualitatively different from the psychosis of schizophrenic diseases. Trials of specific 5HT antagonists in schizophrenia have not been encouraging. Gallant and co-workers (1964) were unable to demonstrate any beneficial effect of methysergide in a controlled study. Holden and co-workers (1971) obtained inconclusive results in a trial of cinanserin, although there were indications of a beneficial effect.

Berlet and co-workers (1965) measured urinary excretion of a number of tryptophan metabolites in chronic schizophrenics. They showed that several, and especially tryptamine metabolites, were considerably increased during periods of exacerbation of symptoms, despite a constant or even reduced dietary intake of tryptophan. However, it is extremely difficult to interpret urinary excretion studies, especially where tryptophan metabolism is concerned. Many of the tryptophan metabolites that have been identified as abnormal in a variety of pathological states can be shown to arise as a result of intestinal bacterial action, and thus to represent gastro-intestinal function rather than true endogenous metabolism.

Epidemiological studies in schizophrenia do not give any evidence for a single dominant genetic defect. Nevertheless there is a strong genetic factor, with a marked familial predisposition to psychotic disease and a greater than expected concordance for schizophrenia in twins (Pollin, 1972). One or more abnormal enzymes or other proteins may be involved in schizophrenia, and there have been several reports of abnormal plasma proteins. One of these is the abnormal α_2-globulin reported by Frohman and co-workers (1969, 1971), which differs in both lipid content and secondary structure from the equivalent protein obtained from control subjects. Among other effects this protein was shown to enhance the uptake of tryptophan into chick erythrocytes in an *in vitro* test, and it was suggested that it might act *in vivo* in a similar way to increase tryptophan uptake into the brain.

Thus there is a considerable body of evidence suggesting that one defect in schizophrenia may be in the metabolism of tryptophan, and perhaps especially in its uptake into the brain and subsequent metabolism to the neurotransmitter amine 5-hydroxytryptamine.

5HT is synthesised by a simple pathway involving two enzymes, tryptophan hydroxylase (L-tryptophan mono-oxygenase, EC 1.14.16.4) and aromatic amino acid decarboxylase (L-aromatic amino acid carboxy-lyase, EC 4.1.1.28). The hydroxylase has a relatively low affinity for its substrate, Kaufman (1974) has quoted a K_m of 50 μmol/l. Since the normal concentration of tryptophan in the brain has been estimated to be about 30 μmol/l (Fernstrom and Wurtman, 1971), this means that under normal conditions the hydroxylase will not be saturated with its substrate, and therefore as the concentration of tryptophan in the brain increases the rate of hydroxylation would also be expected to increase. The second enzyme, aromatic amino acid decarboxylase, is not generally regarded as rate-limiting. It is generally thought that the main regulation of brain 5HT synthesis is by the availability of tryptophan in the brain.

Brain tryptophan uptake is thought to be regulated by two factors: (1) There is a single carrier mechanism at the blood-brain barrier for all the so-called large neutral amino acids, phenylalanine, tyrosine, tryptophan, leucine, isoleucine, valine, methionine and threonine. This means that all these amino acids will compete with each other for uptake into the brain. The affinity of the carrier mechanism for each amino acid is about the same as the plasma concentration of that amino acid, so that any changes of plasma amino acid within the physiological range would be expected to have an effect on brain tryptophan uptake (Pardridge, 1977).

(2) Tryptophan in the blood-stream is mainly bound to serum albumin, rather than in free solution – it is the only amino acid to be bound in this way (McMenamy and Oncley, 1958). It is to be expected that any changes in the binding of tryptophan to albumin would affect the uptake of tryptophan into the brain, since a change in binding would affect the concentration of freely diffusible tryptophan, and it is only the diffusible tryptophan that is *immediately* accessible to the amino acid transport mechanism. There is a great deal of evidence that a number of drug, dietary and other manipulations that alter the binding of tryptophan to albumin (without necessarily altering the total concentration of tryptophan in plasma) alter the uptake of tryptophan into the brain, and the rate of 5HT synthesis ((Tagliamonte *et al.*, 1971; Curzon *et al.*, 1973; Bender and Cockcroft, 1977). However, binding is an equilibrium process, and therefore bound tryptophan can contribute to the pool of the free amino acid. This means that alterations in the binding of tryptophan cannot be translated directly into changes in brain tryptophan uptake of the same magnitude (Etienne *et al.*, 1976; Partridge, 1977).

It thus appears possible to predict the relative rate of brain 5HT synthesis from measurement of serum diffusible tryptophan and competing amino acid concentrations. Obviously, human experiments to confirm this are not possible, but the animal studies cited above indicate that such prediction is possible at least in semi-quantitative terms.

In 1973 we set up a preliminary experiment to measure diffusible serum tryptophan in a group of male chronic schizophrenics treated with chlorpromazine (Bender and Bamji, 1974). We showed that total serum tryptophan was significantly lower than normal, with a greater than normal proportion of tryptophan freely diffusible (see Table 1).

The abnormality in albumin binding that we observed might have been due to a raised level of serum non-esterefied fatty acids (NEFA). It is well established

Table 1 Serum tryptophan binding to albumin in a group of chronic schizophrenics treated with chlorpromazine

	Control subjects (n=21)	*Patients* (n=10)
Total tryptophan μ mol/l	83·6 ± 18·5	44·8 ± 7·7*
Diffusible tryptophan %	11·6 ± 0·9	16·5 ± 1·3*
Diffusible tryptophan μmol/l	8·5 ± 1·8	6·3 ± 1·2*
Tryptophan–albumin complex: K_{diss} l/μmol	0·035 ± 0·027	0·019 ± 0·025
Sites per molecule	0·51 ± 0·09	0·21 ± 0·06*

* Significantly different from control subjects, p<0·001

that variations in NEFA concentration within the physiological range have an effect on tryptophan binding (McMenamy, 1965; Curzon *et al.*, 1974; Bender, Boulton and Coulson, 1975). However, the serum NEFA concentration in the samples from our patients was only marginally higher than in our control subjects and was not sufficient to account for the observed displacement of tryptophan from albumin binding. In some samples we were able to measure the dissociation constant of the tryptophan-albumin complex (K_{diss}), and the concentration of sites available to tryptophan per molecule of albumin. Had the altered binding been due to raised serum NEFA, we would have expected to find a changed K_{diss} (Curzon *et al.*, 1974; Bender, Boulton and Coulson, 1975). As can be seen from Table 1, there was no difference in K_{diss} between the samples from patients and those from controls. However, there was a significant difference in the number of sites available to tryptophan per molecule of albumin; $0{\cdot}51 \pm 0{\cdot}09$ in the control subjects and $0{\cdot}21 \pm 0{\cdot}06$ in the patients. Thus the reduced binding of tryptophan to albumin in the patients appears to be due to a reduction in the number of sites available to tryptophan. It seemed possible that the defective tryptophan binding could be due to an abnormal albumin. However, in none of the patient samples could any abnormality be detected by electrophoresis on cellulose acetate strips.

While these studies were in progress, Manowitz and co-workers reported a similar finding of low total plasma tryptophan in a group of newly hospitalized schizophrenic patients. They also showed that in those patients who responded to drug therapy, clinical improvement was matched by a rise in plasma tryptophan, while in those patients who did not respond there was no change in plasma tryptophan. They did not report any measurement of tryptophan diffusibility (Manowitz *et al.*, 1973; Gilmour *et al.*, 1973). Lovett-Doust and co-workers (1975) have also reported low plasma tryptophan in chronic schizophrenics taking a variety of anti-schizophrenic drugs, while Deniker and co-workers (1976) have shown that in a group of schizophrenics, with or without drug therapy, serum diffusible tryptophan was higher than normal, although total serum tryptophan was normal. However, in a study of patients who had been drug-free for 6 months. Domino and Krause (1974) were unable to show any abnormality of either total or diffusible tryptophan.

The results of our first experiment, and those reported by Manowitz, Lovett-Doust and Deniker and their co-workers were encouraging, in that they indicated a possibly fruitful area of investigation – serum diffusible tryptophan and competing amino acids as predictors of brain tryptophan uptake and 5HT synthesis. As with many studies on schizophrenia, our experiment could be criticised on the grounds that it compared a group of chronically sick hospitalized patients receiving relatively large doses of drugs with a group of healthy, active young men, taking no drugs and receiving a very different diet from that provided for the patients.

A second experiment was therefore set up, in which the patients could be used as their own controls, in that they would be followed for some time, both while relatively well-controlled by chlorpromazine and during a period of placebo administration. In this way it was hoped to be possible to detect any changes in serum chemistry due to changes in drug status and possibly correlated with changes in clinical condition. One blood sample was obtained from each patient before the switch to placebo, one after 3 days on placebo and another after 17 days. A final sample was obtained 14 days later, 3 days after the return to active medication. Unfortunately it was not possible to continue the experiment for longer to observe the long-term effects of restoration of chlorpromazine treatment. The experiment was staggered in such a way that not all the patients were at the same stage at the same time, and samples for analysis were coded in such a way that the laboratory workers could not identify samples with patients or phase of the experiment (Bender, Pigache, Gruzelier and Hammond, 1975).

Table 2 shows the initial biochemical profile of the patients in this study, compared with a group of approximately age-matched normal subjects. As can be seen, total serum tryptophan was significantly lower than normal in the patients at this time. However, there was no difference in tryptophan binding to albumin (unlike the previous group of patients, cited above), so that diffusible tryptophan concentration was also lower than normal. Serum total amino acid concentration (an index of competition for tryptophan transport) was also lower than normal, so that it would be expected that brain tryptophan uptake and 5HT synthesis would be approximately normal.

The effects of drug withdrawal are shown in Figure 1. The first response, at 3 days after the withdrawal of chlorpromazine, was a marked increase in serum total amino acids, together with an increase in the concentration of diffusible tryptophan, due to both an increase in the total tryptophan concentration and a decrease in the proportion bound to albumin. These effects would be expected to balance each other, so that no change in brain tryptophan uptake would be expected.

Seventeen days after the switch to placebo the serum total amino acid concentration had returned to the initial level, while both total and diffusible tryptophan remained elevated, showing either a further increase or only a small decrease compared with the third day after drug withdrawal. Hence at this time a considerable increase in brain tryptophan uptake would

Table 2 Serum amino acids in a group of chronic schizophrenic patients while receiving chlorpromazine

	Control subjects (n=15)	*Patients* (n=7)
Total tryptophan μmol/l	85·0 ± 7·7	64·6 ± 7·1*
Diffusible tryptophan %	12·7 ± 1·9	12·4 ± 1·1
Diffusible tryptophan μmol/l	10·6 ± 2·3	8·0 ± 1·4
Total amino acids mmol/l	3·47 ± 0·34	3·05 ± 0·15

*Significantly different from control subjects, p<0.001

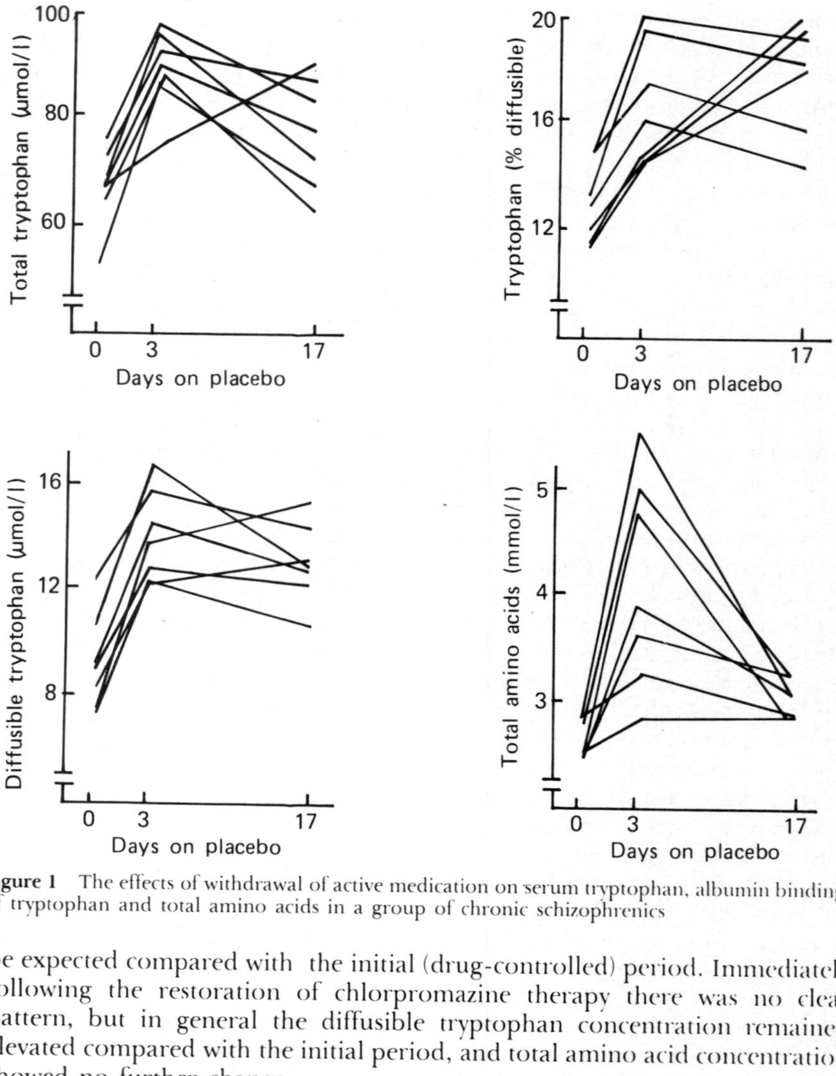

Figure 1 The effects of withdrawal of active medication on serum tryptophan, albumin binding of tryptophan and total amino acids in a group of chronic schizophrenics

be expected compared with the initial (drug-controlled) period. Immediately following the restoration of chlorpromazine therapy there was no clear pattern, but in general the diffusible tryptophan concentration remained elevated compared with the initial period, and total amino acid concentration showed no further change.

Perhaps the most exciting aspect of this experiment was the observation that at 3 days after the withdrawal of drug therapy, when it appeared likely that brain tryptophan uptake would be much the same as during the drug-controlled period, there was no apparent change in the clinical condition of the patients. However, at 17 days after the change in drug status, when a greatly increased brain tryptophan uptake would be predicted, there was a considerable deterioration in the patients' condition, as assessed both by observation and by a nursing rating assessment. Restoration of active medication for only 3 days had no effect on the predictors of brain tryptophan uptake, and the patients remained very disturbed.

From this within-patient study there appears to be some evidence of an association between increased brain tryptophan uptake (and presumably also 5HT synthesis) and exacerbation of schizophrenic symptoms following withdrawal of active medication. No measurement of 5-hydroxy-indoleacetic acid in cerebro-spinal fluid, blood or urine was made, so that although it is probable that brain 5HT synthesis increased during the placebo period, this has not been demonstrated. Furthermore, other tryptophan metabolites could also have been formed in greater amount following increased brain tryptophan uptake.

It is obviously desirable to be able to differentiate between what are the effects of chlorpromazine on tryptophan metabolism and what might be the underlying biochemistry of schizophrenia. No such distinction is possible for the experiment described above. It is difficult to carry out experiments with chlorpromazine or other antipsychotic drugs in non-schizophrenic subjects. There is a considerable difference in sensitivity to chlorpromazine between schizophrenics and non-psychotic patients. The standard dose of chlorpromazine used for pre-medication in surgical patients and as an anti-emetic and sedative for radio-therapy patients is between 25 and 50 mg. A schizophrenic patient can tolerate very much larger doses without signs of more than mild sedation – in the study reported here the patients were receiving between 100 and 800 mg/d (daily mean 4·5±2·8 mg/kg body weight). We therefore carried out a number of animal experiments, using several different phenothiazines: chlorpromazine, prochlorperazine, chlorprothixene and thioridazine as examples of different classes of antipsychotic drugs and promethazine and trimeprazine as two closely related drugs without anti-schizophrenic action.

Administration of chorpromazine to rats at 10 mg/kg body weight (but not at lower doses) led to a considerable fall in serum total tryptophan, together with a considerable increase in the fraction freely diffusible. The combination of these two effects meant that the concentration of diffusible tryptophan was not significantly different from that in control animals. At the same time there was a marked decrease in the concentration of serum total amino acids. This would be expected to lead to an increase in the uptake of tryptophan into the brain, and hence an increase in 5HT synthesis. As can be seen from Table 3, this was so. Although there was no change in the brain tryptophan concentration, there was an increase in the uptake of radioactive tryptophan into the brain, and 4 h after the administration of chlorpromazine brain 5HT concentration was significantly greater than in control animals (Bender, 1976a).

For the other anti-psychotic drugs, preliminary experiments were carried out to determine at what dose they would affect serum total tryptophan concentration. These doses (listed in Table 4) were then used in further studies to assess effects on albumin binding of tryptophan, serum total amino acid concentration and brain tryptophan and 5HT levels. Promethazine and trimeprazine were used at 100 mg/kg body weight – this was the highest dose that was not immediately toxic to the animals, and is very considerably greater than is used in human medication.

Table 3 Effects of chlorpromazine at 10 mg/kg body weight on serum amino acids and brain tryptophan and 5HT in rats

	Saline-treated controls (n=25)	*Chlorpromazine-treated* (n=10)
Serum:		
Total tryptophan μmol/l	96·6 ± 13·5	62·8 ± 10·4*
Diffusible tryptophan %	15·8 ± 3·1	28·3 ± 6·5*
Diffusible tryptophan μmol/l	15·6 ± 2·8	20·4 ± 5·4*
Total amino acids mmol/l	2·2 ± 0·2	1·9 ± 0·3*
Brain		
Tryptophan nmol/g	91·9 ± 12·4	100·0 ± 14·1
Radioactive tryptophan nCi/g	9·9 ± 1·6	12·5 ± 4·2
5HT nmol/g	2·4 ± 0·1	2·8 ± 0·3*

*Significantly different from control animals, p<0·001

As can be seen from Table 4, as well as decreasing serum total tryptophan, all the anti-schizophrenic drugs also led to a displacement of tryptophan from albumin binding. This meant that the concentration of diffusible tryptophan was either no different from that in control animals or only slightly lower. Prochlorperazine increased the serum total amino acid concentration, while all the others, including promethazine and trimeprazine led to a reduction. Promethazine had no effect on serum total or diffusible tryptophan, while trimeprazine led to an increase in the total tryptophan concentration, balanced by a decrease in the diffusible fraction. so that the concentration of diffusible tryptophan was unchanged. As would be expected from the increase in the diffusible tryptophan : total amino acid ratio, all of these drugs led to an increase in brain tryptophan and 5HT (Bender and Cockcroft, 1977).

From this study it seems probable that while reduction in serum total amino acids may be a general effect of phenothiazines, reduction in serum total tryptophan and displacement of tryptophan from albumin binding may be specific to those drugs that have anti-psychotic action. The displacement of tryptophan from albumin binding by these drugs is not a direct effect of the drugs *per se,* since *in vitro* none has any effect on the binding equilibrium (Bender, 1976b). It remains possible that one or more of the many metabolites of the phenothiazines may block the tryptophan binding site on albumin. The effect of phenothiazines in increasing brain tryptophan uptake and 5HT synthesis is somewhat paradoxical, since this seems to be mediated by the same increase in diffusible tryptophan and decrease in total amino acids as has been observed in schizophrenic patients following withdrawal

Table 4 Phenothiazine effects on serum amino acids and brain tryptophan and 5HT in rats

	Saline (n=24)	*Prochlorperazine* (n=8)	*Chlorprothixene* (n=8)	*Thioridazine* (n=8)	*Promethazine* (n=8)	*Trimeprazine* (n=8)
Dose mg/kg		20	40	60	100	100
Serum:						
Total tryptophan μmol/l	96·8 ± 7·7	61·8 ± 17·3*	59·4 ± 8·8*	49·7 ± 6·4*	104·0 ± 8·2	134·1 ± 12·2*
Diffusible tryptophan %	11·4 ± 1·7	17·6 ± 6·6*	26·1 ± 9·9*	36·2 ± 10·2*	11·6 ± 1·6	8·1 ± 1·1*
Diffusible tryptophan μmol/l	11·0 ± 1·6	10·9 ± 3·0	15·5 ± 2·3*	17·9 ± 2·3*	12·1 ± 1·0	10·9 ± 1·0
Total amino acids mmol/l	2·24 ± 0·19	2·52 ± 0·23*	1·53 ± 0·09*	1·82 ± 0·23*	1·50 ± 0·14*	2·02 ± 0·22
Brain:						
Tryptophan nmol/g	96·7 ± 20·2	141·7 ± 31·8*	200·6 ± 46·3*	197·8 ± 26·4*	148·5 ± 28·9*	177·3 ± 26·5*
5HT nmol/g	2·47 ± 0·36	2·99 ± 0·28*	4·44 ± 0·73*	5·60 ± 0·53*	3·23 ± 0·47*	2·81 ± 0·24*

*Significantly different from control animals, $p < 0·02$

of chlorpromazine, and coinciding with the onset of exacerbation of symptoms.

There is some evidence that several of the anti-psychotic phenothiazines may act to blockade the 5HT receptors of the central nervous system. Thus, von Hungen and co-workers (1975) have shown that chlorpromazine will inhibit the 5HT-stimulated adenylate cyclase of brain preparations, as will cyproheptadine, a known 5HT antagonist. Similarly, Bennett and Snyder (1976) have shown that chlorpromazine and fluphenazine will displace 5HT specifically bound to a brain membrane preparation, again an effect shared by known 5HT antagonists. They also showed that promethazine will not displace 5HT except at very high concentrations.

Thus, one possible action of the anti-schizophrenic phenothiazines may be to blockade the brain 5HT receptors. An increase in brain 5HT synthesis might be expected as an attempt to overcome such receptor blockade if there is a neuronal feed-back system between the post-synaptic and pre-synaptic neurons. Some evidence for such regulation has been proposed by Hamon and co-workers (1976). However, it is unlikely that such events could influence peripheral amino acid metabolism and so enhance brain tryptophan uptake. This response to phenothiazine administration in experimental animals remains unexplained.

If 5HT receptor blockade is an important part of the action of anti-schizophrenic drugs then it is possible that schizophrenia involves a relative overproduction of 5HT, or a hypersensitive 5HT receptor. Such a defect would not conflict with either the data reported here or the evidence for a genetic predisposition to psychotic disease, although the failure to demonstrate any beneficial effect of anti-serotonin medication (Gallant *et al.*, 1964; Holden *et al.*, 1971) and the lack of correlation between the anti-psychotic action of phenothiazines and their ability to displace LSD from membrane (receptor) binding do not agree with such a hypothesis.

ACKNOWLEDGEMENTS

I should like to express my thanks to Drs Andrew N. Bamji and Paul M. Cockcroft, who were involved in some parts of this work, and to Mr Robert J. Read for his technical assistance in some of the later animal studies. Parts of this work were supported by grants from The Wellcome Trust.

REFERENCES

Alexander, F., Curtis, C., Sprince, H. and Crosley, A. P. (1963). L-Methionine and L-tryptophan feedings in non-psychotic and schizophrenic patients with and without tranylcypromine. *J. Ner. Ment. Dis.*, **137**, 135

Bender, D. A. and Bamji, A. N. (1974). Serum tryptophan binding in chlorpromazine-treated chronic schizophrenics. *J. Neurochem.*, **22**, 805

Bender, D. A., Pigache, R. M., Gruzelier, J. and Hammond, N. (1975). Changes in serum tryptophan and albumin binding of tryptophan in chlorpromazine-treated chronic schizophrenics on withdrawal and restoration of drug therapy. *Psychol. Med.*, **5**, 397

Bender, D. A., Boulton, A. P. and Coulson, W. F. (1975). A simple method for the study of tryptophan binding to serum albumin by small-scale equilibrium dialysis: application to animal and human studies. *Biochem. Soc. Transact.*, **3,** 193

Bender, D. A. (1976a). The effects of chlorpromazine on serum tryptophan, brain tryptophan uptake and serotonin synthesis in the rat. *Biochem. Pharmacol.*, **25,** 1743

Bender, D. A. (1976b). Changes in serum tryptophan, tryptophan binding to serum albumin and serum total amino acid concentration following administration of neuroleptic drugs to rats. *Biochem. Soc. Transact.*, **4,** 98

Bender, D. A. and Cockcroft, P. M. (1977). Increase in brain tryptophan and 5-hydroxytryptamine on administration of phenothiazines to rats. *Biochem. Soc. Transact.*, **5,** 155

Bennett, J. P. and Snyder, S. H. (1976). Serotonin and lysergic acid diethylamide binding in rat brain membranes: relationship to post-synaptic receptors. *Molec. Pharmacol.*, **12.** 373

Berlet, H. H., Spaide, J., Kohl, H., Bull, C. and Himwich, H. E. (1965). Effects of reduction of tryptophan and methionine intake on urinary indole compounds and schizophrenic behaviour. *J. Nerv. Ment. Dis.*, **140,** 297

Curzon, G., Katamaneni, B. D., Winch, J., Rojas-Bueno, A., Murray-Lyon, E. T. I. and Williams, R. (1973). Plasma and brain tryptophan changes in experimental acute hepatic failure. *J. Neurochem.*, **21,** 137

Curzon, G., Friedel, J., Katameneni, B. D., Greenwood, M. H. and Lader, M. H. (1974). Unesterified fatty acids and the binding of tryptophan in human plasma. *Clin. Sci. Molec. Med.*, **47,** 415

Deniker, P., Loo, H., Zarifian, E., Bousquet, B., Dreux, C. and Escande, C. (1976). Etude du tryptophane libre et total dans le plasma. Son interêt en psychiatrie. *L'Encephale*, **2,** 123

Domino, E. F. and Krause, R. R. (1974). Free and bound serum tryptophan in drug-free normal controls and chronic schizophrenic patients. *Biol. Psychiatr.*, **8,** 265

Etienne, P., Young, S. N. and Sourkes, T. L. (1976). Inhibition by albumin of tryptophan uptake by rat brain. *Nature*, **262,** 144

Fernstrom, J. D. and Wurtman, R. J. (1971). Brain serotonin content: physiological dependence on plasma tryptophan levels. *Science*, **173,** 149

Frohman, C. E., Warner, K. A., Yoon, H. S., Arthur, R. E. and Gottlieb, J. S. (1969). The plasma factor and transport of indoleamino acids. *Biol. Psychiatr.*, **1,** 377

Frohman, C. E., Harmison, C. R., Arthur, R. E. and Gottlieb, J. S. (1971). Conformation of a unique plasma protein in schizophrenia. *Biol, Psychiatr.*, **3,** 113

Gallant, D. M., Bishop, M. P., Steele, C. A. and Noblin, C. D. (1964). Anti-serotonin activity and clinical tranquilisation. *J. Neuropsychiatr.*, **5,** 273

Gilka, L. (1975). Schizophrenia – a disorder of tryptophan metabolism. *Acta Psych. Scand.*, (suppl.), **258,** 10

Gilmour, D. G., Manowitz, P., Frosch, W. A. and Shopsin, B. (1973). Association of plasma tryptophan levels with clinical changes in female schizophrenic patients. *Biol. Psychiatr.*, **6,** 119

Hamon, M., Bourgoin, S., Héry, F., Ternaux, J. P. and Glowinski, J. (1976). *In vivo* and *in vitro* activation of soluble tryptophan hydroxylase from rat brain stem. *Nature*, **260,** 61

Holden, J. M. C., Itil, T., Keskiner, A. and Gannon, P. (1971). A clinical trial of an anti-serotonin compound, cinanserin, in chronic schizophrenia. *J. Clin. Pharmacol.*, **11,** 220

von Hungen, K., Roberts, S. and Hill, D. F. (1975). Serotonin-sensitive adenylate cyclase activity in immature rat brain. *Brain Res.* **84,** 257

Kaufman, S. (1974). Properties of the pterin-dependent aromatic amino acid hydroxylases, In *Aromatic Amino Acids in the Brain,* CIBA Fdn Symp, **22,** pp. 85–115 (Amsterdam: Associated Scientific Publishers)

Lovett-Doust, J. W., Huszka, L. and Lovett-Doust, J. N. (1975). Psychotropic drugs and gender as modifiers of the role of plasma tryptophan and serotonin in schizophrenia. *Compre. Psychiatr.*, **16,** 349

Manowitz, P., Gilmour, D. G. and Racevskis, J. (1973). Low plasma tryptophan in recently hospitalized schizophrenics. *Biol. Psychiatr.*, **6,** 109

McMenamy, R. H. and Oncley, J. L. (1958). The specific binding of L-tryptophan to serum albumin. *J. Biol. Chem.*, **233,** 1436

McMenamy, R. H. (1965). Binding of indole analogues to human serum albumin. *J. Biol. Chem.*, **240,** 4235

Pardridge, W. M. (1977). Kinetics of competitive inhibition of neutral amino acid transport across the blood–brain barrier. *J. Neurochem.*, **28,** 103

Pollin, W., Cardon, P. V. and Kety, S. S. (1961). Effects of amino acid feedings on schizophrenic patients treated with iproniazid. *Science,* **133,** 104

Pollin, W. (1972). The pathogenesis of schizophrenia. *Arch. Gen. Psychiatr.,* **27,** 29

Tagliamonte, A., Tagliamonte, P., Perez-Cruet, J. and Gessa, G. L. (1971). Increase of brain tryptophan caused by drugs which stimulate 5-hydroxtryptamine synthesis. *Nature New Biol.,* **229,** 125

9

Neurochemical findings in the post-mortem schizophrenic brain

E. D. BIRD

INTRODUCTION AND METHODS

The ability to measure neurochemical substances in brain tissue and the realization that a number of these neurochemical substances can be measured many hours after death in the human brain has clarified some of the neurochemical abnormalities that exist in disorders of the central nervous system. The discovery by Ehringer and Hornykiewicz (1960) of decreased concentration of dopamine in the post-mortem brain of patients dying with Parkinson's disease resulted in the rational pharmacological administration of L-dopa which has given relief to patients with this disorder. Similarly, the decreased concentration of the neurotransmitter γ-aminobutyric acid (GABA) by Perry *at al.* (1973) and the decreased activity of the biosynthetic enzyme for GABA, glutamic acid decarboxylase (GAD), by Bird *et al.* (1973) has given us some clearer understanding of the neurochemical defect in Huntington's chorea.

The frequent appearance of schizophrenic-like symptoms before the onset of choreiform movements in Huntington's chorea suggested to this author that the loss of neuroinhibitory control by the neurotransmitter GABA in specific regions of the brain such as the limbic system might be responsible for the schizophrenic-like symptoms in those 'at-risk' subjects who were predestined to develop chorea. It was this observation that led us to examine post-mortem brain tissue from patients who died having had the diagnosis of schizophrenia made during life. The collection of schizophrenic post-mortem brain tissue has been notoriously difficult in the past and, therefore, it seemed logical that we should use the approach we used for collecting post-mortem tissue from patients who die with Huntington's chorea.

We wrote to many of the psychiatrists who had previously been so helpful in informing the next-of-kin of deceased patients of our research. Our second approach was again similar to that used for Huntington's chorea seeking the co-operation of the lay organizations and we visitied a number of chapters throughout the country to explain our research programme. During the past 2 years we have been able to examine 47 post-mortem brain tissue from patients dying having had the diagnosis of schizophrenia made during life. The mean age of death of the patient group was 57 ± 3 years and for the control group was 61 ± 3 years. The time interval between the hour of death and the time in which the corpse was placed in the specially cooled room in the mortuary was $3 \pm 0{\cdot}3$ hours for the patient group and $2 \pm 0{\cdot}3$ hours for the control group. The ability to measure neurochemical substances in post-mortem brain is more dependant upon the rate of cooling after death than upon the time the post-mortem is carried out. The interval from death to brain removal was 39 ± 3 hours in the control group and 40 ± 4 in the patient group. Immediately after the post-mortem the tissues are frozen in a deep-freeze and transported to Cambridge for further dissection. The brain tissues are sub-divided into neuro-anatomical regions and the areas of interest to be discussed are the limbic system which include the nucleus accumbens, amygdala and hippocampus and one region of the basal ganglia, the putamen. The assays carried out were dopamine, as measured by the method of Cuello *et al.* (1973), GAD by the method of Roberts and Simonsen (1963) and choline acetyltransferase (CAT) by the method of Fonnum (1969). Protein was measured by the method of Lowry *et al.* (1951).

RESULTS

Dopamine

There was a significant increase in the dopamine concentration in the nucleus accumbens of the patient group when compared to the controls (see Table 1). There were no differences between patients who had been on neuroleptic treatment until death and a smaller sub-group of nine patients which included three who had not been on any neuroleptics and six that had not been on neuroleptics for the year prior to death. The dopamine concentrations in the putamen of both the control and the patient group were essentially the same (Table 1).

GAD

The activity of GAD was significantly decreased in all areas examined of the patient group when compared to controls (Table 1). There was also a significant decrease in GAD activity in both the amygdala and hippocampus when compared to the control group (Table 2). Again there were no significant differences between the patients who had been receiving neuroleptics and those who had not been receiving neuroleptics.

CAT

There were no differences in CAT activity of the areas examined between the patient and control groups (Tables 1 and 2).

DISCUSSION

A number of authors have directed attention to the limbic system of the brain and suggested that this will be the most likely area in which a defect in schizophrenia will be found (Stevens, 1973; Torrey and Peterson, 1974). The occurrence of a schizophrenia-like illness in disorders associated with temporal lobe epilepsy (Slater and Beard, 1963), encephalitis (Glaser and Pincus, 1969) and tumours (Malamud, 1967) made it imperative that any neuro-

Table 1 Dopamine, GAD and CAT in post-mortem brain

	Controls	*Schizophrenics*
Nucleus accumbens		
DA	9·4 ± 1·49 (26)	13·9 ± 1·4* (26)
GAD	90 ± 9 (23)	50 ± 6*** (27)
CAT	222 ± 13 (24)	182 ± 15 (27)
Putamen		
DA	22 ± 2 (29)	22 ± 2 (33)
GAD	61 ± 5 (27)	42 ± 5* (33)
CAT	340 ± 21 (27)	296 ± 18 (33)

DA in μg/g protein

GAD, CAT } in μmol/g protein

*$p<0·02$; **$p<0·01$; ***$p<0·001$

Table 2 GAD and CAT in post-mortem brain

	Controls	*Schizophrenics*
Amygdala		
GAD+	26 ± 3 (17)	14 ± 2*** (29)
CAT+	35 ± 4 (16)	27 ± 3 (29)
Hippocampus		
GAD +	25 ± 3 (36)	13 ± 2*** (39)
CAT +	15 ± 1 (36)	14 ± 1 (39)

in μmol/g protein

+***$p<0·001$

chemical study of schizophrenia include this region of the brain.

The development of the psychosis following the administration of amphetamine (Angrist and Gershorn, 1970) and the knowledge that amphetamine is involved in both the release of dopamine and stimulation of dopamine receptors would suggest that dopamine might be a key transmitter in the production of schizophrenia. This resulted in the 'dopamine hypothesis' for the cause of schizophrenia (Matthysse, 1973). This is further supported by the fact that phenothiazine agents are potent blocking agents at the dopamine receptor (Iversen, 1975). The present finding of increased dopamine in the nucleus accumbens, therefore, is consistent with the dopamine hypothesis proposed for schizophrenia.

The production of dopamine by dopaminergic cells is under the direct control of the gabanergic neurons that produce GABA. It has also been proposed in the past that there may be a defect in GABA metabolism in schizophrenia (Roberts, 1972). Our finding of decreased GAD activity throughout the limbic system as well as in the putamen is consistent with this hypothesis and may be the cause of increased dopamine production in schizophrenia. It is of interest that the gabanergic activity is decreased in the putamen of the brain from patients with this illness. Since neuroinhibitory gabanergic fibres pass from the putamen to the brain stem terminating on dopamine cell bodies, the decreased GAD activity in the putamen of the patient group was not as marked as that seen thoughout the limbic system of this group.

It is known that the neuroleptic agents when given to animals will alter dopamine metabolism in the brain increasing dopamine production in the first few days after administration (Carlsson and Lindqvist, 1968) but after prolonged administration the dopamine concentration in the striatum will return to normal (O'Keefe *et al.,* 1970) and may even decrease to below normal concentrations (Bird *et al.,* 1979). Although it is conceivable that the dopamine concentrations recorded in this study may be secondary to neuroleptic treatment since nearly all patients received neuroleptic drugs at some time during their life, this would not be consistent with the animal experience. Furthermore, the three patients who had never received neuroleptic treatment and a group of six patients who had not had any neuroleptic treatment during the year prior to death had similar neurochemical changes as the group who had received neuroleptic drugs until the time of death. The neurochemical abnormalities reported here in the limbic system are not too dissimilar to the abnormalities that we previously found in the basal ganglia of the post-mortem brain of patients dying with Huntington's chorea. Neuroanatomical areas outside the basal ganglia of the choreic brain frequently have normal GAD activities. Therefore, I believe that the decreased GAD activity and increased dopamine activity found in the choreic brain are secondary to a primary genetic defect which is as yet undiscovered. Long before the use of neuroleptic agents for schizophrenia many patients with this illness manifested disorders of movement which undoubtedly involved the basal ganglia (Jones and Hunter, 1969). I, therefore, would like to propose that at the present time, these two diseases have, in addition to their clinical similarities, neurochemical similarities with the spectrum of neurochemical disorder in schizophrenia having its greatest abnormality in the limbic system with mild involvement of the basal ganglia, whereas in Huntington's chorea the greatest neurochemical abnormality is found in the basal ganglia with a mild abnormality in some cases in the limbic system. I should indicate to you that we have been sending portions of the post-mortem tissue that we have collected throughout the country to research laboratories in England and the United States and I sincerely believe that in the next few years we shall be proceeding quite rapidly towards the elucidation of the biochemical abnormalities associated with schizophrenia. Dr E. Spokes and Dr L. L. Iversen were my colleagues involved with this study.

ACKNOWLEDGEMENTS

This study could not have been done without the help and co-operation of numerous consultant psychiatrists and pathologists who assisted with the post-mortems and the National Schizophrenia Fellowship. We are grateful to Professor Austin Gresham and his colleagues in the Department of Morbid Pathology, Addenbrooke's Hospital, for assistance with control tissues. We thank Joan Bird for collection of tissues, Jean Gale, Julia Gray, Les Sullivan, Jane Koch and George Ingram for expert technical assistance and Gail Moore for assistance with the clinical records. We would also like to thank the County Coroners for their help and co-operation.

REFERENCES

Angrist, B. M. and Gershorn, S. (1970). The phenomenonology of experimentally induced amphetamine psychosis: preliminary observations. *Biol. Psychiatry*, **2**, 95

Bird, E. D., Mackay, A. V. P., Rayner, C. N. and Iversen, L. L. (1973). Reduced glutamic-acid decarboxylase activity of post-mortem brain in Huntington's chorea. *Lancet*, **i**, 1090

Bird, E. D., Szabo, E. I. and Anton, A. H. (1979). The effect of a phenothiazine on dopamine concentration in the basal ganglia of monkeys. (submitted for publication)

Carlsson, A. and Linqvist, M. (1963). Effect of Chlorpromazine on haloperidol formation of 3-methoxytyramine and normetanephrine in mouse brain. *Acta Pharmacol. Toxicol. (Kobenhaven)*, **20**, 140

Cuello, A. C., Hilley, R. and Iversen, L. L. (1973). Use of catechol *O*-methyl transferase for the enzyme radiochemical assay of dopamine. *J. Neurochem.*, **21**, 1337

Ehringer, H. and Hornykiewicz, O. (1960). Verteilung von noradrenalin und dopamin (3-hydroxytyramin) im gehirn des menshen und ihr verhalten bei erkrankungen des extra-pyramidalen. *Systems Klin. Wochenschr.*, **38**, 1236

Fonnum, F. (1969). Radiochemical micro-assays for the determination of choline acetyltransferase and acetylcholinesterase activities. *Biochem. J.*, **115**, 465

Glaser, G. H. and Pincus, J. H. (1969). Limbic encephalitis. *J. Nerv. Ment. Dis.*, **149**, 59

Iversen, L. L. (1975). Dopamine receptors in the brain. *Science*, **188**, 1084

Jones, M. and Hunter, R. (1969). Abnormal movements in patients with chronic psychiatric illness. In G. E. Crane and R. Gardner Jr. (eds.) *Psychotropic Drugs and Dysfunction of the Basal Ganglia* pp. 53–65. Public Health Publication No. 1938, Chevy Chase, Maryland, U.S.A.

Lowry, O. H., Rosebrough, N. J., Farr, A. L. and Randall, R. J. (1951). Protein measurement with the folin phenol reagent. *J. Biol. Chem.*, **193**, 265

Malamud, N. (1967). Psychiatric disorder with intracranial tumours of limbic system. *Arch. Neurol.*, **17**, 113

Matthysse, S. (1973). Antipsychotic drug actions: a clue to the neuro-pathology of schizophrenia. *Fed. Pro.*, **32**, 200

O'Keefe, R., Sharman, D. F. and Vogt, M. (1970). Effects of drugs used in psychoses on cerebral dopamine metabolism. *Br. J. Pharmacol.*, **38,** 287

Perry, T. L., Hansen, S. and Kloster, M. (1973). Huntington's chorea; deficiency of γ-amino-butyric acid in brain. *N. Engl. J. Med.*, **288,** 337

Roberts, E. (1972). An hypothesis suggesting that there is a defect in the gaba system in schizophrenia. In S. S. Kety and S. Matthysse (eds.), *Prospects for research on schizophrenia. Neurosci. Res. Bull.*, **10,** 468

Roberts, E. and Simonsen, D. G. (1963). Some properties of L-glutamic acid decarboxylase in mouse brain. *Biochem. Pharmacol.*, **12,** 113

Slater, E. and Beard, A. W. (1963). The schizophrenia-like psychoses of epilepsy, **I.** Psychiatric aspects. *Br. J. Psychiatry*, **109,** 95

Stevens, J. R. (1973). An anatomy of schizophrenia? *Arch. Gen. Psychiatry.*, **29,** 177

Torrey, E. F. and Peterson, M. R. (1974). Schizophrenia and the limbic system. *Lancet*, **ii,** 942

POSTSCRIPT

A larger series of post-mortem brains have now been examined and in the schizophrenic group there is a significant increase in dopamine concentration in both the nucleus accumens and the anterior perforated space – another area within the limbic system. However, the activity of the enzyme glutamic acid decarboxylase (GAD) has been noted to be decreased in the post-mortem brain tissue from patients that had bronchial pneumonia prior to death. When only those schizophrenic cases that had an acute death were compared to similar controls, there was no difference in GAD activity in any brain region from the schizophrenic group when compared to the control group.

10

The pineal gland: its possible significance in schizophrenia

J. A. SMITH

Historically, the pineal gland has for at least two centuries been implicated in psychiatry. Since the time Descartes described the gland as the seat of the soul, the pineal body has held a mysterious relationship with mental functioning. Thus, in the early 1900s aqueous pineal extracts were used in the treatment of abnormal mental states with some success. But for a variety of reasons, one of which was the lack of control experiments, the results were viewed with suspicion. It was not until the late 1950s that pineal research began to progress and over the last two decades has mushroomed to the point where the gland is now considered in man as part of the endocrine system. It is a single and compact organ situated medially between the habenular and posterior commisures. If the brain is cut near the median sagittal plane the pineal gland is exposed. Although it is seated in the middle of the brain it is not connected to the rest of the brain neuronally. It receives its nervous supply from the sympathetic nervous system via the posterior fibres from the superior cervical ganglion. It is also situated in close proximity to the third ventricle and so any hormone secretion could pass directly into the ventricular fluid or alternatively drain into the great cerebral vein and thus into the peripheral blood system. There exists no portal blood system between the pineal gland and other parts of the brain such as the hypothalamus or the pituitary.

The human pineal calcifies at puberty and was therefore thought until recently to be vestigial. It is, however, now known to be biochemically active throughout life. The principal metabolite or hormone is called melatonin, so named because of its affect on frog melanocytes in blanching frog skin. Melatonin is synthesized from serotonin first through *N*-acetylation by serotonin *N*-acetyl transferase (SNAT) and then by methylation with hydroxyindole-*O*-methyl transferase (HIOMT)(Axelrod, 1974) (Figure 1). This latter enzyme is very interesting since it is found almost exclusively in the pineal gland in man. Even more fascinating is the fact that pineal metabolism

Figure 1 Biosynthesis of melatonin

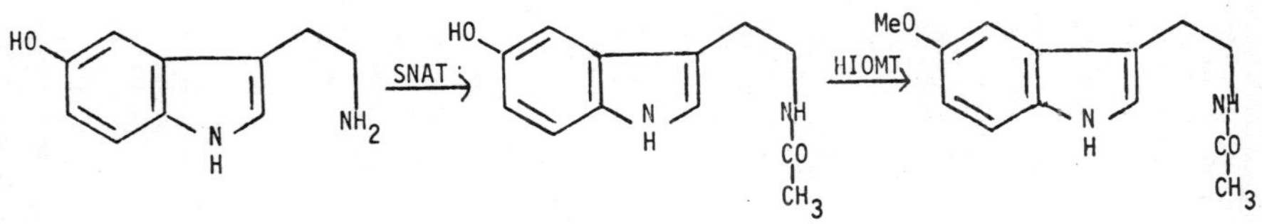

shows a definite circadian rhythm which is controlled by light input. Thus, melatonin synthesis is stimulated in response to light changes perceived by the retina. Nerve impulses are transmitted from the retina via the sympathetic nervous system to the pineal. It has been shown in the pineal of the rat that SNAT (Klein and Weller, 1970) and HIOMT (Axelrod *et al.*, 1965) activities exhibit a diurnal rhythm such that the enzyme activities are highest in the dark and lowest in the light period. Recently our studies with post-mortem human pineal tissue (Smith *et al.*, 1977a) (Table 1) in collaboration with Dr Bird in Cambridge, have shown that similar diurnal rhythms exist in the SNAT and HIOMT enzyme activities taken from post-mortem normal human pineal. The pineal gland acts, therefore, as a neurotransducer. Melatonin is synthesized in response to the lighting regimen and is then secreted into the peripheral blood supply and into the ventricular fluid.

Table 1 **Synchronous synthetic enzyme rhythms in human post-mortem pineal**

	Time of death					
	24–04	04–08	08–12	12–16	16–20	20–24
No. of patients	7	8	4	6	5	4
SNAT pmol h^{-1} mg^{-1} $\pm$SD	1278 ± 100	939 ± 135	755 ± 156	728 ± 46	748 ± 73	1073 ± 182
HIOMT pmol h^{-1} mg^{-1} $\pm$SD	414 ± 40	362 ± 45	344 ± 13	214 ± 31	274 ± 45	367 ± 33

Although the exact function of the pineal is not yet clear, an important normal physiological function of melatonin, and possibly of other related indoles, would appear to be the regulation of gonadal function by controlling hypothalamic releasing hormones (Minneman and Wurtman, 1975). Melatonin has been shown in animals to delay the onset of puberty and indeed in man destruction of pineal tumours are associated with precocious puberty. Further evidence supporting its effect on the gonads is seen in women in that serum melatonin concentrations also show a 28 day rhythm with maximal values at menstruation (Arendt and Wetterberg, 1976).

Another important aspect of melatonin activity is that the pineal may have an effect on brainstem neurons which control variations in sleep and arousal (Quay, 1974). Certainly melatonin induces sleep when administered to human volunteers (Cramer *et al.*, 1974), alters EEG patterns and also increases REM sleep. A further action of melatonin seems to be that it significantly elevates cerebral serotonin particularly in midbrain (Anton-Tay, 1974).

So much for the state of pinealogy in the normal situation. In addition to the historical implication of the pineal in psychiatry, there is more recent biochemical and clinical evidence that the pineal gland may be involved in central nervous disorders (Anton-Tay *et al.*, 1971), particularly the schizophrenias (Jones *et al.*, 1969). From the biochemical viewpoint the transmethylation hypothesis is still the centre of much research into the cause of the disease.

McIsaac (1961) suggested that transmethylation by pineal HIOMT might, if defective, be implicated in the pathogenesis of the schizophrenias by the production of abnormally methylated compounds. He showed that melatonin under physiological conditions would cyclize to form a psychotomimetic compound related to harmaline. *In vivo,* both haloperidol (Naylor and Olley, 1969) and LSD (Diab *et al.,* 1971) have been shown to concentrate more in the rat pineal than in any other part of the brain. Moreover, we have demonstrated that *in vitro,* bovine HIOMT is inhibited by neuroleptics (Smith *et al.,* 1972) and activated by psychotomimetic agents (Smith and Hartley, 1973). However, we were not able to show these effects conclusively *in vivo.*

There was also a report by Greiner (1970) that he thought that skin pigmentation in schizophrenics was due to abnormal pineal metabolism and not to phenothiazine therapy. However, although melatonin blanches frog skin, it has no effect on human pigmentation and Robins (1972) disproved Greiner's theory.

On the clinical side, there is also evidence relating the pineal to the illness in terms of its effect on sleep and the endocrine system. Schizophrenic patients for example often show sleep disturbance and even a reversal of their sleep rhythm (Slater and Roth, 1969). Indeed insomnia may be the first symptom of a relapse whilst changes in REM sleep and in EEG patterns during sleep have been observed in schizophrenic patients (Reich, 1975; Jus, 1973). Also the level of arousal may be altered (Gruzelier, 1975) and the most extreme example of such change is seen in catatonic stupor. Furthermore, schizophrenia is relatively rare in childhood and many patients give a history of onset in adolescence (Sands, 1976). There may also be a delay in sexual maturation and poor development of secondary sexual characteristics. In some patients, however, an increase in sexual activity may occur during the acute stages of the illness (Slater and Roth, 1969).

Although there is much circumstantial evidence linking the pineal gland with schizophrenia, the theories have not been tested. The major problem has been until recently the lack of a sufficiently sensitive method for measuring melatonin in biological samples. In 1976, however, we developed a radioimmunoassay (based on the method of Arendt) (Arendt, 1975) which was specific for melatonin and was sensitive to 10 pg/ml of serum. Up until 1976 there was a dearth of normal pineal data in terms of serum and CSF melatonin concentration. Obviously, before comparisons can be made between pineal metabolism in normal individuals and that in clinically rated schizophrenic patients, the normal parameters must be studied. For the past year, we in Bradford in collaboration with Dr J Barnes and Dr E Bird in Cambridge have been measuring serum and CSF melatonin concentrations in normal and schizophrenic individuals.

We have already seen that in post-mortem pineals from normal individuals, SNAT and HIOMT activity exhibit a diurnal rhythm being highest around 0200 hours and lowest about 1400 hours. We have measured by radioimmunoassay serum melatonin concentration through 24 hours in normal male volunteers (Smith *et al.,* 1977a). We found (Table 2) that the

Table 2 Variation with time of human male serum melatonin concentration (pg ml^{-1})

Time (h)	0200	0600	1000	1400	1800	2200
Normal male ($n = 5$) Average age=35 years±SD	78 ± 25	55 ± 5	35 ± 8	20 ± 8	26 ± 6	46 ± 10
Psychiatric male not treated with chlorpromazine ($n = 5$) ± SD Average age = 42 years	26 ± 10	20 ± 8	14 ± 6	12 ± 2	16 ± 2	18 ± 8
Time (h)	0300	0700	1100	1500	1900	2300
Psychiatric male treated with chlorpromazine (100–400 mg daily) ($n = 5$) Average age = 35 years ±SD	122 ± 34	98 ± 30	80 ± 12	110 ± 29	124 ± 33	136 ± 39

serum melatonin levels also showed a diurnal rhythm which was synchronous with those rhythms of the synthesizing enzymes SNAT and HIOMT. It seems, therefore, that due to this synchrony, the serum melatonin concentration accurately reflects pineal function in man. Thus, in comparing normal melatonin levels with those in a pathophysiological condition, the time of sampling must be taken into account.

We next commenced our preliminary study on 30 schizophrenic patients. The clinical rating of these patients is presently being completed by Dr J Barnes and for the purpose of this book it would be better to simply class them as psychiatric patients. In our preliminary studies only 3 out of 30 psychiatric patients exhibited normal diurnal rhythms in serum melatonin concentration. The remaining 27 divided into two groups (Smith *et al.*, 1977b).

The first group of patients (Table 2) showed lower than normal absolute melatonin levels with a shallow rhythm. If we compare five of this group with five normals, then the night-time melatonin levels at 0200 hours are three-fold less in the psychiatric patients than in the normal individuals. Whether the low shallow melatonin levels are associated with the psychiatric illness or alternatively with some other parameter is not yet established.

The second group of psychiatric patients in our preliminary study (Table 2) on the other hand exhibit very high serum melatonin levels with little rhythm. Like the previous group, the measurements had been carried out blind without the background clinical data. This group of high melatonin levels corresponded to those patients being treated with chlorpromazine in varying dosage. The daytime levels are 4–5 times higher than normal whilst the night-time levels are only slightly higher than normal.A similar elevation of serum melatonin has been reported by Wurtman in rats being given chlorpromazine (Ozaki *et al.*, 1976). This suggests, therefore, that the elevated melatonin levels are due to the drug particularly since the first group who were not being treated with chlorpromazine had much lower than normal levels. However, no dose correlation can yet be made. It will be interesting to find out if the levels before chlorpromazine in these patients are normal, high or low. Whether the effect of chlorpromazine is due to an increased biosynthesis of melatonin, or increased rate of release from the gland or decreased rate of metabolism is unclear. But, since intravenous injection of melatonin in man induces sleep (Cramer *et al.*, 1974), the elevated melatonin concentration may explain the initial tranquillizing effect observed in the clinical use of chlorpromazine before the gradual onset of the antipsychotic action.

At the present time however, we are unable to correlate the abnormal rhythms with type of schizophrenia. We await the clinical rating with interest. We are currently studying the effect of other drugs such as fluphenazine, haloperidol, depixol and pimozide.

As previously mentioned, we think that serum and CSF melatonin measurements may well reflect pineal function in both normal individuals and in psychiatric patients. However, with the availability of post-mortem brain tissue we are now able to study any biochemical changes that might occur in the pineal in schizophrenia and correlate them with the psychiatric serum measurements. Thus in our preliminary study we have found apparent abnormal HIOMT activity in 10 out of 15 such pineals and further investigations are now being made.

In conclusion, I have presented a summary of the circumstantial evidence linking the pineal gland with psychiatry. I have also presented some preliminary findings. The new methodology for the measurement of melatonin in serum and CSF has removed the major obstacle to testing the theories. In addition, the availability of post-mortem brain tissue is providing the means for studying any biochemical abnormalities. Whilst melatonin is probably not the only pineal metabolite of importance, the way is now clear for testing our theories which will finally prove or discount the idea that the pineal gland is implicated in the aetiology of the schizophrenias.

REFERENCES

Anton-Tay, F. *et al.* (1971). On the effect of melatonin on human brain. Its possible therapeutic implications. *Life Sci.*, **10,** 841

Anton-Tay, F. (1974). Melatonin: effects on brain function. *Adv. Biochem. Psychopharmacol.*, **11,** 315

Arendt, J. *et al.* (1975). Melatonin radioimmunoassay. *J. Clin. Endocrinol. Metab.*, **40,** 347

Arendt, J. and Wetterberg, L. (1976). Melatonin in serum and cerebro-spinal fluid in the human. *J. Clin. Endocrinol. Metab.*, **42,** (1) 185

Axelrod, J. *et al.* (1965). Control of hydroxyindole-*O*-methyltransferase activity in the rat pineal gland by environmental lighting. *J. Biol. Chem.*, **240,** 949

Axelrod, J. (1974). The pineal gland: a neurotransducer. *Science,* **184,** 1341

Cramer, H. *et al.* (1974). On the effects of melatonin on sleep and behaviour in Man. *Adv. Biochem. Psychopharmacol.*, **11,** 187

Diab, I. M. *et al.* (1971). ^{3}H lysergic acid diethylamide, cellular autoradiographic localisation in rat brain. *Science,* **173,** 1022

Greiner, A. C. (1970). Schizophrenia and the pineal gland. *Can. Psychiatr. Assoc.*, **15,** 433

Gruzelier, J. H. (1975). Evidence of high and low levels of physiological arousal in schizophrenia. *Psychophysiology,* **12,** (1) 66

Jones, R. L. *et al.* (1969). Metabolism of exogenous melatonin in schizophrenic and non-schizophrenic volunteers. *Clin. Chim. Acta,* **26,** 281

Jus, K. (1973). Sleep EEG studies in untreated long-term schizophrenic patients. *Arch. Gen. Psychiatry,* **29,** (3) 386

Klein, D. C. and Weller, J. L. (1970). Indole metabolism in the pineal gland: a circadian rhythm in N-acetyltransferase. *Science,* **169,** 1093

McIsaac, W. M. (1961). Methoxyharmalan-potent serotonin antagonist which affects conditioned behaviour. *Science*, **134**, 674
Minneman, K. P. and Wurtman, R. J. (1975). Effects of pineal compounds on mammals. *Life Sci.* **17**, 1189
Naylor, R. J. and Olley, J. E. (1969). The distribution of haloperidol in rat brain. *Br J. Pharmacol.*, **36**, 208
Ozaki, Y. *et al.* (1976). Melatonin in rat pineal, plasma and urine: 24-hour rhythmicity and effect of chlorpromazine. *Endocrinology*, **98**, (6) 1418
Quay, W. B. (1974). *Pineal Chemistry in Cellular and Physiological Mechanisms*. pp. 193–194 (Springfield: C. C. Thomas)
Reich, L. (1975). Sleep disturbance in schizophrenia. *Arch. Gen. Psychiatry*, **32**, (1) 51
Robins, A. H. (1972). Skin melanin concentrations in schizophrenia. *Br. J. Psychiatry*, **121**, 613
Sands, D. E. (1976). In D. Richter (ed.) *Endocrine Changes in Schizophrenia*, (New York: Pergamon Press)
Slater, E. and Roth, M. (1969). *Clinical Psychiatry*. p. 285. (London: Ballière, Tindall and Cassel)
Smith, J. A. *et al.* (1972). The inhibition of pineal hydroxyindole-O-methyltransferase by haloperidol and fluphenazine. *J. Pharm. Pharmacol.*, **24**, (suppl.) 100
Smith J. A. and Hartley, R. (1973). The activation of pineal hydroxyindole-O-methyltransferase by psychotomimetic drugs. *J. Pharm. Pharmacol.*, **25**, 751
Smith, J. A. *et al.* (1977a). Synchronous nyctohemeral rhythms in human blood melatonin and in human post-mortem pineal enzyme. *Clin. Endocrinol.*, **6**, 219
Smith, J. A. *et al.*, (1977b). Elevated melatonin serum concentrations in psychiatric patients treated with chlorpromazine. *J. Pharm. Pharmacol.*, **29**, (suppl.) 30

SECTION 4:
Treatment

11
Rational drug treatment in schizophrenia

T. J. CROW

INTRODUCTION

Following the introduction by Delay and Deniker of chlorpromazine in 1952, the major tranquillizers have now been in use in the treatment of schizophrenia for more than 25 years. Although many, like chlorpromazine, have been phenothiazines, two other major groups, the butyrophenones (like haloperidol) and thiaxanthenes (including flupenthixol) are widely used. It seems increasingly likely that they owe their therapeutic effects to a single pharmacological action. Deniker originally suggested that the extrapyramidal side effects were necessary for the antipsychotic action. Although the relationship between these two actions is not perfect (thioridazine has a low incidence of side effects, for example) this hypothesis, at least in an updated form, appears increasingly probable.

Since the work of Hornykiewicz and Carlsson, the parkinsonian side effects have been attributed to dopamine receptor blockade. A number of laboratory studies have shown that dopamine receptor blockade is an excellent predictor of antipsychotic activity. Recently in a clinical trial we have been able to demonstrate that for flupenthixol, which exists in two isomeric forms, the α-isomer, which blocks the dopamine receptor, has therapeutic activity in acute schizophrenia, while the β-isomer, which does not block the receptor, is devoid of such activity.

Since the correlation with extrapyramidal side effects is not perfect it seems likely that the therapeutic effect is occurring elsewhere than in the corpus striatum (which presumably is the site of the parkinsonian effects). However, there are other dopamine-containing areas of brain and some, for example, related to the limbic system, seem more likely sites of the antipsychotic action. Whether or not the primary disturbance in schizophrenia, or in some types of schizophrenic illness, is a disorder of dopaminergic transmission is at present the subject of intensive research.

While for some patients drugs are almost curative, in others they are of limited use, and some patients with apparently typical illnesses do well without them. Since they are far from free of unwanted effects the precise indications for their use is a matter of some importance.

TREATMENT OF ACUTE SCHIZOPHRENIA

Drug trials in the early 1960s established the value of neuroleptics in recent onset or relapse. In the NIMH trial of 1964, for example, 75% of patients given a phenothiazine were well after 4 weeks compared to 25% on placebo. One half of the placebo-treated group and only 5% of the drug-treated group were judged unchanged or worse. Analysis of the results of this trial showed that the drug-placebo differences were similar for many of the symptoms of the disease, and that drugs had as great a beneficial effect on some 'negative' features (e.g. social withdrawal and lack of self-care) as on the more characteristic 'positive' symptoms of delusions, hallucinations and thought disorder. From this type of finding it is sometimes argued that drug therapy may be more than merely symptomatic and may somehow be reversing the underlying disturbance.

Drugs have been compared with other therapies. In California P. R. A. May conducted a large scale trial of drugs against drugs plus psychotherapy, against psychotherapy alone, against ECT, and against routine ward care. On nearly all indices drugs were the most effective treatment and were also the cheapest since patients were discharged more quickly. The benefits of psychotherapy at best were marginal and this treatment delayed discharge. ECT was less effective than regimens including drug treatment, but more so than psychotherapy alone or ward care. Thus the use of neuroleptic drugs appears to be the most effective ingredient in the treatment of acute schizophrenia.

PREVENTION OF RELAPSE

More than 24 controlled studies of neuroleptic medication of schizophrenic out-patients have shown that patients on medication are less likely to relapse. The findings of a recent study by Hogarty and Goldberg (Figure 1) which attempts to assess the role of drug therapy and social casework in schizophrenic patients in the community are of particular interest.

Patients were randomly allocated to drug or placebo treatment with or without social casework (MRT – major role therapy, directed mainly at returning the patient to his or her job or major role, e.g. as housewife). The figure shows the percentage of patients having relapsed at various points during the 24 months of the trial. Findings of particular interest are:

(1) At 24 months 80% of placebo-treated and 48% of drug-treated patients had relapsed.

(2) Although in placebo-treated patients social work support was of little value, in patients on drug therapy this was helpful, and the effect appeared to increase with time.

(3) Although 80% of patients on placebo relapsed, by 24 months the curve had flattened out. This suggests that a proportion of patients (perhaps 15 to 20%) will do well without drug treatment. Unfortunately there is little indication of how such patients are to be identified.

(4) In spite of drug therapy at 24 months 48% of patients have relapsed. This indicates again that drugs are not a cure for the condition.

Despite drugs some patients become long-term inmates of mental institutions. The value of drugs in treating such patients is probably much less

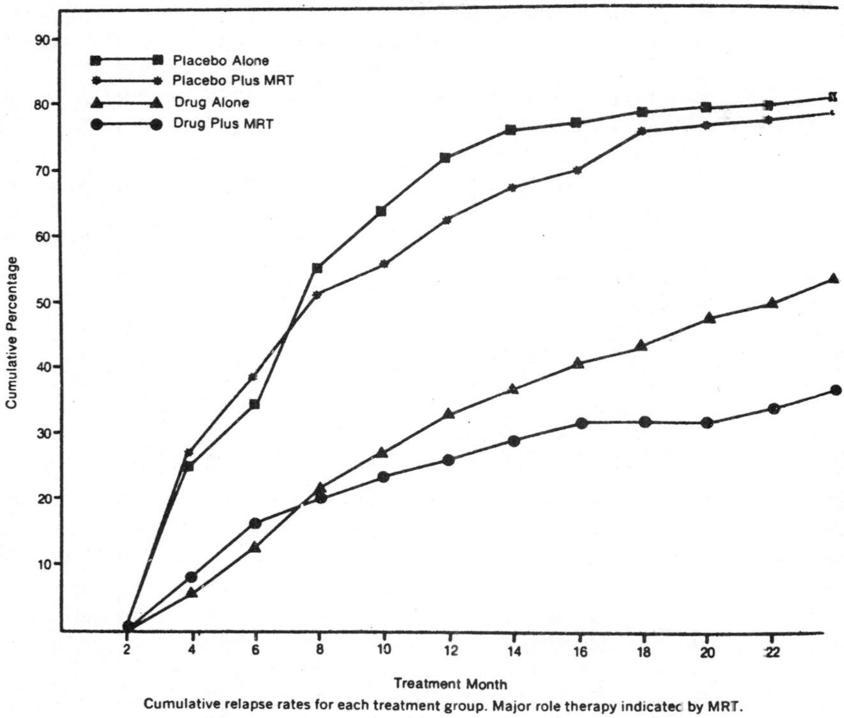

Figure 1 Cumulative percentage relapse rates in out-patients with schizophrenia treated with or without neuroleptic drugs and with or without social casework follow-up (MRT – major role therapy). (From Hogarty, G. E. *et al.* (1974). *Arch. Gen. Psychiat.*, **31,** 603)

than in the acute phase of the illness and in preventing relapse. Indeed some trials in long-stay inpatients have failed to show significant drug effects at all. Whether this is because some severe schizophrenic illnesses are drug-resistant from the outset, because they progress to a drug resistant phase, or because patients in institutions are protected from environmental stresses which would otherwise exacerbate their florid symptoms, remains to be established.

The choice of drugs is very wide. There is no really convincing evidence that particular drugs are selective to particular symptoms. On the other hand side effects do vary. Some drugs such as thioridazine cause relatively few extrapyramidal side effects, probably because they possess a high degree of anticholinergic potency, and for this reason may possess 'in-built' antiparkinsonian activity. However, such anticholinergic activity may have unwanted effects of its own, e.g. in producing a dry mouth, a particular disadvantage in the elderly. Many patients are well maintained on the standard depot injections of flupenthixol and fluphenazine. Perhaps partly because this mode of administration allows relatively constant blood levels to be maintained, and perhaps partly because the depot clinic milieu allows closer supervision of progress, this has proved a satisfactory treatment regime for many otherwise resistant patients.

The hazards of neuroleptic medication are mostly well established but some are of increasing concern. The acute extrapyramidal effects (parkinsonian symptoms, akathisia, dystonias) are probably little influenced by the *routine* administration of anti-parkinsonian drugs which should therefore be avoided. A reduction of neuroleptic dosage is often the best management of such symptoms. Of more insidious onset and a greater potential hazard is tardive dyskinesia, the syndrome of repetitive involuntary oro-facial movements sometimes accompanied by choreoathetoid limb and trunk movements which appears to be a consequence of long continued drug administration, and may be commoner with high dosage and combined anticholinergic medication.

HOW LONG SHOULD MEDICATION BE CONTINUED?

On the question of how long medication should be continued opinions vary widely. Probably this is partly because the disease does too. Some patients will do badly in spite of drugs and some will do well without them. The potential hazards must be weighed against the benefits. Many patients in institutions are probably better off without medication. For out-patients it is suggested that the question of drug withdrawal or reduction for a trial period should be kept under review. Obviously such decisions will have to take into account the unwanted effects the patient experiences, his own views on medication and the possible consequences, often not inconsiderable, of relapse.

REFERENCES

Drug and Therapeutics Bulletin (1977). **15,** 57
Lancet (1976). **ii,** 563

12

Investigations into serum folate and B_{12} concentrations in psychiatric in-patients with particular reference to schizophrenia

M. W. P. CARNEY

INTRODUCTION

The various haematological, neurological and psychiatric manifestations of vitamin B_{12} deficiency are well documented. However, the clinical effects of folate deficiency are much more obscure. They are thought to include megaloblastic anaemia, a neurological syndrome like sub-acute combined degeneration of the cord and mental symptoms (Reynolds, 1976a). Folic acid in the central nervous system is involved in nucleoprotein synthesis, as a methyl donor in transmethylation, in monoamine metabolism (notably serotonin) and in synaptic events, possibly as a neurotransmitter. Folate has excitatory and convulsant properties and counteracts the inhibitory effects of γ- amino-butyric acid. Reynolds (1976b) states that the neuropsychiatric expressions of B_{12} deficiency are due to a block in folic acid metabolism.

In this paper I wish to describe studies I made of serum folate and B_{12} values in two large groups of mentally ill patients admitted under my care; and also the results of treating some of these patients with very low serum concentrations of the vitamin, with the appropriate vitamin supplements. I must stress that my investigations cannot answer the question whether folate and B_{12} deficiency *cause* mental illness. I can only provide pointers. Nevertheless the two surveys I shall describe are among the most extensive carried out of serum folic acid and B_{12} in mental illness and thus may have some value.

RESULTS

In the sixties methods of assay for serum folate, employing *Lactobacillus casei* (Waters and Mollin, 1961) and B_{12} using *Lactobacillus leichmanii* (Meynell *et al.*, 1957) became generally available. In view of several reports, especially those of Gough and his colleagues (Gough *et al.*, 1963) linking low folate with psychiatric conditions and Reynolds (1967) implicating it in the schizophrenia-like complications of epilepsy treated with long-term anti-convulsants, I performed (Carney, 1967; Carney, 1969; Carney, 1970) serum folate and B_{12} estimations on all patients newly-admitted to a general hospital psychiatric unit over a 2 year period in the hope of spotting deficiencies and possibly doing something to correct them. At that time the range of normal serum folate values was in doubt so we also measured serum folate in normal control volunteers – ambulance drivers, nurses, doctors, etc.

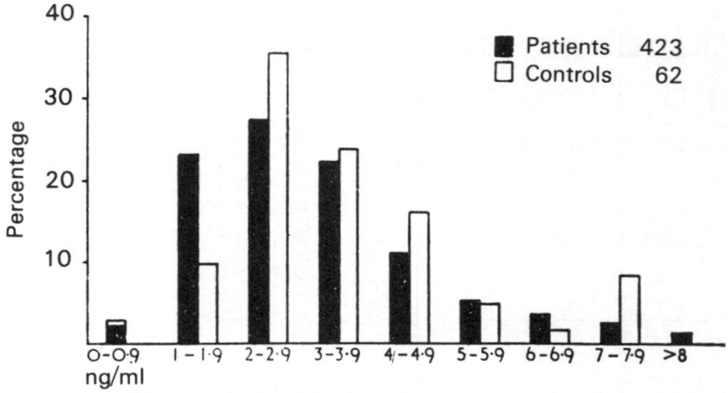

Figure 1 Serum folate levels: psychiatric patients compared with normal controls

There were 423 patients of mean age 54 years and 62 controls of mean age 39. Though this is a significant age difference, as I did not find any clear correlation between age and vitamin levels in either survey I feel it can safely be ignored. Figure 1 compares serum folate values for patients and controls. There is a clustering of values below 2ng/ml in the case of the patients but not the controls. This difference between the two groups was significant $\chi^2=6{\cdot}89$; df=1; $p<0{\cdot}01$ and we took values below 2 ng/ml as being low folate. In fact there were 105 patients or 23% with low folate values. Table 1 compares the mean serum folate values for various age groups. Thus there is no consistent trend here.

Table 1 Mean serum folate levels for various age groups

	Age in years							
	10–29	30–39	40–49	50–59	60–69	70–79	80+	*Overall mean*
Mean serum folate (ng/ml)	3.2	3.6	3.1	3.4	3.0	3.0	3.1	3.2

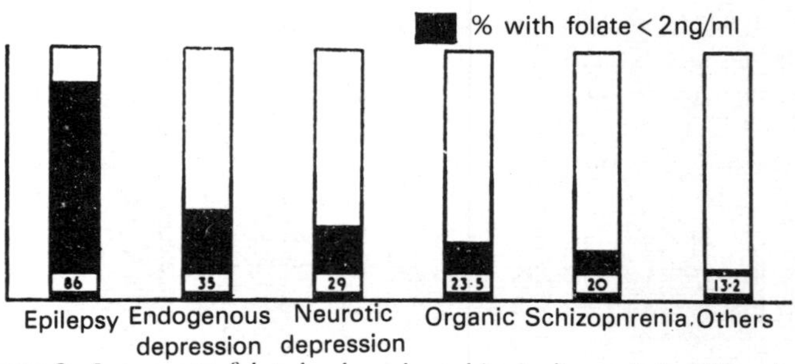

Figure 2 Low serum folate levels and psychiatric diagnosis in 317 patients

In regard to psychiatric diagnosis, Figure 2 shows the proportions of the common diagnostic groups with low folate (low B_{12} patients excluded). As many as 86% of the epileptics, over 30% of the depressed patients, 24% of those with organic psychoses and 20% of the schizophrenics, had low folate compared with 13% of the remaining patients (significantly different from normal folate patients: $X^2 = 13{\cdot}55$; df = 4; $p < 0{\cdot}01$).

Figure 3 shows the percentages of the diagnostic groups with low B_{12}. We took values of less than 150 pg/ml as being low. These were 14% of the whole group. Low values are clustered among the organic and endogenous depressive patients rather than among the others. This distribution differs significantly from that of the normal B_{12} patients ($X^2=16{\cdot}78$; df=4; $p < 0{\cdot}01$).

We looked more closely at the low folate patients with a view to identifying extrinsic folate-lowering factors which would account for the surprising frequency of low serum concentrations in this series. Table 2 shows that 75% had had drugs of various kinds in the 3 weeks before admission. This finding suggests, but by no means proves, a link between drugs and low folate. However, a history of drugs in the 3 weeks before admission was significantly more frequent in the low folate than in the low B_{12} patients ($X^2 = 13{\cdot}89$; df = 1; $p < 0{\cdot}001$). Four patients had had a gastrectomy and three were pregnant. We concluded that these were not important aetiological factors. Of the low folate group 23% were grossly undernourished including

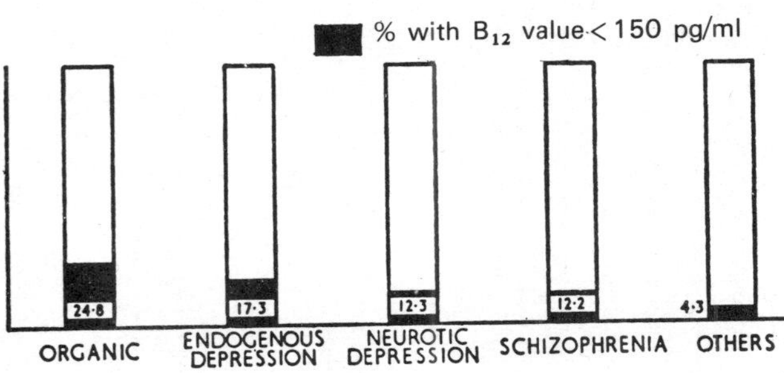

Figure 3 Low serum vitamin B_{12} and psychiatric diagnosis in 377 patients

Table 2 Drugs and low serum folate and vitamin B_{12} levels

	No. of cases	*Drugs*	*No drugs*
Serum folate <2ng/ml and normal serum B_{12}	86	68	18
Serum B_{12} <150pg/ml and normal serum folate	34	15	19
Total	120	83	37

$X^2 = 13.89$; d.f. = 1; $p < 0.001$

six patients with nutritional oedema and two food cranks, and 17% were physically ill on admission.

Thus, there was little evidence that any one of these factors alone could have accounted for all the low folate values observed. On the other hand, only 21 patients were free of all these circumstances. Of these five had low serum B_{12} so that only 16 were free of any recognised or suspected cause of folate deficiency. These could be expected to show in 'pure culture' a link (if any) between low folate and any particular form of mental illness. However this hope was not realised, the patients coming from a broad spectrum of psychiatric conditions. However, we did find that no fewer than 44% of the low folate patients had been ill virtually continuously for more than 3 years. In other words this was a far more chronic population than anticipated and this was possibly a relevant finding.

Following the completion of this earlier survey in 1967 serum folate and B_{12} estimations continued to be done by the same methods of assay on those patients newly-admitted to the general hospital psychiatric unit who were considered to be at risk, namely the elderly, the alcoholics and those suffering from severe illness, like endogenous depression, schizophrenia and organic psychosis. In fact 272 of 477 new patients admitted under my care during 1972 and 1973 had these investigations (Carney, 1970). The proportion, 21%, with low folate was remarkably similar to the 23% of the first survey. Figure 4 shows the pattern of psychiatric diagnosis among these – once more low folate seemed unusually common among the depressed or organic psychotics. Again, the distribution is significantly different from that of the normal folate patients ($X^2=7{\cdot}94$; df=1; $p<0{\cdot}01$).

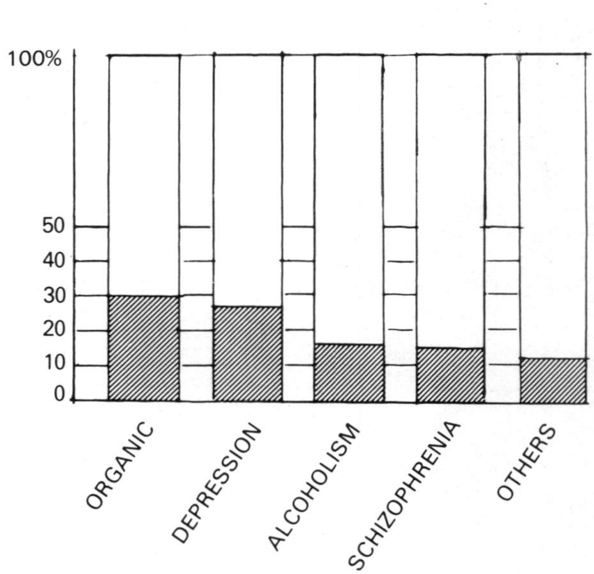

Figure 4 Diagnostic distribution of low folate

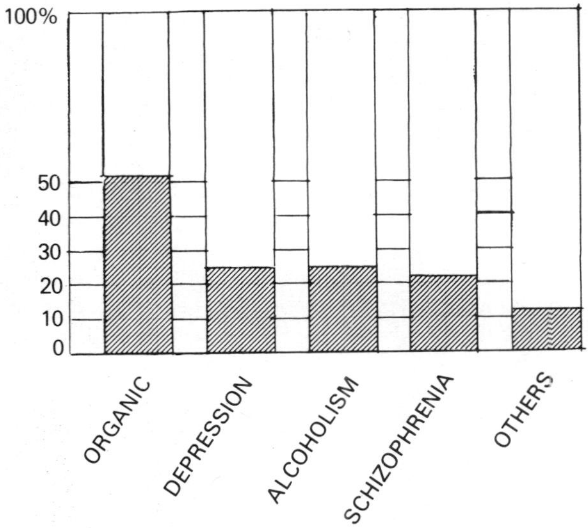

Figure 5 Diagnostic distribution of low B_{12}

Figure 5 compares the incidence of low and normal B_{12} among the various diagnoses. Again, the distributions differ, organic psychosis predominating among the low B_{12} group. The mean ages of the low folate and low B_{12} patients did not differ radically from those with normal values. Once more we confirmed the frequency of pre-admission drug treatment among them. We also noted the frequency of malnutrition and physical illness among the low folate but not among the low B_{12} patients Indeed 49% of the depressives, organic psychoses patients and alcoholics taken together were undernourished (i.e. substantial weight loss, clinical signs of avitaminosis or nutritional oedema) or physically ill compared with only 19% of the remainder ($X^2 = 23{\cdot}9$; df = 1; $p < 0{\cdot}001$). Low serum folate was also found to be significantly associated with several abnormalities in the haemogram – low red cell count, low white cell count, low haemoglobin. Low B_{12} was linked with low RBC and low WBC. Unexpectedly we did not find macrocytosis to be significantly more common among low folate or B_{12} patients than among the others. However, the presence of one or more abnormalities on the haemogram correctly predicted low folate in 76% and low B_{12} in 79%, but these were also found in 40% of the normal folate and 41% of the normal B_{12} patients. Lest it be thought that we found macrocytosis to have no predictive value no fewer than 67% of the alcoholics had elevated MCV (mean corpuscular volume) compared with a very much lower proportion of the other patients. This finding has also been reported by other investigators (Carney and Sheffield, 1977) and elevated MCV may well prove to be a useful screening test for otherwise occult alcoholics (Wu, Chanarin and Levi, 1974).

We made a retrospective survey of replacement therapy in the low folate and B_{12} patients. During the first survey 102 of the 105 low folate patients were discharged from hospital. Of these 39 were put on folic acid before discharge, and 63 were not. Apparently the decision as to whether or not to treat depended on random factors like whether the serum folate and B_{12} results were back or not. In the case of the low B_{12} patients 52 of 53 were discharged and of these 15 were given cyanocobalamin and 37 were not. Treated and untreated patients were found not to differ significantly on age and sex distribution. All were continued, however, on appropriate conventional psychiatric treatment. Thus, quite fortuitously, a virtually randomized trial of each vitamin in these low serum level patients had been set up. The case notes of these patients were examined and grades of clinical well-being at discharge awarded retrospectively as follows:

(a) Symptom free and socially recovered,
(b) Socially recovered with residual symptoms,
(c) Improved without full social recovery,
(d) Slightly or not improved.

Table 3 shows the proportion of (a) and (b) grades in folate-treated and untreated patients divided into diagnostic sub-groups. Only the schizophrenics, endogenous depressives and organic psychotics show improvement and on X^2 test this is significant ($X^2 = 3{\cdot}9$; df $= 1$; $p < 0{\cdot}05$). However, when the treated and untreated low B_{12} patients were combined there was little difference between them (Table 4). It could be said with some justice that these results are suspect because the method of assessment was retrospective and therefore liable to be subject to observer bias. I therefore looked for an independent criterion of an improvement. Time in hospital is a stable objective measure. Of course the date of discharge tends to be determined by a whole set of social factors as well as the patient's clinical state. Nevertheless, a shorter time in hospital for folate and B_{12} treated patients would suggest that these patients improved more rapidly than the untreated patients.

Table 5 shows that overall the folate-treated patients tended to have a shorter period in hospital than the untreated patients, but the difference does not reach significance. If, however, schizophrenia, endogenous

Table 3 Outcome at discharge: folate-treated and untreated patients compared

	No.	*Social recoveries (A + B) (expressed as percentage of each category)*	
		Folate	*Non-folate*
Endogenous depression/schizophrenia	36	12 (92.3)†	16 (69.6)
Organic psychoses	24	5 (56)	1 (6.7)
Epilepsy	5	1 (20)	0 (0)
Others	37	6 (50)	18 (72)
Total	102	24 (61.5)	35 (55.6)

* Three patients still in hospital excluded
† Figures in parentheses are percentages

Table 4 Outcome at discharge: cyanocobalamin-treated and untreated patients compared

	No.	Social recoveries (A + B) (expressed as percentage of each category)	
		Cyanocobalamin	Non-cyanocobalamin
Endogenous depression/schizophrenia	21	5 (83.3)*	11 (73.3)
Organic psychoses	18	1 (20)	1 (7.7)
Others	13	3 (75)	5 (55.5)
Totals	52	9 (60)	17 (45.9)

* Figures in parentheses are percentages

Table 5 Mean length of stay: folate-treated and untreated patients compared (patients with less than 10 days in hospital excluded)

Diagnosis	Folate		Non-folate	
	No.	Time in hospital (days)	No.	Time in hospital (days)
Endegenous depression	10	23.3	8	32.9
Schizophrenia	3	44.3	10	70.1
Organic psychoses	7	76.3	12	99.6

depression and organic psychoses are considered separately, then there was indeed a significant difference, the folate-treated patients being discharged more quickly (Mann-Whitney u-test; $u=203$; $Z=1{\cdot}922$; $p=0{\cdot}027$ (one-tailed)). When the B_{12} treated or untreated patients, however, are compared for time in hospital there is no appreciable difference between them, either overall or between sub-groups.

CONCLUSIONS

Both surveys show that a surprisingly high proportion of patients ill enough to need admission to hospital had low serum folate or B_{12}. This consistency occurs despite the surveys being held at different times and in different hospitals. Of course the same methods of assay were used in each. Though the incidence of low B_{12} was higher in the second survey than in the first, that of low folate was fairly constant throughout. Other investigators (Edwin *et al.*, 1965; Hunter and Matthews, 1965; Shalman, 1967; Hallstrom, 1969) have also found low levels of these vitamins to be common in psychiatric patients.

A low serum value for either substance does not automatically reflect a deficiency state. In the case of folate many drugs, e.g. anticonvulsants, antibiotics and cytotoxic agents may depress the level and barbiturates can apparently lower both serum folate and B_{12} within a matter of hours. Moreover, falsely low results can arise because of inhibition of the test organism *in vitro* by drugs present in the serum, e.g. the effect of chlorpromazine on *E. gracilis* (Herbert *et al.*, 1965).

However, two facts suggest that these low concentrations were not merely artefacts but were physiologically meaningful: (1) Both low folate and low B_{12} were linked with different patterns of psychiatric diagnosis from normal concentrations of the vitamins. (2) Both sets of low results were associated with haematological abnormality.

If subnormal folate and B_{12} did indeed reflect deficiency states, what aetiological factors can be recognised? The medical disorders usually implicated – pernicious anaemia, intestinal malabsorption, rheumatoid arthritis, tuberculosis, stomach operations and the like – were infrequent or absent. Pregnancy was rare. On the other hand, malnutrition, chronic physical illnesses and all kinds of psychotropic drugs and barbiturates were common. Many patients, especially the schizophrenics, had psychiatric illnesses of long duration.

The diagnoses most commonly associated with low folate were epilepsy, organic psychoses and endogenous depression, and with low B_{12}, organic psychoses. These associations were not substantially accounted for by age, malnutrition or physical illness. Low folate was found in 13–20% of the schizophrenics and low B_{12} in 12–20% of the schizophrenics.

The question arises of whether low folate and low B_{12} were of causal significance or were merely secondary to the impaired nutrition so frequent in the mentally ill. (1) It has to be admitted that in those few patients in whom any recognizable extrinsic causes of low folate were absent – the idiopathic group – who could be expected to show in 'pure culture' the links, if any, there was no typical syndrome or mode of presentation. (2) Furthermore the conditions with most low values, e.g. depression or organic psychoses, tended to be those characterized by poor nutrition. (3) However, the drug addicts and alcoholics, possibly the worst nourished patients, yielded no excess of low serum concentrations, whereas if one considers another vitamin, thiamine, deficiency of this is more common in these categories than in other psychiatric patients (Carney *et al.*, 1976). This paradox suggests that not all low folate values were merely secondary to malnutrition due to mental distrubance. (4) Moreover in low folate schizophrenics, endogenous depressives and organic psychotics, treatment with folate was followed by a better mental state at discharge and a shorter time in hospital. Of course this trial was not controlled and the numbers were small. Nevertheless, others (Reynolds, 1967; Botez *et al.*, 1976; Manson and Runcie, 1976) have also reported improvement in mental state with folic acid therapy. Obviously, properly controlled trials are required.

Thus the issues of whether low folate causes mental illness and, if so, of what kind, remain unresolved. However, Reynolds (1967) has implicated folic acid deficiency in the schizophrenia-like psychoses of epileptics on long-term anticonvulsants (most of our epileptics had low serum folate but no characteristic psychiatric disorders) and Strachan and Henderson (1967) attributed dementia to folic acid deficiency. However, if the role of folate in the genesis of major mental illness remains problematical, there can be no doubt about its causal significance in the mental retardation linked with inborn errors of folate metabolism. Indeed it would be surprising if a substance so intimately concerned with central nervous system metabolism did not influence psychological phenomena. Nevertheless I must admit that in most of our low-folate patients, the low folate probably reflected dietary deficiency. There is of course a third possibility: that mental illness impaired nutrition, leading to folate deficiency and hence to further mental deterioration and still further deficiency, linked in a vicious circle.

Traditional medical teaching listed organic brain damage as one of the consequences of pernicious anaemia. Shulman (1967) found memory disturbance rather than other mental symptoms to yield to B_{12} replacement therapy. Therefore our finding that organic psychoses were the characteristic accompaniment of low B_{12} is not surprising, and low B_{12} probably was a primary phenomenon in many of these patients.

What are the practical implications of these results? If even a proportion of these subnormal results indicated true deficiency states, then there is a strong case for doing serum folate and B_{12} estimations on every patient on admission to hospital. It is argued that macrocytosis alone will identify such deficiency. However it is well known that the CNS effects of B_{12} deficiency can anticipate by many months haematological signs. In the present series 24% of the low folate and 21% of low B_{12} patients would have been missed if sole reliance had been placed on the haemogram, and if something is worth detecting there are good ethical and medical grounds for using the widest possible detecting net – in the way that mass radiography is used to detect pulmonary TB. To say that all this is costly does not diminish the force of this argument. Naturally serum folate and B_{12} should always be estimated together to avoid giving folate alone to patients with occult B_{12} deficiency.

What is the picture as it relates to schizophrenia? Low serum levels of folate and B_{12} are common (about 15–20%). Most are due to malnutrition. However, some may be causal, and this is supported by: (1) the schizophrenia-like psychoses of low-folate epileptics, (2) the occasional occurence of schizophreniform symptoms in patients with inborn errors of folate metabolism or those treated for meningeal leukaemia with the folate antagonist methotrexate and (3) the improvement in mental state reported in low folate schizophrenics after folic acid therapy. However, it would be rash to claim that folic acid is a major therapy in the disease.

REFERENCES

Botez, M. I., Cadotte, M., Beaulieu, R., Pichette, L. P. and Pison, C. (1976). Neurologic disorders responsive to folic acid therapy. *Can. Med. Assoc. J.*, **115,** 217

Carney, M. W. P. (1967). Serum folate values in 423 psychiatric patients. *Br. Med. J.*, **4,** 512

Carney, M. W. P. (1969). Serum B_{12} values in 374 psychiatric patients. *Behav. Neuropsych.*, **19,** 1

Carney, M. W. P. and Sheffield, B. F. (1970). Associations of abnormal serum folate and vitamin B_{12} values and effects of replacement therapy. *J. Nerv. Ment. Dis.*, **150**, 404

Carney, M. W. P., Leigh, D., Vyas, I. and Williams, D. (1976). Blood pyruvate concentrations in newly admitted psychiatric patients. *IRCS Med. Sci.*, **4**, 377

Carney M. W. P. and Sheffield, B.F. (1977a). Serum folate and B_{12} concentrations and haematological status of 272 psychiatric in-patients. *Psychol. Med.* (in press).

Carney, M. W. P. and Sheffield, B. F. (1977b). Serum folate and B_{12} and haematological status of in-patient alcoholics. *Br. J. Add.* (in press)

Edwin, E., Holten, K., Norum, K. R., Schrumpf, A. and Skaug, O. E. (1965). Vitamin B_{12} hypovitaminosis in mental disease. *Acta Med. Scand.*, **177**, 689

Gough, K. R., Read, A. E., McCarthy, C. F. and Waters, A. H. (1963). Megaloblastic anaemia due to nutritional deficiency of folic acid. *Q. J. Med.*, **32**, 243

Hallstrom, T. (1969). Serum B_{12} and folate concentrations in mental patients. *Acta Psychiatr. Scand.*, **45**, 19

Herbert, V., Gottlieb, C. W. and Altshcule, M. D. (1965). Apparent low B_{12} levels associated with chlorpromazine. *Lancet*, **ii**, 1052

Hunter, R. and Matthews, D. M. (1965). Mental symptoms in vitamin B_{12} deficiency. *Lancet*, **ii**, 738

Manzow, M. and Runcie, J. (1976). Folate-responsive neuropathy: report of 10 cases. *Br. Med. J.*, **1**, 1176

Meynell, M. J., Coke, W. T., Cox, E. V. and Gaddie, K. (1957). Serum cyanocobalamin levels in chronic intestinal disorders. *Lancet*, **i**, 901

Reynolds, E. H. (1967a). Schizophrenia-like psychoses of epilepsy and disturbances of folate and vitamin B_{12} metabolism and mental symptoms. *Br. J. Psychiatry*, **113**, 911

Reynolds, E. H. (1967b). Effects of folic acid on the mental state and fit frequency of drug-treated epileptic patients. *Lancet*, **i**, 1086

Reynolds, E. H. (1976a). The neurology of vitamin B_{12} deficiency. *Lancet*, **ii**, 832

Reynolds, E. H. (1976b). Neurological aspects of folate and B_{12} metabolism. *Clin. Haematol.*, **5**, 661

Shulman, R. (1967a). A survey of vitamin B_{12} deficiency in an elderly psychiatric population. *Br. J. Psychiatry*, **113**, 241

Shulman, R. (1976b). Psychiatric aspects of pernicious anaemia: a prospective controlled investigation. *Br. Med. J.*, **3**, 260

Strachan, P. W. and Henderson, J. G. (1967). Dementia and folate deficiency. *Q. J. Med.*, **34**, 303

Wu, A., Chanarin, I. and Levi, A. J. (1974). Macrocytosis of chronic alcoholism. *Lancet*, **i**, 829

Waters, A. H. and Mollin, D. L. (1961). Studies in the folic acid activity of human serum. *J. Clin. Pathol.*, **14**, 335

13

Propranolol and schizophrenia: Objective evidence of efficacy

J. H. GRUZELIER and N. J. YORKSTON

The treatment of schizophrenic patients with drugs is not without controversy. There is little doubt that a way to check violent and deranged outbursts quickly and dependably has provided a sense of security for those involved in day-to-day caring for patients. The means to control socially disruptive behaviour has permitted more humane conditions for treatment. Through drugs patients have become accessible to refined non-pharmacological approaches such as dietary programmes and psychotherapies. However, the benefits of antipsychotic drugs go hand in hand with undesirable effects, notably parkinsonian tremors. To tranquillize mood or behaviour may be to lose vitality and blunt the experience of happiness and joy. More serious side effects are those like oro-facial dyskinesias which may be irreversible, continuing after the drug is withdrawn.

From another standpoint, drug therapy has advanced our understanding of the pathogenesis of schizophrenia. Research with animals has shown that most antipsychotic drugs reduce dopamine transmission (Carlsson and Linqvist, 1963; Crow *et al.*, 1976; Hornykiewicz, 1966; Iverson, 1975; Matthysee, 1973; Seeman and Lee, 1975; Seeman *et al.*, 1976; Snyder *et al.*, 1974). A blocking of dopamine in the brain's limbic regions is thought to reduce psychotic behaviour, while undesirable Parkinsonian effects stem from blocking dopamine synapses in striatal regions. Treatment may be advanced when this knowledge is further refined and when drugs are found to act more selectively on the brain mechanisms responsible for psychosis.

The present report concerns research with one of a class of drugs new to the treatment of schizophrenia. Preliminary observations and now objective, controlled evidence indicate that while sharing the benefits of conventional treatment fewer disadvantages have been encountered and additional benefits may accrue.

Like many scientific discoveries the application to psychosis of the drug in question was accidental. In a case of porphyria accompanied by rapid pulse rate and florid psychotic symptoms the pulse returned to normal and psychosis disappeared after propranolol, a drug known to lower pulse rate, was given in what was at the time a high dose (Atsmon and Blum, 1970). Subsequently propranolol treatment was examined in seven acute and five chronic cases of schizophrenia. Little success was found in chronic patients but five of the acute cases were considered 'much improved'. Improvement was associated with high urinary catecholamine levels, particularly MHPG

(Atsmon *et al.*, 1971). Later 13 excited and emotionally labile cases with acute psychotic episodes were found to improve or lose all symptoms on propranolol, some within 24 hours (Atsmon *et al.*, 1972). In another study ten cases of post-partum psychosis were administered either propranolol or chlorpromazine. Those on propranolol were discharged on average in 61 days compared with 104 days (perhaps an unusually long time) on chlorpromazine. With propranolol there was noticeable improvement after 3 days compared with 55 days on chlorpromazine (Steiner *et al.*, 1973).

Two investigations followed in which the drug was administered to schizophrenic patients with little success. In one, eight patients who had been resistant to treatment for a year were examined on conventional medication which was then withdrawn and replaced first with placebo for 4 weeks and then propranolol for between 6 and 10 weeks in daily doses up to 720 mg. While most patients were reported as calmer on propranolol the drug had no reliable antipsychotic effects (Gardos *et al.*, 1973). In the second investigation three compounds were tried: (1) propranolol in its racemic form ((±)-propranolol) as used by other investigators; (2) the dextro isomer (+)-propranolol) which has less of the hypotensive effects of the racemic form; (3) oxprenolol, a drug of the same class of β-adrenergic blocking agents. These were administered to cases of schizophrenia, mania and organic psychosis. The two cases of organic psychosis and two/four cases of mania who completed the course of treatment were noticeably improved on ±-propranolol. In six cases of schizo-affective psychosis there was slight improvement and in three cases of schizophrenia no improvement (Rackensperger *et al.*, 1974; Van Zerssen, 1976).

The equivocal nature of the results apart, the early applications of the drug encountered drawbacks in the form of toxic side effects., Fortunately, subsequent studies in Britain with 55 cases of florid schizophrenia showed that toxic effects could be avoided by increasing dose in a more gradual fashion. Excessive and possibly toxic doses were also avoided by withholding increments in dose at signs of impending toxicity or clinical improvement (Yorkston *et al.*, 1976b). With this regimen lower doses of the drug were effective about 1·0 g compared with 2–4 g used by others. In 28 of the 55 cases florid symptoms remitted at least temporarily and others showed some improvement. Improvement and loss of all symptoms were found with chronic as well as acute cases, some of whom lost all schizophrenic symptoms after more than 20 years illness. In some chronic cases remission of symptoms took as long as a year, indicating that it was worth persisting with treatment even when in the early stages there was minimal improvement (Yorkston *et al.*, 1974; Yorkston *et al.*, 1976a).

With a safe method for administering propranolol a controlled study with cases of chronic schizophrenia was conducted in which either propranolol or a matching placebo of identical appearance and taste were added to conventional neuroleptic medication. Results with the first 14 cases have now been analysed and published (Yorkston *et al.*, 1977). This was the first controlled study of the efficacy of propranolol in treating schizophrenia. Details of the patient sample are shown in Table 1.

Table 1 Patient characteristics in the controlled comparison of propranolol and placebo added to existing antipsychotic medication

Variables	*Propranolol* (n=7)	*Placebo* (n=7)
Sex (male:female)	3:4	2:5
Age (mean)	39 years 9 months	40 years 9 months
Age of onset (mean)	32 years 5 months	26 years 7 months
Years in hospital (mean)	4 years 9 months	10 years 7 months
Number of whole years' remission (mean)	0·6	1·0
Number of episodes (mean)	1·3	1·9
Length of current episode (mean)	5 years 11 months	11 years 6 months
Daily phenothiazine dose expressed as the chlorpromazine equivalent	972 mg	1371 mg
Modal dose experimental drug at week 12	436 mg	448 mg

Clinical improvement was evaluated with a modified version of the Brief Psychiatric Rating Scale (Overall and Gorham, 1962) and by nurses' ratings of ward behaviour. Grouping the psychiatric scales (BPRS) according to schizophrenic thought disorder, remaining schizophrenic symptoms and non-schizophrenic symptoms both groups were shown to improve. However, by the twelfth week patients with propranolol improved more on the schizophrenic subscales than patients who had placebo added to existing medication (F=3·06, df=3·36, p<0·04) (Figures 1 and 2). Differential improvement was also found on a psychiatrist's global rating of improvement (F=11·20, df=1,12, p<0·005) and this was already marginally significant as early as the fourth week (F=3·57, df=1,12, p<0·1), suggesting that there were clinical signs not covered by the BPRS that differentiated the groups (Figure 3). This inference was supported by the ward ratings of nurses where from among 24 items the scale relating to 'how well the patient looks' best discriminated the groups, (F=9·63, df=1,12, p<0·01). Of the individual items rated by the psychiatrists at week 12 the patients on propranolol manifested less 'unusual thought content' (F=7·18, df=1,12, p<0·05) and tended to be less 'grandiose' (F=3·20, df=1,12, p<0·1) and 'conceptually disorganized' (F=3·96, df=1,12, p<0·1) than patients on placebo. In addition to higher ratings of 'well being' the nurses found less 'violence' and 'incoherent speech' in patients on propranolol compared with placebo.

Despite the hypotensive effects of propranolol differences between the groups in pulse and blood pressure were not readily apparent. This was borne out by the virtually identical rate at which the dose of placebo and

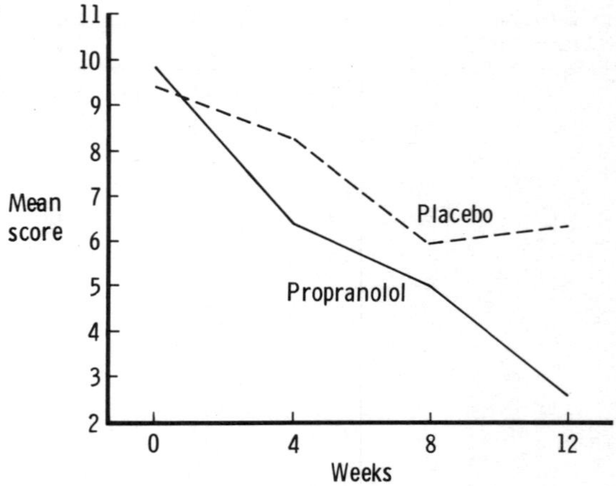

Figure 1 Schizophrenia thought disorder subscale ratings with the BPRS

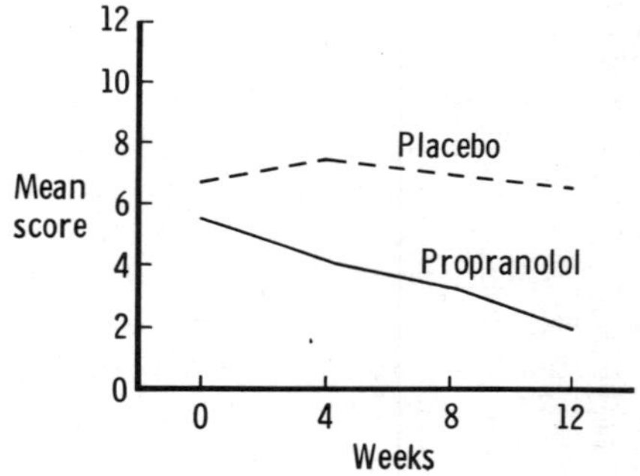

Figure 2 Schizophrenia non-thought disorder subscale ratings with the BPRS

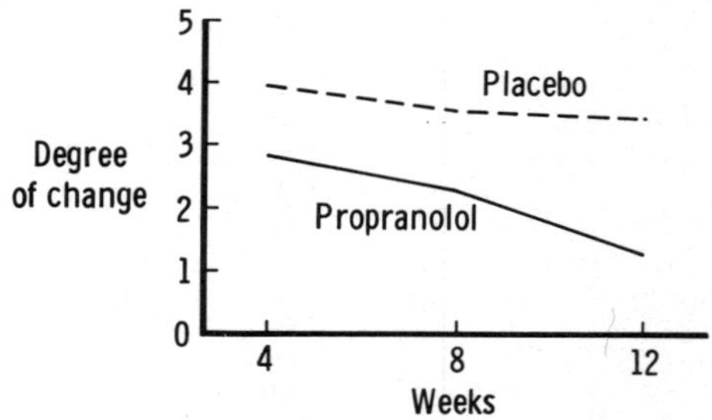

Figure 3 Psychiatrist's global ratings of change

propranolol was increased (t values $<0 \cdot 25$ for t-tests at weeks 4, 8 and 12); the cardiovascular measures being the most influencial factors in permitting an increase in dose. There was further support from the overlap in the means and standard deviations of pulse in individual patients (Figure 4) and the non-significant differences in blood pressure (Table 2). The hypotensive effects of phenothiazines with respect to blood pressure are likely to have provided camouflage and may have restricted the doses of propranolol which on average reached only 500 mg/day by the 12th week, a lower modal dose than was necessary to bring about symptom remission in earlier studies.

Soon after the controlled trial began laboratory measures were recorded of an aspect of patients' autonomic nervous system function previously shown to be atypical in schizophrenia and some other psychiatric disorders. Measures were taken of the arousal reaction to an irrelevant sound presented through headphones at irregular intervals between 20 and 40 secs. The technical name for the arousal reaction to incidental stimuli is the orienting reflex, or 'what is it?' reflex as it was termed by the Russian physiologist Pavlov (1941). A reaction to novelty is necessary for the survival of the organism and reflects a fundamental aspect of selective attention (Sokolov, 1963). The physiological index recorded here was the electrodermal response, a measure of the transient increase in the electrical conductivity of the skin that accompanies sweating (Prokasy and Raskin, 1973). Phasic, discrete electrodermal responses are sensitive to emotional and cognitive connotations of the stimulus. These contrast with the generalized increases in sweating that accompany physical exertion or states of anxiety.

The phasic electrodermal orienting response and the rate at which it disappears with stimulus repetition, a process termed habituation, have relevance to localizing central nervous system disturbance in schizophrenia.

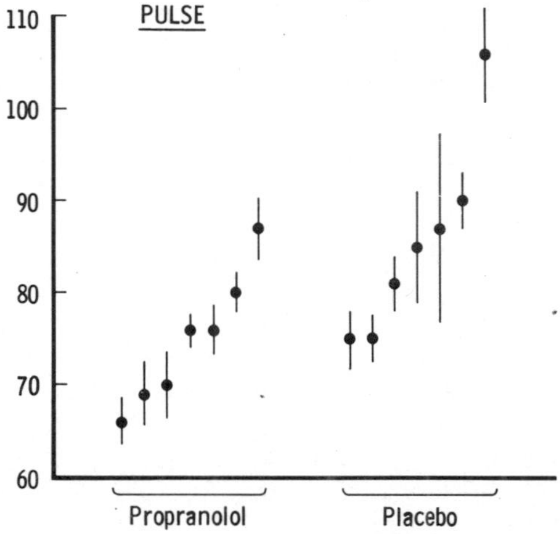

Figure 4 Means and standard deviations of individual patients' pulse rates

Table 2 t-Test comparisons of blood-pressure at weeks 0, 4, 8 and 12

Week	*Systolic*		*Diastolic*	
	t	*p*	*t*	*p*
0	0·97	ns	0·23	ns
4	0·70	ns	1·55	ns
8	0·98	ns	0·64	ns
12	0·61	ns	1·07	ns

It has been shown that primates with lesions of structures such as the amygdala and hippocampus in limbic regions of the brain have disordered electrodermal orienting reflexes to irrelevant sounds (Bagshaw *et al.*, 1965; Bagshaw and Benzies, 1968; Pribram and McGuiness, 1975). In the case of lesions of the amygdala two opposite abnormalities are found – animals are either over-responsive, so that their responses are slow to habituate, or they are under-responsive. Animals with lesions of the hippocampus show an over-responsive pattern. In the light of the neurophysiological data, and the accumulating evidence that schizophrenia involves a disorder of limbic and temporal lobe structures, the electrodermal orienting reflexes of schizophrenic patients were examined in a series of investigations (Gruzelier, 1973; Gruzelier and Venables, 1972, 1974; Gruzelier and Hammond, 1976). Over-responsive and under-responsive orienting patterns were found in about equal numbers in large groups of schizophrenic patients on phenothiazine medication (Gruzelier and Venables, 1972, 1974). These results have been replicated by others (Patterson, 1976; Rubens and Lapidus, 1978), and one report of a discrepant finding (Zahn, 1976) appears to have arisen for methodological reasons (O'Gorman, 1978). The same over- and under-responsive patterns were found in patients on placebo when withdrawn from chlorpromazine and therefore cannot be attributed to phenothiazines (Gruzelier and Hammond, 1976, 1977).

In view of the evidence suggesting that the anti-psychotic effect of neuroleptics is achieved by blocking dopamine transmission in the limbic system, it was of interest to explore whether propranolol might affect measures of orienting and habituation in schizophrenic patients. If this was the case it would imply that propranolol may act more directly on limbic structures than phenothiazines which do not reinstate responses in non-responders, nor increase rates of habituation in over-responsive patients.

In the first experiment three different groups of patients were compared, one was on no drug either before treatment or after drug withdrawal, another was on phenothiazines in standard clinical doses and a third was on propranolol either as the sole drug or combined with phenothiazines. In addition a group of normal volunteers was tested. There were 36 subjects in each group; of those on propranolol 17 received it as sole drug and 19 had it combined with phenothiazines. In order to be included in the study all patients had to have responded clinically to their medication whether it was propranolol or phenothiazines. This was confirmed by

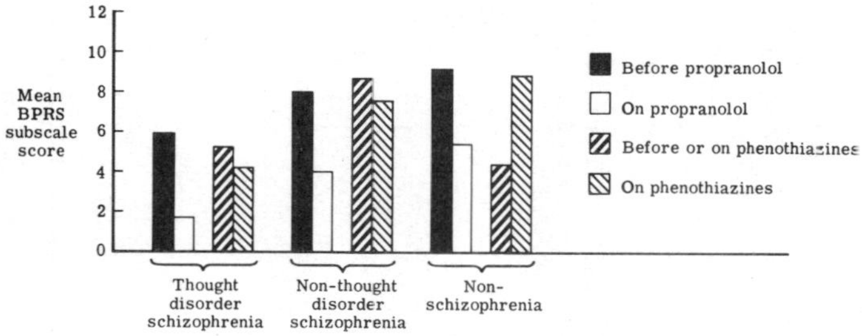

Figure 5 BPRS subscale ratings when ill and later after response to treatment of patients in psychophysiological studies

comparing ratings on the schizophrenia subscales of the BPRS taken prior to treatment and at the time of testing, see Figure 5.

All patients were diagnosed unambiguously schizophrenic by the hospital psychiatrists. The patients' sex and the means and ranges of their age, age at first onset of schizophrenia, number of hospital admissions and total length of time in hospital are shown in Table 3, and drug doses in Table 4. In addition a control group of 18 male and 13 female healthy volunteers was examined. Their mean age was 32 years, range 29 to 47 years and their scores on the Eysenck Personality Inventory Scale of Neuroticism ($\bar{x}$ 6·67, σ 4·27) classified them as a stable group. Additional details of the patients, methods and procedures are reported elsewhere (Gruzelier, 1978).

The orienting responses of most patients on propranolol were distinguished from those of patients on no drug or phenothiazines. Most strikingly none of the patients on propranolol showed deficits of habituation.

Table 3 Characteristics of patients whose orienting responses were examined when on propranolol, no drug or phenothiazines

Variables		*Groups*		
		Propranolol	*No drug*	*Phenothiazines*
Sex	Male	22	26	31
	Female	14	10	5
Age in years	$\bar{x}$	35	38	39
	range	18–59	18–57	22–52
Age in years at first onset	$\bar{x}$	25	27	25
	range	16–56	15–50	16–45
Number of hospital admissions	$\bar{x}$	5	3	5
	range	1–13	1–13	1–24
Length of total time in hospital	$\bar{x}$	7 yrs 23 wks	8 yrs 20 wks	11 yrs 5 wks
	range	4 wks–30 yrs	1 wk–30 yrs	3 wks–26 yrs

Table 4 Propranolol and phenothiazine doses in mg/day

Group	*Mean*	*Range*
Propranolol alone	605	160–1920
Propranolol with	420	160–1500
phenothiazines	355	50–1071
Phenothiazines	779	74–2976

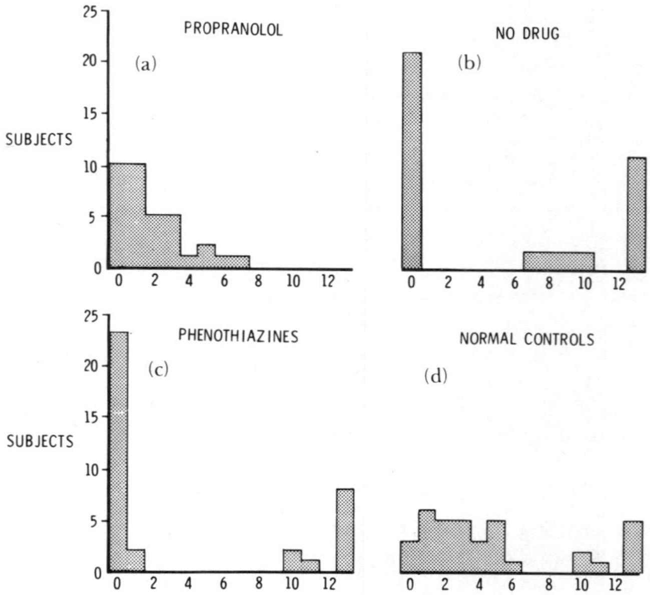

Figure 6 Trials to habituation of schizophrenic patients on propranolol (a), no drug (b) or phenothiazines (c) and of the normal volunteers (d)

All habituated by trial seven, see Figure 6a. Only ten of the patients were non-responders, half the number found in patients not on drugs (Figure 6b) and less than half the number of non-responders on phenothiazines (Figure 6c). The number of trials to habituation in patients on propranolol was more similar to that of the normal controls (see Figure 6d). The conventional three successive no responses was used as the criterion of habituation. In one respect reactions were more appropriate in the patients on propranolol insofar as none of the patients were slow in habituating compared with eight (22·2%) of the controls. However, at the other extreme of the distribution there were still more non-responders (10) in the propranolol treated patients than in the control group (2).

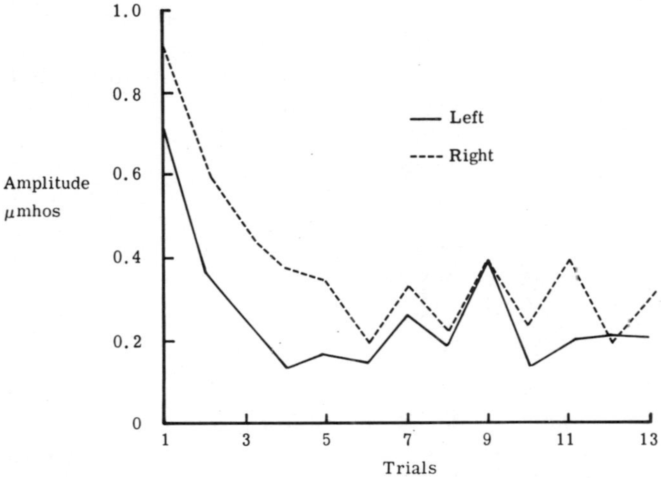

Figure 7 Bilateral orienting response amplitudes across trials for the patients on no drugs

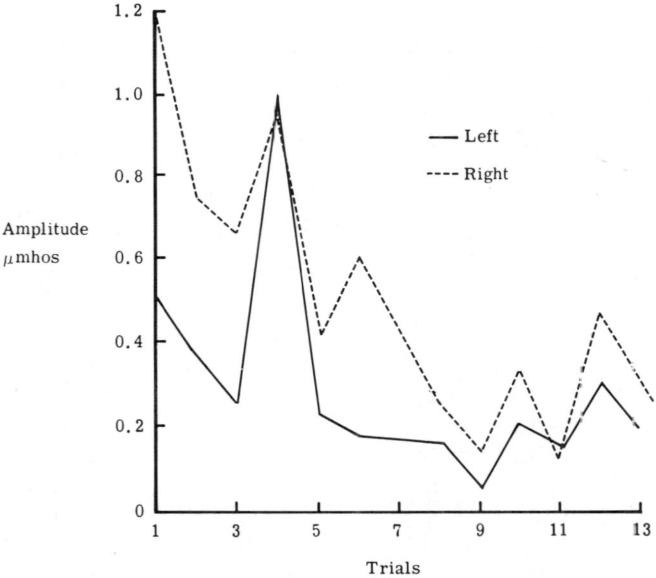

Figure 8 Bilateral response amplitudes of patients on phenothiazines

Other features of the orienting reaction examined here were the amplitude of the response and the symmetry in the response amplitudes of the two hands. In earlier investigations it was found that schizophrenic patients have larger and more frequent reactions to irrelevant sounds on the right hand than the left, whereas responses of normal controls tend to be similar on both hands (Gruzelier, 1973; Gruzelier and Venables 1974; Gruzelier and Hammond, 1977). Interestingly, depressed patients showed the opposite asymmetries, namely higher left than right hand amplitudes (Gruzelier and Venables, 1974), cf. Flor-Henry (1974). The asymmetries in schizophrenic patients were similar to those found with neurological cases with lateralized tumours and animals with unilateral lesions in whom responses ipsilateral to the lesion are reduced and contralateral responses are augmented (Luria and Homskaya 1963; Sourek, 1966). This supports other evidence that schizophrenia may primarily represent a disorder of the hemisphere dominant for speech (Boklage, 1977; Flor-Henry, 1969, 1974, 1976; Gruzelier, 1973, 1974a, b; Gruzelier and Venables, 1974; Gruzelier and Hammond, 1976, 1978; Gur, 1977; Hammond and Gruzelier, 1978; Venables, 1977).

In support of earlier evidence the amplitudes of responses across trials were higher on the right than the left hand for the patients on no treatment or on phenothiazines (Figures 7 and 8). Propranolol when prescribed alone did not correct the response asymmetries, right hand responses remained higher (Figure 9). However, when propranolol was combined with phenothiazines (Figure 10) there were no bilateral differences in responses (F=0·95, df=1,11 ns), as was the case with the normal volunteers (F=0·57, df=1,34, ns), see Figure 11. The magnitude of the responses of patients receiving the combined medication were more like the response amplitudes of the control group (F=0·85, df=1,45, ns) than those of patients receiving phenothiazines (F=11·59, df=1,45, p<0·001). Patients on propranolol alone appeared midway between these groups.

In summary, patients who were over-responsive to incidental sounds before receiving propranolol habituated more reliably when on propranolol than the normal controls. In addition there were 50% fewer patients in the propranolol group who were unresponsive to the sounds compared with patients on no drug or phenothiazines. Some aspects of orienting activity, however, remained abnormal in those taking propranolol. The incidence of non-responders remained higher than in the control group. When propranolol was the sole drug, the magnitude of the reaction to the first few sounds remained exaggerated and bilateral differences in responsivity were unaffected. Nevertheless none of the facets of orienting activity corrected by propranolol were affected by phenothiazines. It was of interest therefore to find that when phenothiazines and propranolol were combined, the remaining aspects not corrected by propranolol returned to normal, patients no longer over-reacted to sounds and responses became bilaterally symmetrical.

A drug which reinstates both the responses of some under-responsive patients, and the habituation of responses in many non-habituators is unique in its action on orienting activity. Typically drugs suppress or increase responding. Propranolol's powerful effect on response habituation cannot be attributed to a blocking of the peripheral sweat mechanism. With the exception of the skin conductance levels of the patients on combined medication, the levels were higher in patients than in normal controls. In fact propranolol may have a

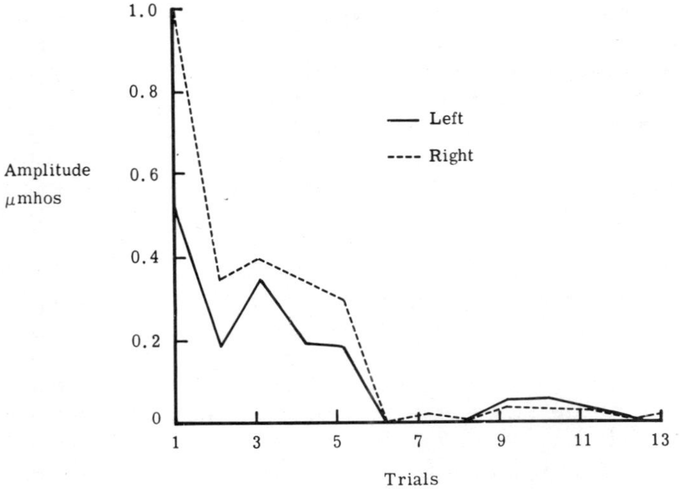

Figure 9 Bilateral response amplitudes of patients on propranolol as sole drug

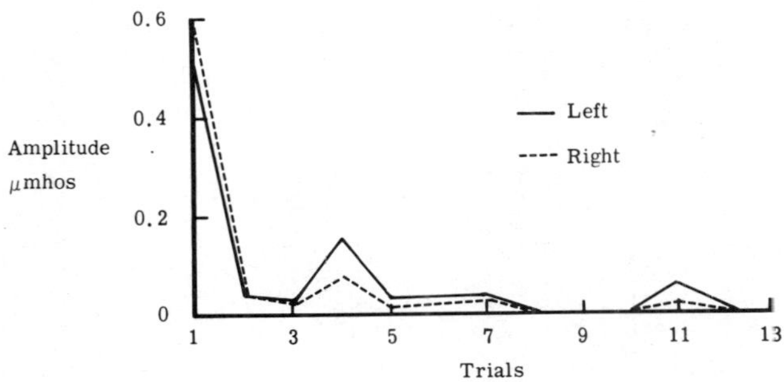

Figure 10 Bilateral response amplitudes of patients on propranolol and phenothiazines

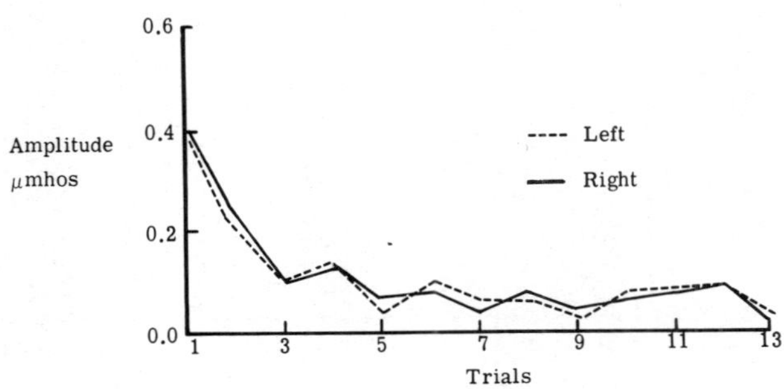

Figure 11 Bilateral response amplitudes of normal volunteers

tendency to increase levels of sweating (see Figure 12). Levels were highest in patients on propranolol alone. Here too the combined medication tended to return measures closer to the normal range. Skin conductance levels were lowest in those on combined drugs and this effect approached significance when contrasted with patients on propranolol alone (F=3·41, df=1,34, p<0·07). Similarly, spontaneous fluctuations in skin conductance, alternatively termed non-specific responses, were not reduced by propranolol and did not differentiate patients on propranolol from the other groups (see Figure 13). Thus propranolol's action in modulating the orienting reflex implies a specific central action.

A second replication experiment was designed with 14 patients who were examined both before and after treatment with propranolol and were compared with 14 patients tested either before and after phenothiazines (4) or twice on phenothiazines (10). There was a minimum retest interval of 4 weeks. As in the first experiment it was necessary for all patients to have shown a positive clinical response to treatment whether with phenothiazines or propranolol. Details relating to age, sex, age of first onset, number of hospital admissions, length of current time in hospital and drug doses are shown in Tables 5 and 6. The conditions of testing were the same as in Experiment 1.

All features above of the differential effects of drugs on trials to habituation and the incidence of responding were replicated (see Figure 14). Both groups when first tested as well as the phenothiazine group on the second test

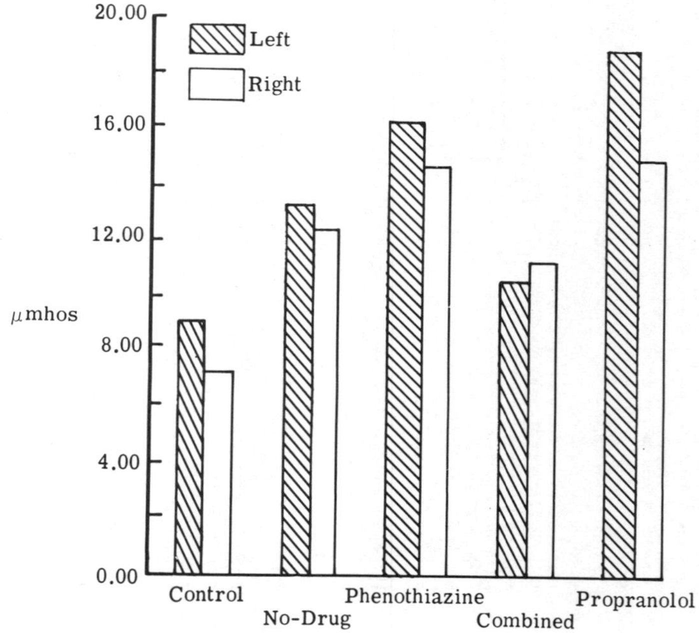

Figure 12 Bilateral skin conductance levels

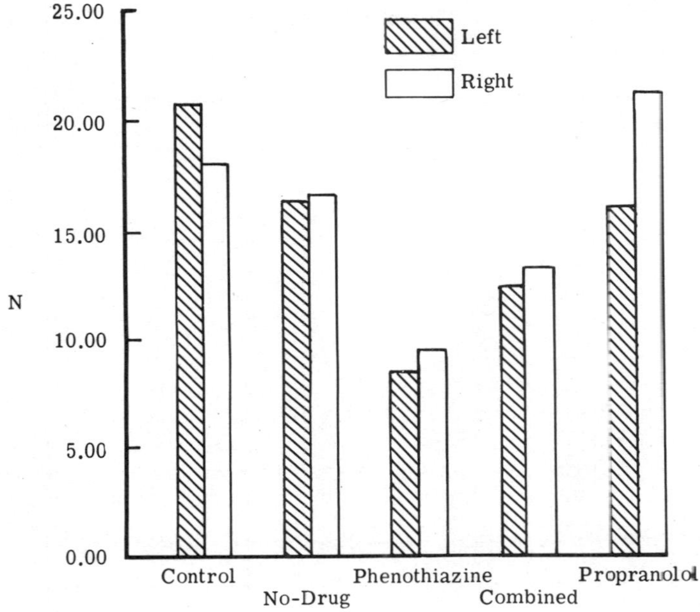

Figure 13 Bilateral spontaneous fluctuations in skin conductance

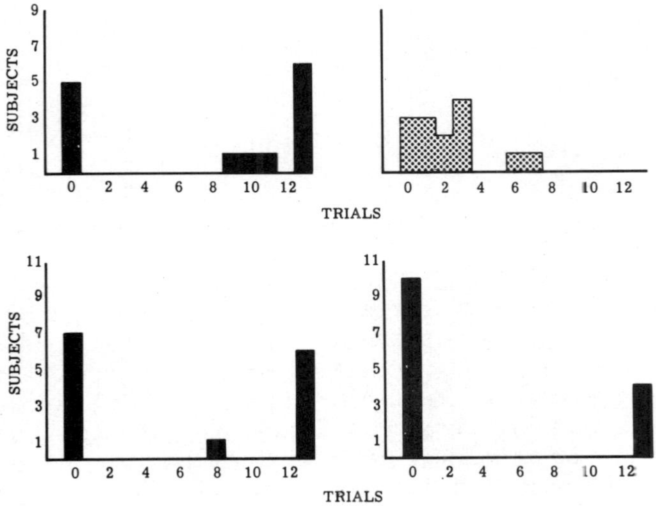

Figure 14 Trials to habituation for patients in replication experiment. Group I (top) before and after the addition of propanolol to no drug or phenothiazines. Group II (bottom) phenothiazines on both occasions

Table 5 Patient characteristics in the replication orienting response study

		Groups	
		Propranolol	*Phenothiazines*
Sex (male : female)		8 : 6	11 : 3
Age in years	$\bar{x}$	37	42
	range	18–52	22–56
Age in years at first onset	$\bar{x}$	22	25
	range	16–33	18–38
No. of hospital admissions	$\bar{x}$	5	3
	range	1–13	1–11
Length current time in hospital	$\bar{x}$	7 years	8 years
	range	1 wk–12 yrs	1 wk–15 yrs

Table 6 Propranolol and phenothiazine doses in mg/day for the replication study

Group	*Session*			
	I		*II*	
Propranolol alone ($n=7$)	—	—	$\bar{x}$	568
			range	160–1080
Propranolol with phenothiazines ($n=7$)	—	—	$\bar{x}$	550
			range	120–1360
	$\bar{x}$	524	$\bar{x}$	524
	range	100–986	range	100–986
Phenothiazines ($n=5$)	—	—	$\bar{x}$	499
			range	100–814
Phenothiazines ($n=9$)	$\bar{x}$	514	$\bar{x}$	556
	range	99–1172	range	177–1302

occasion showed a bimodal distribution, either no responses or delayed habituation of responses. In contrast, on propranolol there were no persistent responders who were slow in habituating. The number of non-responders was reduced to 60% of the number found before treatment or in the phenothiazine group. The effects of propranolol were further clarified by comparing the response patterns of patients on propranolol alone with those on propanolol combined with phenothiazines. Response distributions are shown in Figure 15. Whereas propranolol by itself normalised both orienting ($p<0{\cdot}005$) and habituation ($p<0{\cdot}0006$) the results with those on combined medication did not reach significance. This suggests that phenothiazines may militate against the reinstatement of responses in non-responders by propranolol.

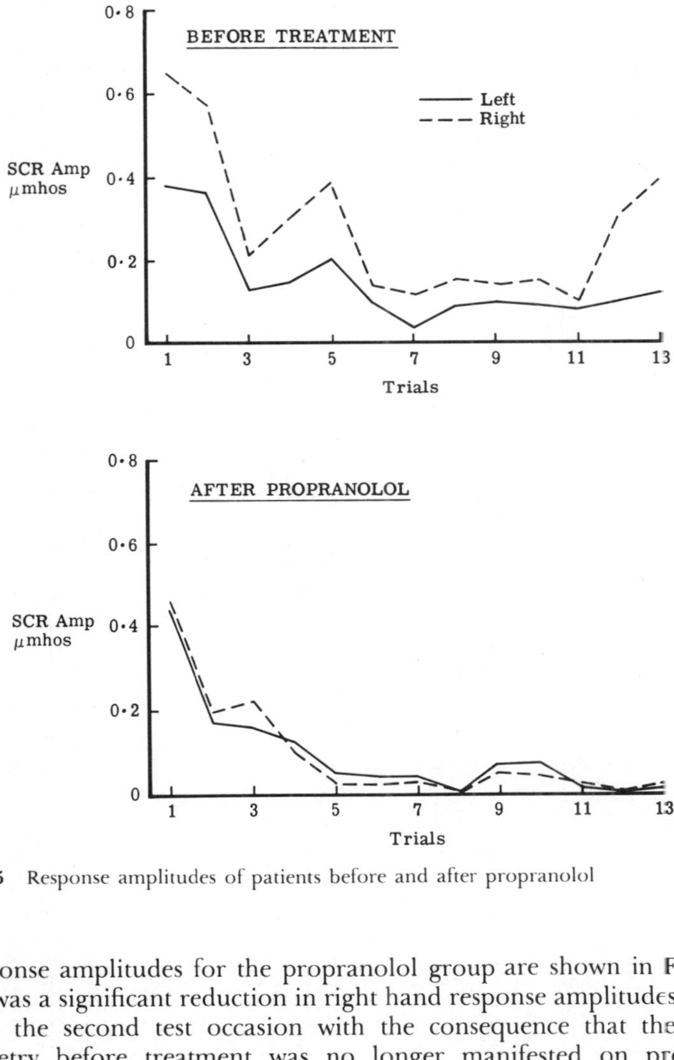

Figure 15 Response amplitudes of patients before and after propranolol

Response amplitudes for the propranolol group are shown in Figure 15. There was a significant reduction in right hand response amplitudes from the first to the second test occasion with the consequence that the bilateral asymmetry before treatment was no longer manifested on propranolol ($F=7{\cdot}88$, df$=1{,}6$. $p<0{\cdot}03$). There were too few patients (3) in the phenothiazine group who showed responses on both test occasions to carry out a reliable statistical analysis. As in the first experiment, propranolol did not alter levels of skin conductance ($F=0{\cdot}90$, df$=1{,}13$, ns) nor spontaneous fluctuations in skin conductance ($F=0{\cdot}00$, df$=1{,}13$, ns).

The differential effects of propranolol and phenothiazines on the orienting response are consistent with the impression that propranolol has novel therapeutic effects in treating schizophrenic patients. These are reflected in the quality of recovery on propranolol and the fact that patients have improved and remitted on the drug, sometimes after failing to respond to conventional

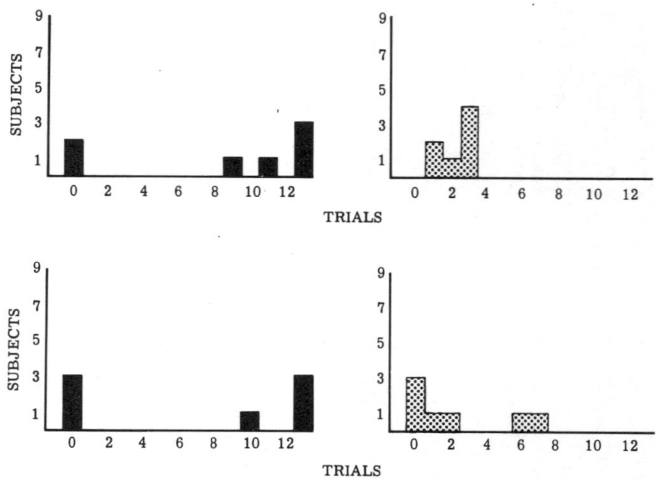

Figure 16 Trials to habituation of patients on propranolol as sole drug (above) or combined with phenothiazines (below)

treatment for more than 20 years. To what extent the changes in the orienting responses on propranolol underlie clinical recovery is the subject of current longitudinal studies where propranolol is prescribed under double-blind conditions.

The drug's powerful effect on response habituation may be thought to be due to its anxiolytic properties in view of evidence that habituation of electrodermal orienting responses is delayed in anxiety states (Lader and Wing, 1966). An anxiolytic action would provide a rationale for the drug's growing applications in psychiatry in view of the fact that anxiety appears to be a syndrome that many disorders share (Jefferson, 1974).

However, correction of response habituation without reducing levels of sweating suggests involvement of a central, psychological component of anxiety rather than the somatic component, a view currently in vogue (Tyrer, 1976). On the other hand the possibility that anxiety may play a central role in schizophrenia should not be overlooked (Mednick, 1958; Prick, 1969; Leff, 1976).

Anxiety may be inextricably linked with the psychotic process, especially in florid cases. In this regard two investigations have shown that the number of trials to habituation of the electrodermal orienting response correlates with the severity of positive psychotic symptoms (Meares and Horvath, 1973, Frith *et al.*, 1976). Furthermore groups of schizophrenic non-habituators have been distinguished from schizophrenic non-responders by nurses' ratings. The scales that distinguished them were anxiety, mania, psychotic belligerence, attention demanding and assaultive behaviour. All these were higher in the over-responsive group (Gruzelier, 1976). Questions of the role in schizophrenia aside, enhanced electrodermal response with habituation with propranolol is an effect not shared by phenothiazines. This suggests a novel and direct central action of propranolol on processes of habituation important in anxiety.

Schizophrenic patients without orienting responses typically represent a less behaviourally active group with few symptoms of florid psychosis. The finding that more than half showed a reinstatement of orienting responses in propranolol is worthy of further research as reviews of the efficacy of conventional antipsychotic drugs indicate that no drug as yet benefits this large group of patients (May, 1968; Crow, this volume). The precise relation of the reinstatement of orienting responses to clinical improvement is currently being examined. If verified this has important implications for the treatment of schizophrenic patients as does preliminary evidence that propranolol reduces and sometimes controls tardive dyskinesias (Yorkston *et al.*, in preparation).

At a neurophysiological level limbic systems centred on the amygdala and hippocampus are implicated in the regulation of the electrodermal orienting response and its habituation with stimulus repetition. The postulated relevance of these structures to schizophrenia (Gruzelier and Venables, 1972; Heath, 1964; MacLean, 1970; Malamud, 1967; Smythies, 1969; Torrey and Peterson, 1974; Venables, 1973) has found recent support in studies of neurotransmitter concentrations in post-mortem brains of schizophrenic patients (Bird *et al.*, 1977; Bird, 1977, and this volume). Current neuropharmacological theory proposes that the antipsychotic properties of drugs result through common action on dopamine synapses in the limbic system. Here propranolol and phenothiazines which both reduced psychotic symptoms in the patients tested had differential effects on the orienting response, suggesting a more direct action by propranolol on limbic mechanisms that modulate the response. Other evidence supports this view. Only in unusually high doses were phenothiazines found to influence the electrical activity of the amygdala and hippocampus in animals (Grossman, 1967). On the other hand autoradiographic studies have shown that in mouse and rabbit, propranolol remained localized in the hippocampus long after it disappeared from the cerebral cortex, thalamus and brain stem nuclei (Masuoka and Hanssen, 1967). Parallels have been drawn between the effects of propranolol and behaviour and the behavioural functions of the amygdalae (Richardson, 1974).

The results also provided support for evidence of hemisphere asymmetries of function in schizophrenia and the correction of aspects of those asymmetries with antipsychotic drugs. Evidence of an association between left-sided foci and schizophrenic psychoses first arose from a survey of patients who had temporal lobe epilepsy with schizophrenic-like psychoses (Flor-Henry, 1969). Evidence of a similar statistical nature has consistently implicated a left hemisphere limbic disturbance in schizophrenia from bilateral recordings of electrodermal orienting responses (Gruzelier, 1973; Gruzelier and Venables, 1974; Gruzelier and Hammond, 1977; Gruzelier, 1978). Neuropsychological testing (Flor-Henry, 1976; Gruzelier and Hammond, 1976) and auditory tests (Gruzelier and Hammond, 1976, 1978; Hammond and Gruzelier, 1978) provide further support. A higher incidence of left-handedness in schizophrenic patients also suggests that disorders of functional organisation of the two hemispheres may exist in schizophrenia (Lishman and McMeekan, 1976; Gur, 1977). Discordance for handedness was found related to the incidence and severity of psychosis in monozygotic twins with schizophrenia (Boklage, 1976). That the therapeutic action of drugs may stem in part from a correction of brain asymmetries is the further implication from a small body of evidence (Serafetinides, 1972, 1973; Gruzelier, 1978a,b; Hammond and Gruzelier, 1978) as well as the combined action of propranolol and phenothiazines reported here. It is hoped that future studies of the neuropsychophysiology of schizophrenic patients will further clarify the nature of the disorder and so provide guide lines to better forms of treatment.

ACKNOWLEDGEMENTS

We wish to thank the many colleagues and patients who participated in the research and the Sir Jules Thorn Medical Research Endowment Trust and ICI Pharmaceutical Division for financial support. The manuscript was written while the first author was in receipt of a grant from the Scottish Rite Schizophrenia Research Programme, Massachusetts.

REFERENCES

Atsmon, A. and Blum, I. (1970). Treatment of acute porphyria variegata with propranolol. *Lancet,* **i,** 196

Atsmon, A., Blum, J., Wijsenbeck, H., Maoz, B., Steiner, M. and Ziegelman, G. (1971). The short term effects of adrenergic blocking agents in a small group of psychotic patients. *Psychiatr. Neurol. Neurochir.,* **74,** 251

Atsmon, A., Blum, I., Steiner, M., Latz, A. and Weisenbeck, H. (1972). Further studies with propranolol in psychotic patients. *Psychopharmacology,* **27,** 249

Bagshaw, M. H., Kimble, D. P. and Pribram, K. H. (1965). The GSR of monkeys during orienting and habituation and after ablation of the amygdala, hippocampus and inferotemporal cortex. *Neuropsychologia,* **3,** 111

Bagshaw, M. H. and Benzies, S. (1968). Multiple measures of the orienting reaction and their dissociation after amygdalectomy in monkeys. *Exp. Neurol.,* **20,** 175

Boklage, C. E. (1977). Schizophrenia, brain asymmetry development and twinning: Cellular relationships with etiological and possibly prognostic implication. *Biol. Psychiatry,* **12,** 19

Bird, E. D., Spokes, E. G., Barnes, J., MacKay, A. V. P., Iversen, L. L. and Shepherd, M. (1977). Increased brain dopamine and reduced glutomic acid decarboxylase and choline acetyl transferase activity in schizophrenia and related psychoses. *Lancet,* **i,** 1157

Carlsson, A. and Lindqvist, T. M. (1965). Effect of chlorpromazine and haloperidol on formation of 3-methoxytyramine and normetanephrine in mouse brain. *Acta Pharmacol.,* **20,** 140

Crow, T. J., Deakin, J. F. W., Johnstone, E. C. and Longden, A. (1976). Dopamine and schizophrenia. *Lancet,* **ii,** 563

Douglas, R. J. (1967). The hippocampus and behaviour. *Psychol. Bull.,* **67,** 416

Flor-Henry, P. (1969). Psychosis and temporal lobe epilepsy: a controlled investigation. *Epilepsia,* **10,** 363

Flor-Henry, P. (1974). Psychosis, neurosis and epilepsy: development and gender-related effects and their aetiological contributions. *Br. J. Psychiatry,* **124,** 144

Flor-Henry, P. (1976). Lateralised temporal-limbic dysfunction and psychopathology. *N. Y. Acad. Sci.,* **280,** 777

Frith, C. D., Baker, H. F., Deakin, J. F. W., *et al.* Brain noradrenaline metabolism and psychophysiological variables in chronic schizophrenia. 1st annual conference of the Brain Research Association, Bath 1976

Gardos, G., Cole, J. O., Volicer, L., Orzack, M. H. and Oliff, A. (1973). A dose response study of propranolol in chronic schizophrenics. *Curr. Ther. Res.*, **15**, 314

Grossman, S. P. (1968). Behavioural and electrophysiological effects of intracranial micro-injections of phenothiazines. *Comm. Beh. Biol.*, **1**, 9

Gruzelier, J. H. (1973). Bilateral asymmetry of skin conductance orienting activity and levels in schizophrenia. *J. Biol. Psychol.*, **1**, 21

Gruzelier, J. H. (1976). Clinical attributes of schizophrenic skin conductance responders and non-responders. *Psychol. Med.*, **6**, 245

Gruzelier, J. H. (1978a). Propranolol acts to modulate autonomic orienting and habituation processes in schizophrenia. In E. Roberts and P. Amacher (eds.). *Propranolol and Schizophrenia.* (New York: A. R. Liss)

Gruzelier, J. H. (1978b). Bimodal states of arousal and lateralised dysfunction in schizophrenia. The effect of chlorpromazine upon psychophysiological, information processing and endocrine measures. In L. Wynne, R. Cromwell and S. Matthysee (eds.) *Nature of Schizophrenia: New Findings and Future Strategies.* (New York: Wiley)

Gruzelier, J. H. and Hammond, N. V. (1976). Schizophrenia: A dominant hemisphere temporal-limbic disorder? *Res. Comm. Psychiatry. Beh.*, **1**, 33

Gruzelier, J. H. and Hammond, N.V. (1977). The effect of chlorpromazine upon bilateral asymmetries of bioelectrical skin reactivity in schizophrenia. *Studia Psychol.*, **19**, 40

Gruzelier, J. H. and Hammond, N. V. (1978a). The effect of chlorpromazine on psycho-physiological, endocrine and information processing measures in schizophrenia. *J. Psychiatr. Res.* (in press)

Gruzelier, J. H. and Hammond, N. V. (1978b). Gains, losses and lateral differences in the hearing of schizophrenic patients. *Br. J. Psychol.* (in press)

Gruzelier, J. H. and Venables, P. H. (1972). Skin conductance orienting activity in a hetero-generous sample of schizophrenics: Possible evidence of limbic dysfunction. *J. Nerv. Ment. Dis.*, **155**, 277

Gruzelier, J. H. and Venables, P. H. (1974). Bimodality and lateral asymmetry of skin conductance orienting activity in schizophrenics: Replication and evidence of lateral asymmetry in patients with depression and disorders of personality. *Biol. Psychiatry*, **8**, 55

Gur, R. E. (1977). Motoric laterality imbalance in schizophrenia. *Arch. Gen. Psychiatry*, **34**, 33

Hammond, N. V. and Gruzelier, J. H. (1978). Laterality, attention and rate effects in the auditory temporal discrimination of chronic schizophrenics: The effect of treatment with chlorpromazine. *Q. J. Exp. Psychol.*

Heath, R. G. (1964). Developments toward new physiologic treatments in psychiatry. *Neuro-psychiatry*, 318

Hornykiewicz, O. (1966). Dopamine (3-Hydroxytyramine acid). *Pharmacol. Rev.* **18**, 925

Iversen, L. L. (1975). Dopamine receptors in the brain. *Sciences*, **188**, 1984

Jefferson, J. W. (1974). Beta-adrenergic blocking drugs in psychiatry. *Arch. Gen. Psychiatry*, **31**, 673

Kimble, D. P. (1968). Hippocampus and internal inhibition. *Psychol. Bull.*, **70**, 285

Lader, M. H. and Wing. I. (1966). *Physiological Measures, Sedative Drugs and Morbid Anxiety.* Institute of Psychiatry, Maudsley Monographs, **14** (London: Oxford University Press)

Leff, J. (1976). Assessment of psychiatric and social state. *Br. J. Clin. Pharm.*, **3**, (suppl. 2), 385

Lishman, W. A., McMeekan, E. R. I. (1976). Hand preference patterns in psychiatric patients. *Br. J. Psychiatry*, **129**, 159

Luria, A. R. and Homskaya, E. D. (1963). Le trouble du role regulateur du langage au course des lesions au lobe frontal. *Neuropsychologia*, **1**, 9

MacLean, P. D. (1970). The limbic brain in relation to psychoses. In P. Black (ed.) *Physiological Correlates of Emotion.* (New York: Academic Press)

Malamud, N., (1967). Psychiatric disorders with intracranial tumors of the limbic system. *Arch. Neurol.*, **17**, 113

Masuoka, D. and Hanssen, E. (1967). Autoradiographic distribution studies of adrenergic blocking agents. II 14C – propranolol a β-receptor-type blocker. *Acta Pharmacol. Toxicol.*, **25**, 477

Matthysse, S. (1973). Antipsychotic drug actions: a clue to the neuropathology of schizophrenia? *Fed. Proc.*, **32**, 200

May, P. R. A. (1968). *Treatment of Schizophrenia: A comparative study of five treatment methods* (New York: Science House)

Mednick, S. A. (1958). A learning theory approach to research in schizophrenia. *Psychol. Bull.*, **55**, 316

Meares, R. and Horvath, T. (1973). A physiological difference between hallucinosis and schizophrenia. *Br. J. Psychiatry,* **122,** 687
O'Gorman, J. G. (1978). Method of recording: A neglected factor in the controversy over the bimodality of electrodermal responsiveness in schizophrenic samples. *Schizophrenia Bull.,* **4,**
Overall, J. E. and Gorham, D. R. (1962). The brief psychiatric rating scale. *Psychol. Rep.,* **10,** 799
Patterson, T. (1976). Skin conductance responding/non-responding and pupillometrics in chronic schizophrenia: A confirmation of Gruzelier and Venables. *J. Nerv. Ment. Dis.,* **163,** 200
Pavlov, J. P. (1941). *Conditional Reflexes and Psychiatry.* translated by Gantt (New York: Internat. Univ. Press)
Pribram, K. H. and McGuinness, D. (1975). Arousal, activation and effort in the control of attention. *Psychol. Rev.,* **82,** 116
Prick, J. J. G. (1969). The role of anxiety in psychosis. In M. M. Lader (ed.), *Studies of Anxiety.* (London: Royal Medico-Psychological Association)
Prokasy, W. F. and Raskin, D. C. (eds.). *Electrodermal Activity in Psychological Research.* (New York: Academic Press)
Rackensperger, W., Gaupp, R., Mattke, D. J., Schwarz, D. and Stutte, K. H. (1974). Treatment of acute schizophrenic psychosis with beta-adrenergic blocking agents. *Arch. Psychiatr. Nervenkr.,* **219,** 29
Richardson, J. S. (1974). Basic concepts of psychopharmacological research as applied to the psychopharmacological analysis of the amygdala. *Acta Neurobiol. Exp.,* **34,** 543
Rubens, R. I. and Lapidus, I. B. (1977). Arousal patterns and stimulus barrier functioning in schizophrenia. *J. Abnormal Psychol.* (in press)
Seeman. P. and Lee, T. (1975). Antipsychotic drugs: Direct correlation between clinical potency and presynaptic action on dopamine neurons, *Science,* **188,** 1217
Seeman, P., Lee, T., Chan-Wong, M. and Wong, K. (1976). Anti-psychotic drug doses and neuroleptic/dopamine receptors. *Nature (London)* **261,** 717
Serafetinides, E. A. (1972). Laterality and voltage in the EEG of psychiatric patients. *Dis. Nerv. Syst.,* **33,** 622
Serafetinides, E. A. (1973). Voltage laterality in the EEG of psychiatric patients. *Dis. Nerv. Syst.,* **34,** 190
Smythies, J. R. (1969). The behavioural physiology of the temporal lobe. In R. N. Herrington (ed.). *Current Problems in Neuropsychiatry.* (London: Royal Medico-Psychological Association)
Snyder, S. H., Banerjee, S. P., Yamamura, H. J., Greenberg, D. (1975). Drugs, neurotransmitters and schizophrenia. *Science,* **184,** 1243
Sokolov, E. M. (1963). *Perception and the Conditioned Reflex* (New York: MacMillan)
Sourek, K. (1965). *The Nervous Control of Skin Potential in Man.* (Prague: Nakladatelstvi Ceskoslovenska Academic Ved.)
Steiner, M., Blum, J., Wijsenbeek, H. and Atsmon, A. Propranolol versus chlorpromazine in the treatment of psychoses associated with child bearing. *Psychiat. Neurochir.,* **76,** 421
Torrey, E. S. and Peterson, M. R. (1974). Schizophrenia and the limbic system. *Lancet,* **ii,** 942
Tyrer, P. J. (1976). *The Role of Bodily Feelings in Anxiety.* Institute of Psychiatry. Maudsley Monographs (London: Oxford University Press)
Van Zerssen, D. (1976). Beta-adrenergic blocking agents in the treatment of psychoses. A report on 17 cases. *Adv. Clin. Pharmacol,* **52,** (Suppl. 4), 105
Venables, P. H. (1973). Input regulation and psychopathology. In Hammer, M., Sutton, S. and Zubin, J. (eds.). *Psychopathology: Contributions from the Social, Behavioural and Biological Sciences* (London: Wiley)
Venables, P. H. (1977). The electrodermal psychophysiology of schizophrenics and children at risk for schizophrenia: Controversies and developments. *Schizophrenia Bull.,* **3,** 28
Yorkston, N. J., Gruzelier, J. H., Hollander, D., Zaki, S. A., Pitcher, D. and Sergeant, H. S. (1977). Propranolol as an adjunct to the treatment of schizophrenia. *Lancet,* **i,** 575
Yorkston, N. J., Zaki, S. A., Malik, M. K. U., *et al.* (1974). Propranolol in the control of schizophrenic symptoms. *Br. Med. J.,* **4,** 633
Yorkston, N. J., Zaki, S. A., Themen, J. F. A., *et al.* (1976a). Propranolol to control schizophrenic symptoms: 55 patients. *Adv. Clin. Pharmacol.,* **12,** 91
Yorkston, N. J., Zaki, S. A., Themen, J. F. A. and Harvard, C. W. H. (1976b). Safeguards in the treatment of schizophrenia with propranolol. *Postgrad. Med. J.,* **52,** (Suppl. 4), 175
Zahn, T. P. (1976). On the bimodality of the distribution of electrodermal orienting response in schizophrenic patients. *J. Nerv. Ment. Dis.,* **162,** 195

SECTION 5:
Dietary Factors

14

The effect of diet on brain neurotransmitters

R. J. WURTMAN

The hypothesis that I will be describing derives largely from experiments done initially on rats. The data obtained therefrom seem also to predict what happens in people: that is to say, a good correlation between rat and man is found when measuring changes in plasma constituents and neurotransmitter synthesis.

The hypothesis goes briefly as follows: the main point is that nutrition normally affects the brain, and the brain components that most markedly exhibit the effect of nutrition are the neurotransmitters. They are the compounds that serve to carry a signal from one nerve cell to the next nerve cell. We do not begin to know the nature of all the neurotransmitters – most neurobiologists would agree, I think, on a list of seven or eight compounds that do serve this function in the brain, but I would add that there must be many more. The point I will try to make is that the ability of brain neurones to synthesize at least two, and probably more, neurotransmitters is normally controlled by nutritional states. In the case of one of these transmitters, serotonin, 5-hydroxytryptamine, it will be shown that what the animal or the human eats in a particular meal, the composition of each meal, determines whether an hour or so later brain serotonin synthesis will increase or decrease, and, probably, whether corresponding changes occur in the amounts of serotonin released into synapses. The other neurotransmitter that responds so dramatically to diet is acetylcholine. It will be shown that if animals consume diets that contain greater or lesser, but still normal, amounts of choline for as little as 2 or 3 days, there are dramatic variations in acetylcholine levels within all brain regions, but especially the basal ganglia. We also have some evidence that under certain conditions the ability of the brain neurones to synthesize dopamine and noradrenaline can be influenced by dietary composition. The effects of particular foods are specific, and depend on both the composition of the food and the nature of the metabolic and hormonal responses that are induced by the act of eating. Most eating induces insulin secretion, and as we will see, insulin, by changing plasma amino acid patterns, has marked effects on brain serotonin synthesis.

Now what is the potential significance of these observations for schizophrenia? I think it is several-fold. Firstly, we now have a way of trying to explain how the consumption of particular foods might affect brain function: that is, by affecting neurotransmitter levels in the brain, or neurotransmitter synthesis, or neurotransmitter release. These chemicals, the neurotransmitters, constitute the *language* of the brain, or its 'message units'. Therefore if diet, or stress, or hormones, or drugs, or any environmental or physiological factor is going to affect brain function in important ways, it should be possible to correlate the effect of this factor with changes in the neurotransmitters. The data that will be described indicate, I think, that this has already been done with a variety of particular foods. It has not yet to my knowledge been done with gluten or gliadin. However, it should be and undoubtedly will be.

Secondly, as described previously some foods seem to interact with drugs to modify their therapeutic efficiency in schizophrenics. Since many drugs that are used in treating psychoses apparently produce their effects by increasing or decreasing the release of neurotransmitters, or the interaction of transmitters with their receptors, it seems highly likely that the consumption of foods which modify the amounts of transmitters that are there to be released, or there to interact with the receptor, will affect the efficacy of these drugs.

One last introductory comment: I find it remarkable, 5 years into this work, that certain brain neurones should constitute as open a system as appears to be the case, in that the ability of these neurones to make their transmitters and to function should to such a striking extent be manipulable by food choice. When I went to medical school I was taught that the brain is a terribly important organ, so important that it gets first crack at everything it wants, all the oxygen, all the blood, etc. The brain was thought to be relatively immune to changes in the composition of the blood, such as follow the consumption of foods. This turns out *not* to be the case, and I think a very interesting teleological question remains: Why should evolutionary mechanisms have allowed the brain, or allowed certain brain neurones at least, to remain as open as appears to be the case? Perhaps there will be time to come back to this question later.

I would like now to present the evidence that brain serotonin synthesis is food-dependent, and then the likelihood that acetylcholine synthesis is similarly food-dependent. Serotonin, or 5-hydroxytryptamine, is synthesized from a dietary amino acid, namely tryptophan (Figure 1). Tryptophan cannot be made in the body, and must be obtained from dietary protein. The conversion of tryptophan to serotonin, which by the way occurs in the gut and the pineal as well as in the brain, involves two enzymes, i.e. tryptophan hydroxylase, which converts this compound to a different amino acid, 5-hydroxytryptophan (5-HTP), and DOPA decarboxylase, which converts

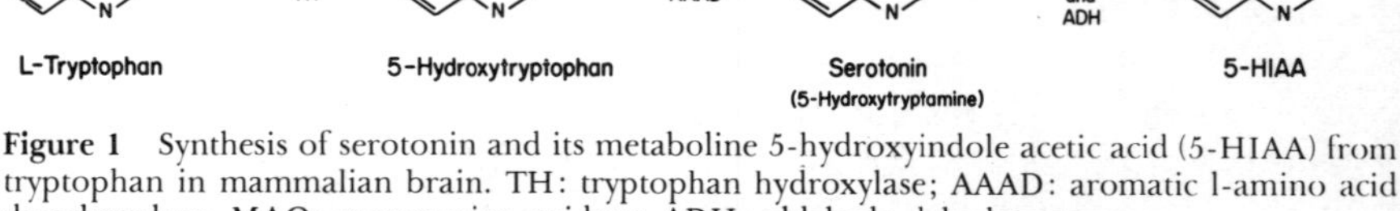

Figure 1 Synthesis of serotonin and its metaboline 5-hydroxyindole acetic acid (5-HIAA) from tryptophan in mammalian brain. TH: tryptophan hydroxylase; AAAD: aromatic l-amino acid decarboxylase; MAO: monoamine oxidase; ADH: aldehyde dehydrogenese

the 5-HTP to an amine, serotonin, by removing its carboxyl group. The major pathway by which serotonin is destroyed involves its deamination by monoamine oxidase. Our thesis will be that the ability of brain neurones to make serotonin depends on brain levels of its precursor, tryptophan. (Wurtman and Fernstrom, 1975 and Fernstrom and Wurtman, 1974). Now those of us who learned biochemistry initially on the model of *E. coli* and other bacteria have been led to believe that when the body wants to increase or decrease the rate at which it makes something, it does so by making more or less of an enzyme, or by making an enzyme more or less active. What I am suggesting here in the case of these neurones is that this is not always true; the control of serotonin synthesis resides not in the amount or activity of a rate-limiting enzyme, but rather in the amount of the precursor. This is the case because there are more of the enzymes present in the serotonin neurones than can normally be used. The enzyme is normally not saturated with its substrate, tryptophan. So by increasing or decreasing the amount of its substrate present in the brain cell one can increase or decrease the amount of material that goes through the enzymatic process to make serotonin. This will be a very important generalization. The enzymes that produce some of the neurotransmitters are not saturated with their substrates, the dietary precursors for the transmitters. Therefore changes in the amount of precursor, changes that follow food consumption for example, can determine the net overall rate of formation of the transmitter.

Most of the brain neurones that utilise serotonin as their transmitter have their cell bodies in the brain stem within several structures known as the Raphe nuclei. Axons originating from these neurones are distributed throughout the brain and the spinal cord. When we observe that food consumption increases whole brain serotonin levels it becomes important to know just where in the brain these increases occur. If they were confined to the region of the cell bodies they would not be terribly important, because they probably would not affect the amount of serotonin that the neurone releases into the synapse. Fortunately this is not the case: diet increases serotonin (and acetylcholine) levels within nerve terminals as well as in cell bodies, hence diet can control the amount of the transmitter that is released into synapses.

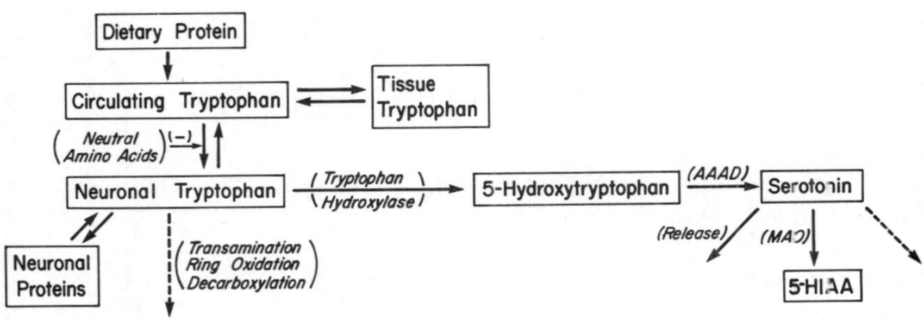

Figure 2 Control of serotonin synthesis in brain neurones. AAAD: aromatic L-amino acid decarboxylase; MAO: monoamine oxidase; --- indicates unproved pathway

As mentioned earlier, tryptophan is not synthesized by mammals, and must thus be obtained from dietary protein. Protein is consumed, and broken down in the gut to its constituent amino acids; these are absorbed into the portal and then the systemic circulation (Figure 2). Tryptophan is unusual in several ways. For one, not all the tryptophan that comes in to the body as food manages to make it, as it were, into the general circulation. The reason is that there is an enzyme in the liver, tryptophan pyrrolase, that destroys a portion of the tryptophan en route to the general circulation. Tryptophan is also interesting because of its scarcity. If one analyses any dietary protein for its constituent amino acids one finds that the limiting or scarcest amino acid is almost always tryptophan. It is a scarce amino acid, and the effect of tryptophan pyrrolase in the liver is to take an already scarce compound and make it all the scarcer. (If one wants some particular amino acid to control a metabolic process in the body it makes good teleological sense to have the amino acid which is most scarce to be the controlling amino acid.)

Once tryptophan gets in to the circulation, it travels as two pools: a portion travels like any other amino acid, as a free compound: the larger portion travels bound to albumin. Now the binding to albumin tends to be of a low affinity, high capacity type. It means that tryptophan rather easily couples to the albumin, and just as easily comes apart from the albumin. The binding of tryptophan to albumin does not interfere, as we shall see, with the availability of tryptophan to the brain. But it has an important function in that it enables tryptophan to respond differently to food consumption from any other neutral amino acid. As we will see, this difference in response is why the consumption of food can affect brain serotonin synthesis. The circulating tryptophan goes into equilibrium with tryptophan in the tissues, muscle, liver, etc. but the portion that concerns us now is taken up into brain neurones. Now, the uptake of tryptophan into the brain is mediated by a transport system at the blood/brain barrier level, and this transport system is not specific to tryptophan. Rather it is shared by a whole family of neutral amino acids, those which, like tryptophan, are neutral (i.e. not acidic or basic) in the body. As a result, the ability of the brain cells to take up tryptophan depends not only on the amount of tryptophan in the blood, but also on the amounts of such other neutral amino acids as leucine, isoleucine, valine, tyrosine and phenylalanine (Partridge, 1977). For example if a rat, or for that matter a human, consumes a single meal containing large amounts of protein, even though the protein delivers some tryptophan to the blood stream, tryptophan is so scarce in the protein, and the other neutral amino acids are so abundant, that the net effect of the meal is to cause a major increase in the other neutral amino acids. These other amino acids compete with tryptophan for uptake into the brain and actually *lower* the tryptophan level in the brain. *Therefore*, as will be shown below, the proportion of protein in a meal determines whether brain tryptophan levels (and thus brain serotonin synthesis) are increased or decreased. The brain's response varies inversely with the proportion of protein.

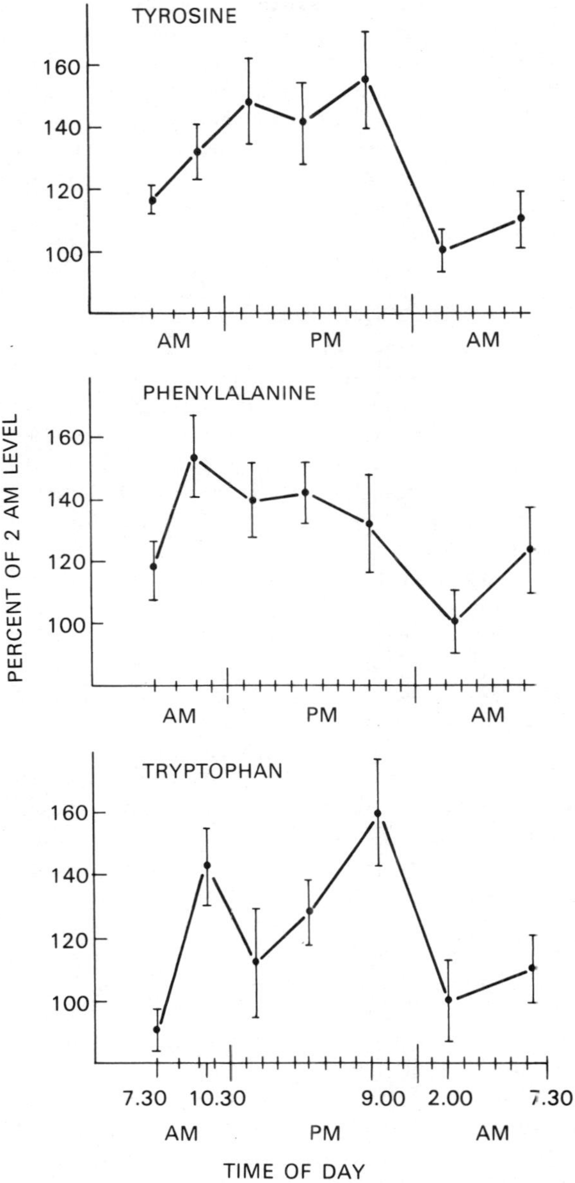

Figure 3 Variations in the plasma concentrations of tyrosine, phenylalanine and tryptophan with time of day among six healthy male subjects given the 'House Diet' (approximately 1.5 g of protein per kg of body weight). The 2.00 a.m. concentrations of the amino acids were: tyrosine, 12.20±0.94 μg/ml: Phenylalanine 8.14±0.85 μg/ml: tryptophan, 9. 3±1.22 μg/ml. (From Wurtman, R. J., Rose, C. M., Chou, C. and Larin, F. F. (1968). *N. Engl. J. Med*., **279,** 171) *Med*., **279,** 171)

Once tryptophan is present in brain neurones, most neurones utilise it only for making their own proteins. The neurones that most concern us now are the ones that have the necessary enzymes to convert tryptophan to the neurotransmitter serotonin. Our interest in tryptophan and brain serotonin developed some 6 or 7 years ago as an offshoot of some clinical studies on the fates of amino acids in people. We had discovered that if one collected blood from people at various times of the day and night, and measured the levels of a particular amino acid in the blood (for example tryptophan, phenylalanine or tyrosine), these levels were not constant but varied predictably as a function of time of day (Figure 3). The mechanism that causes these temporal variations is not some sort of intrinsic biological clock, but rather feeding. Feeding affects blood amino acid levels in two ways. First, by directly contributing some of the amino acids in dietary protein to the blood stream, and secondly (and more importantly) by causing insulin to be released. Insulin causes most of the amino acids (not including tryptophan) to pass from the blood into skeletal muscle and other tissues. Eating *per se* acts via insulin secretion to lower the plasma levels of all the neutral amino acids except tryptophan. Hence these levels tend to fall for a few hours after a meal and to remain lower until the things you have eaten have been digested; then they go up again.

Having thus shown that plasma amino acid levels normally rise and fall each day, we wondered 'So what?' Were there any physiological consequences to these changes in plasma composition? Did it matter that food consumption could change the levels of amino acids in the circulation? How would one know whether an increase or a decrease in, for example, plasma tryptophan had any significance? Well, it seemed reasonable to Dr. Fernstrom and myself that if these changes were indeed important we might detect this by showing that the rate at which the body used an amino acid for some purpose (for example for synthesizing neurotransmitters like serotonin) *also* went up and down in parallel with the changes in plasma amino acid levels. We decided to see whether or not daily rhythms in the plasma tryptophan levels were at all parallel to brain tryptophan rhythms, if indeed such brain rhythms actually existed, and to rhythms in the synthesis of serotonin.

In initial experiments we took brain and blood samples from rats killed at different hours of the day and night. Rats tend to consume most of their food during the hours of darkness. Plasma tryptophan levels exhibited a clear daily rhythm in rats, just as they had in people (Figure 4). We also noted a parallel rhythm in brain tryptophan, actually a two-fold daily rhythm. Tryptophan levels rose from 3 micrograms per g to about 6, soon after the onset of darkness. Brain tryptophan went up at the same time as plasma tryptophan was going up. Brain serotonin levels also varied rhythmically, rising after the onset of darkness. Hence when blood and brain tryptophan levels started to rise, brain serotonin also increased. Thus, perhaps daily rhythms in plasma amino acid levels might be important after all. Perhaps they could influence the ability of the brain to make neurotransmitters and other compounds. Next, we took animals at noon, the time of day when blood and brain tryptophan levels are normally at their lowest, and gave

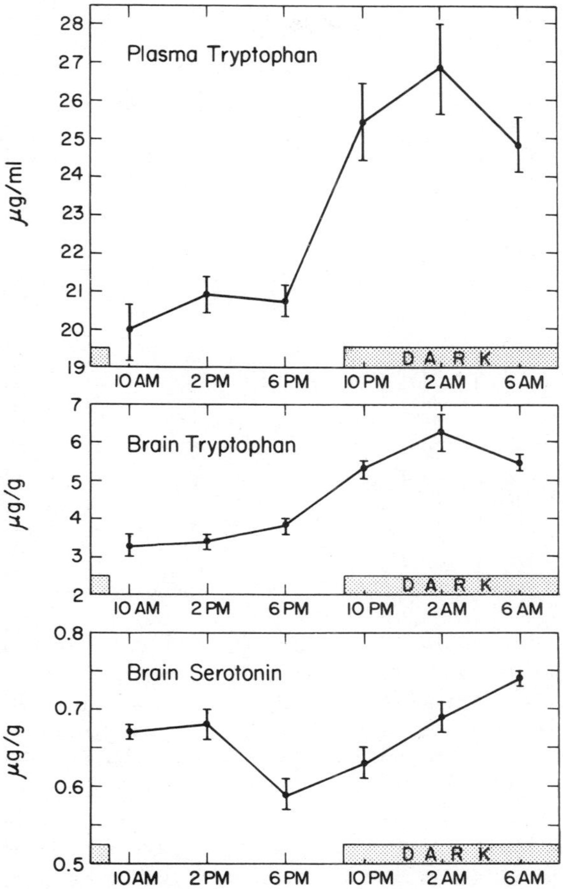

Figure 4 Daily rhythms in plasma tryptophan, brain tryptophan and brain serotonin. Groups of ten rats kept in darkness from 9 p.m. to 9 a.m. were killed at intervals of 4 hours. Vertical bars indicate standard errors of the mean

them a dose of tryptophan which would raise tryptophan levels but not to levels beyond their normal daily range. Could such an increase in tryptophan, *within the normal daily range*, produce an increase in the levels of brain serotonin? Indeed it could. If one gave a low dose of tryptophan (i.e. about 5–10% of the amount that the animal normally eats each day) there were dose-related changes in brain tryptophan and serotonin levels (Figure 5). This effect was most dramatic when low doses of tryptophan were used, further suggesting that similar changes occur normally when food consumption modifies plasma tryptophan levels. So it seemed the system of serotonin neurones was designed by Nature in such a way that changes in the amount of its precursor, tryptophan, produce changes in neurotransmitter synthesis.

Now, having shown that giving tryptophan could raise brain tryptophan levels, and thereby accelerate serotonin synthesis, the next question was what

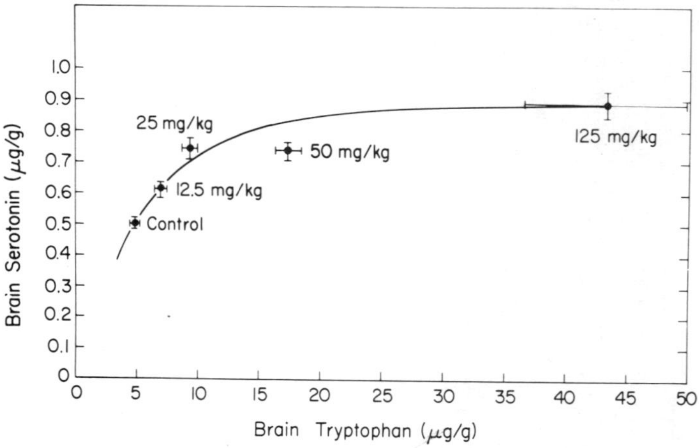

Figure 5 Dose-response curve relating brain tryptophan and brain serotonin. Groups of ten rats received L-tryptophan (12.5, 25, 50 or 125 mg/kg. intraperitoneally) at noon, and were killed one hour later. Horizontal bars represent standard error of the mean for brain serotonin. All brain tryptophan levels were significantly higher than control values ($p<0.001$). All brain serotonin levels were significantly higher than control values ($p<0.01$). Plasma tryptophan rose 22% over control levels in rats injected with the 12.5 mg/kg dose ($p<0.02$)

happens if one lowers brain tryptophan? Does one also decrease serotonin synthesis? At that time there was no way known to lower brain tryptophan levels. However, we guessed (incorrectly as it turned out) that tryptophan would behave like any other amino acid such that if we administered insulin to an animal, it would lower plasma tryptophan levels and thereby would lower brain tryptophan levels. This turned out not to be the case. As Dr Fernstrom showed, the administration of insulin to animals, in doses that lowered blood glucose markedly, did not lower, but actually raised blood tryptophan levels (Figure 6) and, in parallel, raised brain tryptophan and brain serotonin. Even though this experiment was a failure in one perspective (i.e. it did not allow us to produce the low brain tryptophan levels that we had wanted) it did confirm that treatments which increased brain tryptophan also elevated brain serotonin.

At this point we began to do experiments involving nutrition. We decided that, instead of giving animals large doses of insulin, which causes major reduction in blood glucose, we would instead make the animal secrete its own insulin. We did this by fasting the animal overnight and then allowing it to eat a carbohydrate meal or a carbohydrate-fat meal. The consumption of carbohydrate would elicit insulin secretion, and if insulin was really causing increases in plasma and brain tryptophan then they should also occur following the meal. In fact, exactly the same thing happened as after insulin injection: if animals were fasted, then given a carbohydrate meal and killed after 1, 2 or 3 hours, increases were observed in plasma tryptophan and brain serotonin (Fernstrom and Wurtman, 1971). Let me point out here something that is encoutered throughout this entire story. The meal

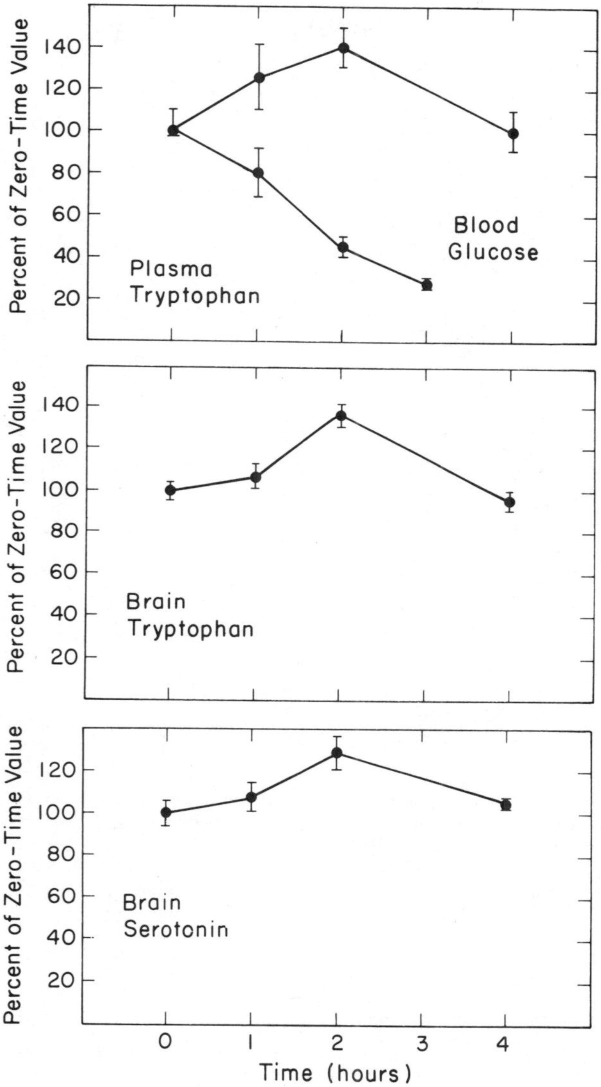

Figure 6 Effects of insulin administration (2 unit/kg intraperitoneally) on plasma tryptophan, blood glucose, brain tryptophan and brain serotonin concentrations. Groups of six to ten rats were killed at 1 hour intervals after insulin was administered. Vertical bars indicate standard errors of the mean

that is most effective in raising brain tryptophan and brain serotonin is a meal that *lacks* protein and so *lacks tryptophan*! The reason for this paradox is that any natural protein contains such higher amounts of the *other* neutral amino acids which compete with tryptophan for uptake into the brain that it actually *lowers* brain tryptophan levels.

At this point we anticipated that if a protein-free meal could cause an increase in brain serotonin then an even larger rise would occur if the meal happened also to contain some protein. We were mistaken; if animals fasted overnight were given access to a meal containing 18–20% protein, brain

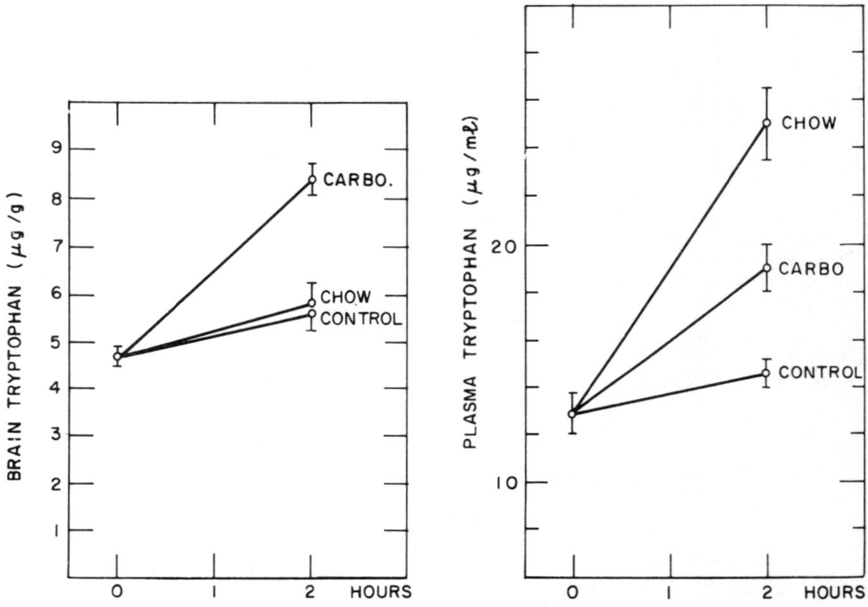

Figure 7 Changes in brain and plasma tryptophan concentrations following the consumption of different foods. Groups of six rats were killed 1 or 2 hours after diet presentation. Vertical bars represent standard errors of the mean. Two hour plasma tryptophan levels were significantly greater in rats consuming either diet than in fasting controls (chow, $p<0.001$; carbohydrate, $p<0.01$). Two hour brain tryptophan levels were significantly elevated above controls only in rats consuming the carbohydrate plus fat diet ($p < 0.001$)

tryptophan – and serotonin – failed to rise even though the increase in plasma tryptophan was now greater than in rats eating the carbohydrate meal (Figure 7). (We later noted that if we gave animals a meal containing a *very* high proportion of protein, 40–50%, even though plasma tryptophan levels increased many-fold, brain tryptophan actually fell. This is what led us to recognise that the entry of tryptophan into the brain depends not only on plasma tryptophan levels, but also on plasma levels of other competing neutral amino acids.) What had happened of course was that consumption of carbohydrate by eliciting insulin secretion raised tryptophan and lowered the plasma levels of the other competing neutral amino acids: in contrast the consumption of a mixed carbohydrate–protein meal raised plasma tryptophan more, but not nearly so much as it raised the neutral amino acid concentrations in the plasma.

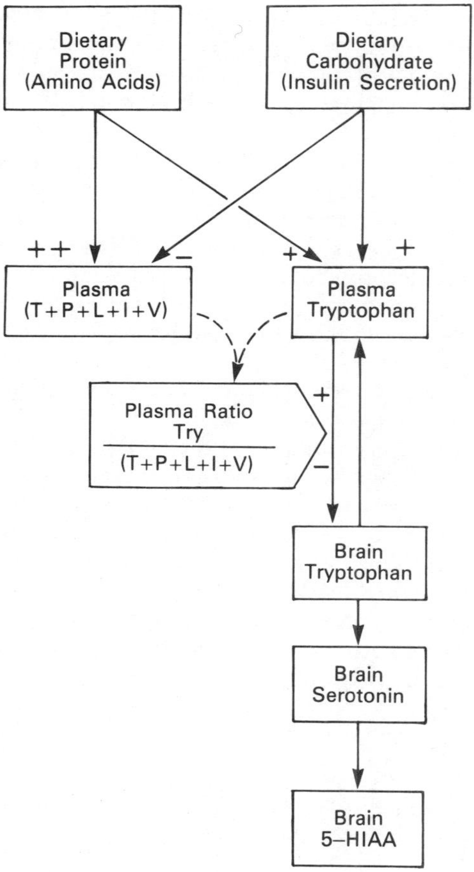

Figure 8 Proposed sequence describing diet-induced changes in brain serotonin concentration in the rat. The ratio of tryptophan to tyrosine (T) plus phenylalanine (P) plus leucine (L) plus isoleucine (I) plus valine (V) in the plasma is thought to control the tryptophan concentration in the brain

On the basis of these studies we developed a model (Figure 8) that is 6 years old now but still seems to be true, a longevity that is already remarkable in the brain sciences. When the animal consumes a carbohydrate meal, the carbohydrate causes insulin to be released. This elevates the plasma tryptophan level and depresses the plasma levels of these other five amino acids (tyrosine, phenylalanine, leucine, isoleucine and valine) which compete with tryptophan for entry to the brain. As a consequence the ratio of the plasma tryptophan concentration to the sum of the concentrations of these other competitors goes up. The numerator goes up and the denominator goes down, so the ratio goes up. Consequently the brain tryptophan concentration rises so more serotonin is synthesized and more is released, forming more of its metabolite 5-hydroxyindole acetic acid. In contrast, when the animal consumes a high protein meal, even though plasma tryptophan levels rise, there is a greater rise in its competitors: thus the ratio does not go up as much, and it may not go up at all, or may even decrease. Brain tryptophan and serotonin levels change in parallel. If you'll pardon an MIT term, serotonin-containing brain neurones appear to function as *variable ratio sensors*. They sense the ratio of tryptophan to its competitors in the plasma: this in turn depends on the ratio of carbohydrate to protein in the meal.

As already mentioned, tryptophan is largely bound to albumin in the plasma. For a while it seemed to some of us that this binding to a plasma protein would keep tryptophan from being available to the brain. It made very good sense on paper, but it turned out not to be the case at all, largely because the affinity of albumin for tryptophan is too low to retard tryptophan's entry into the brain. Numerous experiments have been done to show that albumin binding does not impede the entry of tryptophan into the brain. Let us summarise two of them. In one, animals are fasted overnight, and then given meals that contain various amounts (0–45%) of fat. Now the more fat in the meal, the higher the level in the plasma of non-esterified fatty acids. The non-esterified fatty acids compete with tryptophan for binding to albumin, so as these levels rise the proportion of tryptophan that is bound to albumin goes down, and plasma-free tryptophan levels go up quite considerably. But there is no correlation between this rise and brain tryptophan or serotonin levels (Madras *et al.*, 1974).

Recently, Dr Fernstrom has given animals a whole array of diets and followed the effect of each on total serum tryptophan, on the portion not

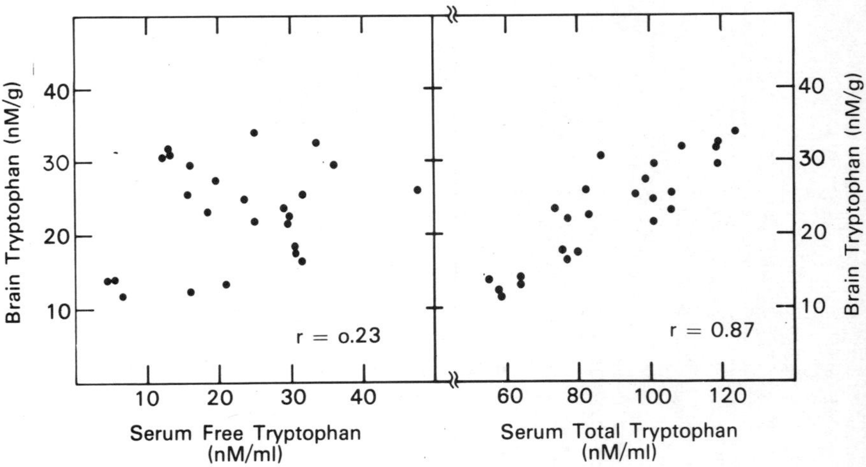

Figure 9 Correlations between brain tryptophan concentrations and (a) free or (b) total serum tryptophan levels in individual rats consuming single meals. Groups of rats deprived of food overnight were given access to one of the following diets and killed two hours later: carbohydrate without fat, carbohydrate plus 40% fat, carbohydrate plus large neutral amino acids without fat, and carbohydrate plus large neutral amino acids plus 40% fat. Values for fasted control animals are also included. For (a) r=0.23, and for (b) r=0.87. (From Fernstrom, J. D., Hirsch, M. J. and Faller, D. V. (1976). *Biochem. J.*, **160,** 589

bound to albumin ('free tryptophan') and on brain tryptophan levels. There is a striking correlation between brain tryptophan and total serum tryptophan (Figure 9) but only a very poor one with 'free tryptophan'. (Fernstrom *et al.*, 1976).

What difference does it make to a human or animal if brain serotonin levels change after eating? It would be very nice if we could measure directly the amounts of serotonin that are released into synapses, and see if there is a correlation between the levels present in the neurones and the amounts that transmit signals from one neurone to another. Alas, we cannot do so. There is no available way of collecting the fluid from within a synapse, much less of measuring transmitter content. We can, however, get an idea as to the amounts of serotonin that are being released by examining various physiological functions and behaviours. By now various scientists have shown that if one gives animals meals that raise or lower brain serotonin levels, one can thereby modify their behaviour. For example, Anderson in Toronto has shown that the tendency of an animal to choose a particular

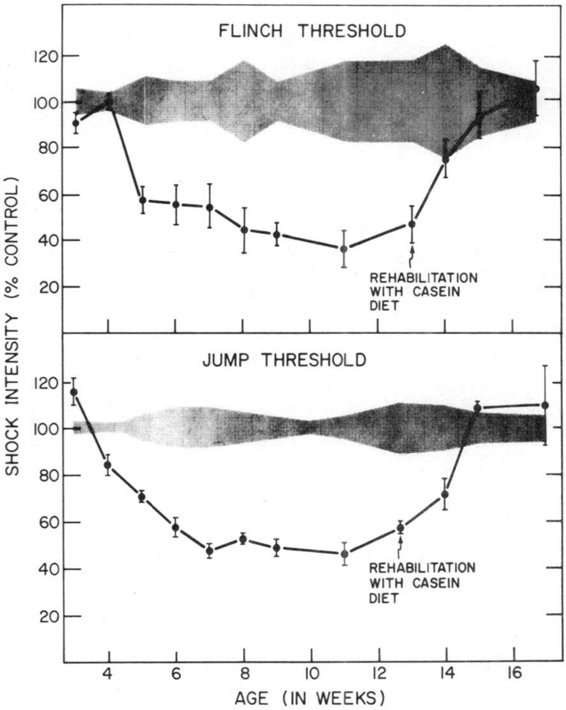

Figure 10 Animals were placed on tryptophan-deficient corn diets (closed circles, solid lines) or on amino acid balanced casein control diets (shaded areas) beginning at week three of life. After 10 weeks on the corn diet, rats were rehabilitated by feeding them the 18% casein diet (beginning at week 13 after birth). All values are the percentages (means±SE) of the shock intensities in the controls for eliciting the flinch or jump response. (From Lytle, L. D., Messing, R. B., Fisher, L. and Phebus, L. (1975) *Science,* **190,** 692

diet shows an extraordinary degree of correlation with the effect of that diet on the ratio of plasma tryptophan to the other neutral amino acids. If the meal causes that ratio to go up (i.e. a meal containing a tryptophan-rich protein), the animal will consume less of it. If the meal causes the ratio to go down, the animal will consume more of it (Ashley and Anderson, 1975).

On the basis of this sort of observation one can speculate that the meal modifies the amino acid composition of the plasma, which, in turn, modifies brain serotonin synthesis: the serotonin-containing neurones then act to influence food selection. One of our MIT associates, Dr Lytle, has studied another function thought to be related to serotonin neurones, that is pain sensitivity. A rat is placed on an electric grid and given very mild electric shocks: Dr Lytle measures the length of time until the animal jumps off the grid. This test is simple and provides a good index of pain sensitivity. If animals are given a corn-based diet that is very low in tryptophan for a few weeks, then the amount of electricity needed to get an animal to flinch or jump decreases (Figure 10). The animal becomes much more sensitive to

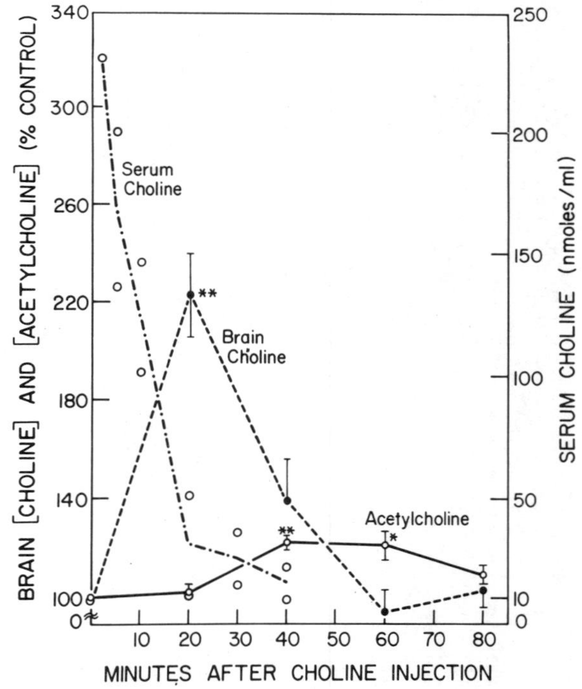

Figure 11 Groups of 150–200 g male rats received choline chloride (60 mg/kg, i.p.) in saline, or the diluent alone. The animals were killed at various times after injection by microwave irradiation of the head. Serum and brain choline and brain acetylcholine concentrations were measured by a radioenzymatic assay. (Serum choline levels were measured in groups of animals killed by decapitation, inasmuch as the blood coagulates too rapidly to be sampled in microwaved animals.) Data are presented as percents of control means for brain choline and acetylcholine; vertical bars represent standard errors of the means. (Redrawn from Cohen, E. L. and Wurtman, R. J. (1975). *Life Sci.*, **16**, 1095

pain. If the animal is then rehabilitated with casein, a high tryptophan protein, or if it is given a single injection of tryptophan, or of an antidepressant drug (chlormipramine) that potentiates brain serotonin, pain sensitivity rapidly returns to normal. The point of all this is that the nutritionally induced changes in pain sensitivity really do, we think reflect and result from changes in the brain serotonin level.

Now let us consider acetylcholine. Acetylcholine is used as a neurotransmitter both within and outside the brain, a fact that makes it much easier to study than serotonin. The same kind of relationship between precursor levels and neurotransmitter synthesis, and between nutrient consumption and precursor levels, as was described for tryptophan and serotonin also exists for choline and acetylcholine. For example, if one gives animals an injection of choline, and kills them after 40 or 60 min, brain choline levels attain their peak after 20 min and then return to normal (Figure 11). Brain acetylcholine levels are significantly elevated after 40 min, remain elevated at 60 min and then come back down (Cohen and Wurtman, 1975). This effect can also be produced by varying the choline content of the diet (Cohen and Wurtman, 1976). In a typical study animals were given meals containing different amounts of choline (20 or 129 mg/day) for 7 or 8 days. Major changes were seen in brain acetylcholine levels (Figure 12). Now this variation in dietary choline is entirely within the range of normal human food con-

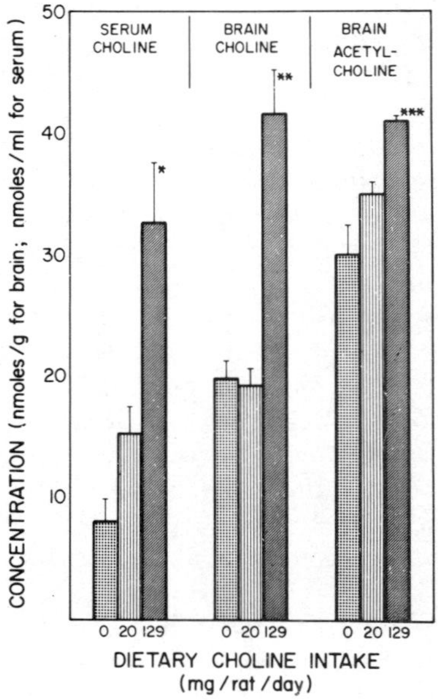

Figure 12 Effect of dietary choline content on serum and brain choline, and on brain acetylcholine concentrations. Groups of rats consumed diets having an average of 0, 20 or 129 mg of choline per day for 11 days. Data are presented as the means ± standard errors of the mean. Differences from corresponding concentrations in rats consuming no choline are indicated by $^{*}p < 0.05$, $^{**}p < 0.01$, $^{***}p < 0.001$

sumption. Choline is not evenly distributed in all of our foods. If we eat liver or eggs we ingest large amounts of choline (mostly as lecithin). In contrast, many foods lack significant amounts of choline. So dietary choline levels probably do normally affect brain acetylcholine levels. The brain nucleus (the caudate nucleus) affected in Parkinson's disease normally has the highest brain concentration of acetylcholine. This is also the region that appears to be most responsive to dietary choline levels. About 3 months after we published our first observations showing that choline administration could raise brain acetylcholine levels in rats, other investigators showed that this effect might have some therapeutic utility in a human disease, tardive dyskinesia. (Tardive dyskinesia is a complication that not infrequently occurs in people that have been taking high doses of such antipsychotic drugs as the phenothiazines and haloperidol. It is characterized by abnormal and very uncomfortable movements.) A patient with tardive dyskinesia received high doses of choline and reportedly showed a marked improvement in his dyskinetic movements (Davis *et al.,* 1975). No other treatment had helped. Now a number of laboratories and clinical centres are investigating the utility of choline in tardive dyskinesia, and in other neurological disorders. While choline is certainly not yet a 'wonder drug', it may become quite useful in treating patients with diseases that result from inadequate brain acetylcholine. We have affirmed the efficacy of choline in a double-blind, crossover study (Gordon *et al.,* 1977) and have also described therapeutic effects of lecithin (Growdon *et al.,* 1978). In the same sense, if Dr Singh or other investigators believe that increasing acetylcholine levels might have some therapeutic effect in some types of psychosis (or, for that matter, if decreasing acetylcholine levels might help), nutritional manoeuvres are now available to produce these desired changes. Obviously, all such experiments should be supported by, at the very least, measurements of blood choline level, so that the investigator can show that a diet designed to increase choline's availability actually did elevate blood choline levels. This is not difficult to do, and a lot of laboratories are now doing it.

Now we have seen two neurotransmitters, serotonin and acetylcholine, whose levels in the brain and rates of synthesis are controlled by precursor availability. As I said with serotonin, one question has been 'so what?' When serotonin levels are raised or lowered by nutritional means, does this mean that more of the transmitter, or perhaps less of it, is being released? It is very hard to study serotonin release directly. With acetylcholine it is a lot easier, for the reason I mentioned, namely, that there are many cholinergic neurones outside the brain. For example, acetylcholine is the neurotransmitter of nerves that go to the adrenal gland and cause the release of adrenalin. Recently, Dr Ulus, one of our associates, has shown that if one gives animals the same sort of choline treatments that I have described, acetylcholine levels in the adrenal medulla also increase. Subsequently changes are observed in the biochemistry of the adrenal cells, specifically a major increase in the activity of an enzyme, tyrosine hydroxylase, present in the chromaffin cells (Ulus *et al.,* 1978). Similarly, one can increase tyrosine hydroxylase activity in the dopamine cells of the caudate nucleus by giving choline, and one can block this effect by giving atropine, a cholinergic blocking agent. (Ulus and Wurtman, 1976). The point of these studies is that tyrosine hydroxylase activity provides a 'read-out', as it were, of the release of acetylcholine into the synapse. In order for choline to produce these changes in tyrosine hydroxylase, it must actually modify the amount of acetylcholine being released into the synapse. Hence I think that we now do have pretty good evidence that in cholinergic neurones the nutritional levels of choline really do modify the amounts of acetylcholine that are released.

Most recently, we have started studying the relationship between brain levels of tyrosine, another nutritionally derived amino acid, and the synthesis and release of the catecholamine neurotransmitters noradrenaline and dopamine. We find that both compounds depend on brain tyrosine noradrenaline generally so (Gibson and Wurtman, 1978), and dopamine in animals receiving antipsychotic drugs (Scally *et al.,* 1977).

In summary, what might the utility of this information be to people interested in the pathogenesis and treatment of schizophrenia? One could mention a fairly long list of possibilities, some of which have already been discussed. Firstly, since the brain is open-loop in this regard, if the physician decides it really is a good thing to increase acetylcholine release, or really is a good thing to increase or decrease serotonin release, it ought to be possible for him or her to design diets that will have the desired effect on the neurotransmitters. Secondly, it becomes possible to determine if the effects of particular diets on schizophrenics can be explained in biochemical terms by analysing their effects on brain neurotransmitters. Thirdly, a host of drugs that are used in the treatment of schizophrenia seem to work by modifying the release of, or the responsiveness of receptors to, neurotransmitters, thus one suspects that nutritional strategies designed to increase or decrease brain neurotransmitter levels may be useful in potentiating the action of the drugs. One could go on and on.

I think we are fortunate the brain works this way, because its responsiveness to the diet gives us a handle on it, something that we can manoeuvre. But I am still rather surprised to find it *does* work this way . . . I never would have believed it.

ACKNOWLEDGMENTS

I am indebted to my colleague Dr John Fernstrom on whose data much of the discussion in this chapter is based.

REFERENCES

Ashley, D. V. M. and Anderson, G. H. (1975). Correlation between the plasma tryptophan to neutral amino acid ratio and protein intake in the self-selecting weanling rat. *J. Nutr.*, **105,** 1412

Cohen, E. L. and Wurtman, R. J. (1975). Brain acetylcholine: Increase after systemic choline administration. *Life Sci.*, **16,** 1095

Cohen, E. L. and Wurtman, R. J. (1976). Brain acetylcholine synthesis: Control by dietary choline. *Science,* **191,** 561

Davis, K. L., Berger, P. A. and Hollister (1975). Choline for tardive dyskinesia. *N. Engl. J. Med.*, **293,** 152

Fernstrom, J. D. and Wurtman, R. J. (1971). Brain serotonin content: Increase following ingestion of carbohydrate diet *Science,* **174,** 1023

Fernstrom, J. D. and Wurtman, R. J. (1974). Nutrition and the brain. *Sci. Am.*, **230,** 84

Fernstrom, J. D., Hirsch, M. J. and Faller, D. V. (1976). Tryptophan concentration in rat brain: Failure to correlate with serum-free tryptophan, or its ratio to the sum of other serum neutral amino acids. *Biochem. J.*, **160,** 589

Gibson, C. J. and Wurtman, R. J. (1978). Physiological control of brain norepinephrine synthesis by brain tyrosine concentration. *Life Sci.*, **22,** 1399

Growdon, J. H., Gelenberg, A. J., Doller, J., Hirsch, M. J. and Wurtman, R. J. (1978). Lecithin can suppress tardive dyskenesia. *N. Engl. J. Med.*, **298,** 1029

Growdon, J. H., Hirsch, M. J., Wurtman, R. J. and Wiener, W. (1977). Oral choline administration to patients with tardive dyskinesia. *N. Engl. J. Med.*, **297,** 524

Madras, B. K., Cohen, E. L., Messing, R. Munro, H. N. and Wurtman, R. J. (1974). Relevance of serum-free tryptophan to tissue tryptophan. *Metabolism,* **23,** 1107

Pardrige, W. M. (1977). Regulation of amino acid availability to the brain. In *Nutrition and the Brain.* (R. J. Wurtman and J. J. Wurtman, eds.) Volume 1. (New York: Raven Press)

Scally, M. C., Ulus, I. and Wurtman, R. J. (1977). Brain tyrosine level controls striatal dopamine synthesis in haloperidol-treated rats. *J. Neural Trans.* **41,** 1

Ulus, I. and Wurtman, R. J. (1976). Choline administration: Activation of tyrosine hydroxylase in dopaminergic neurones of rat brain. *Science,* **194,** 1060

Ulus, I. H., Scally, M. C. and Wurtman, R. J. (1978). Enhancement by choline of the induction of adrenal tyrosine hydroxylase by phenoxybenzamine, 6-hydroxydopamine, Insulin, or exposure to cold. *J. Pharmacol. Exp. Ther.*, **204,** 676

Wurtman, R. J. and Fernstrom, J. D. (1975). Control of brain monoamine synthesis by diet and plasma amino acids. *Am. J. Clin. Nutr.*, **28,** 638

15

Schizophrenia: are some food-derived polypeptides pathogenic?

Coeliac disease as a model

F. C. DOHAN

INTRODUCTION

The first purpose of this paper is to present some evidence supporting the hypothesis that one or more components of cereal grains (and possibly other foods) are the major environmental factor which evokes schizophrenia in those hereditarily susceptible to it.

The second purpose is to urge careful testing by others of this, the principal hypothesis, since additional studies by independent investigators are necessary before it can be either accepted or rejected. If it is fully confirmed, the treatment, prevention, diagnosis, and understanding of schizophrenia should be substantially improved.

The third purpose is to present four testable subsidiary hypotheses concerning pathogenic mechanisms. Figure 1 shows the first two subsidiary hypotheses: (1) One or more of the polypeptides produced by peptic–pancreatic digestion of certain glutamine–proline rich food proteins are psychotoxic (for example, one or more of those found in glutens of cereal grains); (2) They reach the brain of the schizophrenic patient because the small gut, and possibly other, barrier systems (immunological, enyzmatic, mem-

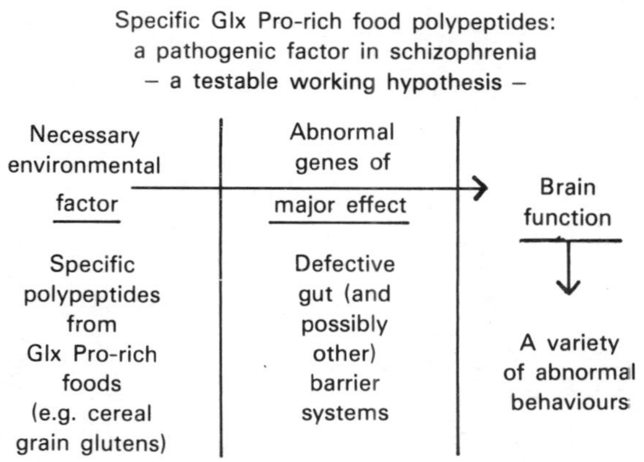

Figure 1 Schizophrenia: Glx Pro-rich polypeptides from food as a pathogenic factor. Glx= glutamine and/or glutamic acid: Pro=proline

branous, other) suffer hereditary defects of an unknown nature. The two other subsidiary hypotheses concern the possible genetic relationship of schizophrenia and coeliac disease: (1) The gut barrier defects are due to one or more abnormal genes common to coeliac disease and schizophrenia; (2) The differences in the two diseases are determined by the dissimilar components of the genotypes.

ARE CEREAL GRAINS PATHOGENIC IN SCHIZOPHRENIA?

Experimental evidence

The possible genetic relationship of coeliac disease (gluten enteropathy) and schizophrenia and epidemiological evidence of a relationship between cereal grain consumption and schizophrenia (see below) encouraged us to test the effects of cereal grain-free diets in relapsed schizophrenics (Dohan *et al.*, 1969; Dohan, 1969). An entire locked ward was used for a series of dietary experiments lasting more than 2 years. The aides and nurses were trained in the dietary and other aspects. All patients entering this locked ward from an open ward or from outside the hospital as a new admission or as a readmission were assigned by randomization to eat either a totally cereal grain-free milk-free diet or a high cereal grain diet. Milk was omitted because some coeliacs are made worse by milk. Its effect, if any, in schizophrenia is unknown. Neuroleptics and other usual treatments were administered as ordered by the three psychiatrists in charge of the patients.

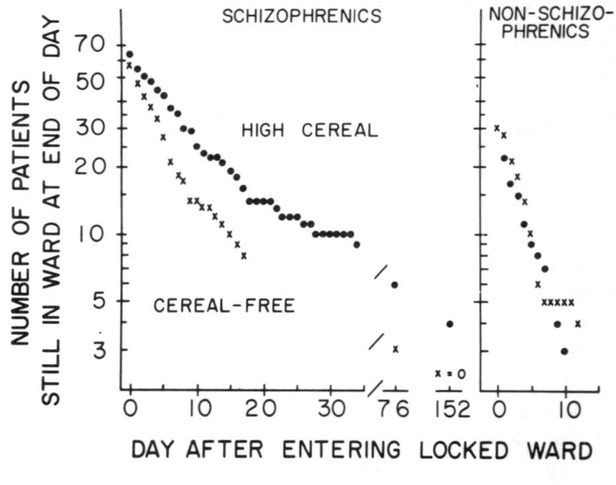

Figure 2 Effect of cereal grain-free milk-free diet versus high cereal grain diet on release from a locked to an open ward

Figure 2 shows the rate of release from the locked ward to an open ward of relapsed schizophrenic male patients. The majority of patients released from the locked ward after the first day are considered improved by the psychiatrist. The schizophrenics on the cereal grain-free diet were released considerably faster than those on the high cereal diet ($p<0.01$). In the next experimental period, as a control for the possible non-specific psychological effect of the diet, we added gluten (about 19 g/d) to the cereal grain-free milk-free diet without either the patients or ward staff knowing about it. During this period (not shown) there was no difference in the release rates of the schizophrenics on the high cereal and cereal-free plus gluten diets. Furthermore, diet had no effect on the release rate of the non-schizophrenic patients (Figure 2).

We also had an opportunity to make an intra-individual comparison of the effect of the cereal-free diet compared to the high cereal diet (Dohan, unpublished). Twenty schizophrenics were sent to the locked ward twice within 90 days because their behaviour worsened. In 16 of the 20 intra-individual comparisons the locked ward stay was longer when assigned to the high cereal diet than when assigned to the cereal grain-free diet (binomial $p<0.01$).

We continued our study so we could test the effect of diet only on those relapsed schizophrenics who were directly admitted to the locked ward from outside the hospital (Dohan and Grasberger, 1973). This time we used as our index of improvement the number of days from admission until discharged, improved, from the hospital. Relapsed schizophrenics who were on the cereal grain-free diet while they were in the locked ward were discharged from the hospital much more rapidly than those randomized to the high cereal grain diet (Figure 3, upper portion). Thus, by 90 days after admission to the hospital, 22 of the 59 relapsed schizophrenics who had the cereal grain-free

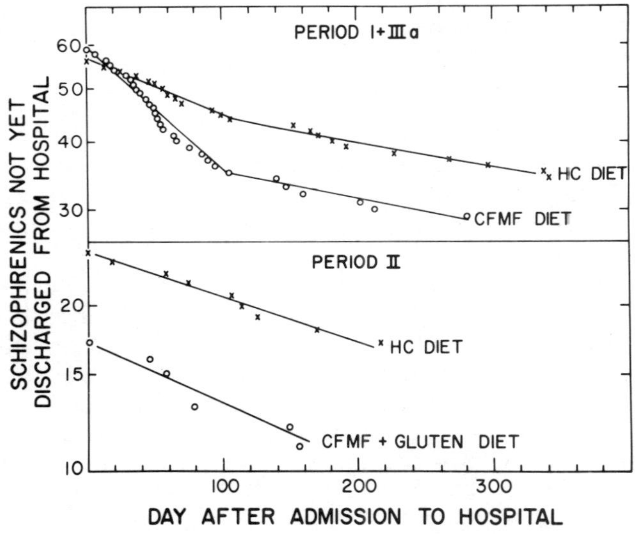

Figure 3 Effect of diet in locked ward on discharge from the hospital. Period I + IIIa – cereal grain-free milk-free (CFMF) diet vs. high cereal grain (HC) diet. Period II – CFMF + gluten diet vs. HC diet

milk-free diet while in the locked ward had been discharged compared to only 9 of the 56 who had been randomized to the high cereal grain diet during their stay in the locked ward (37% vs. 16%, $p<0.01$).

Examination of the effect on relapsed schizophrenics of secretly adding wheat gluten to the locked ward cereal grain-free milk-free diet showed that there was no difference in the rate of discharge from the hospital of the cereal grain-free plus gluten diet group from that of the high cereal diet group (Figure 3, lower portion). It thus seems unlikely that purely 'psychological factors' affecting staff or patients can account for such results. Evidence that the effects of the diet changes are *not* due to alterations in the effectiveness of neuroleptics has been summarized elsewhere (Dohan, 1973).

The recent study by Singh and Kay (1976) has provided evidence that the major symptoms of schizophrenics on a cereal grain-free milk-free diet are significantly exacerbated by ingestion of wheat gluten. The agreement of their experimental results with ours is encouraging but additional trials of the effect of diet are obviously necessary.

Since wheat gluten (i.e. glutenin plus gliadin) may have a psychotoxic effect on schizophrenics my co-workers and I (Dohan, Levitt and Kushnir, 1976) have done some preliminary testing of the effects of gliadin polypeptides on the behaviour of normal rats. Abnormal perseverative behaviour occurred several hours after intracerebral injection of small doses of the ultrafiltered acidic fraction (nominal mol.wt $>500<10\,000$ daltons) of the glutamine, glutamic acid, proline-rich peptides produced by digestion of gliadin with pepsin, trypsin, and other pancreatic enzymes. A patterned convulsive seizure or a catalepsy-like condition has also been occasionally noted. Many control studies remain to be done (e.g. injection of structurally modified specific polypeptides). Administration by other routes is planned. At this time the significance of these preliminary experiments is uncertain.

Epidemiological evidence

Because of a possible association of schizophrenia and coeliac disease and the ill effect of some cereal grains on coeliac patients I decided, about 14 years ago, to determine if the occurrence of schizophrenia is related to the ingestion of cereal grains (Dohan, 1966). I obtained, by diagnostic category, the annual number of women admitted to mental hospitals during the period before and during World War II. Figure 4 shows the percentage change in admissions for schizophrenia in four of the five countries studied. The number of admissions during the prewar period is considered as 100%. There was a marked decrease in admissions of women with schizophrenia in Finland and in Sweden and a small decrease in Canada during the first three war years but an increase in the United States. In addition (not charted), we obtained the average values for 5-year periods for first admissions to Norwegian hospitals. First admissions of women with schizophrenia in Norway decreased 40% during World War II. Each of the other psychoses increased.

Figure 5 shows the high positive correlation between the percentage change in weighted wheat and rye consumption from prewar levels and the equally

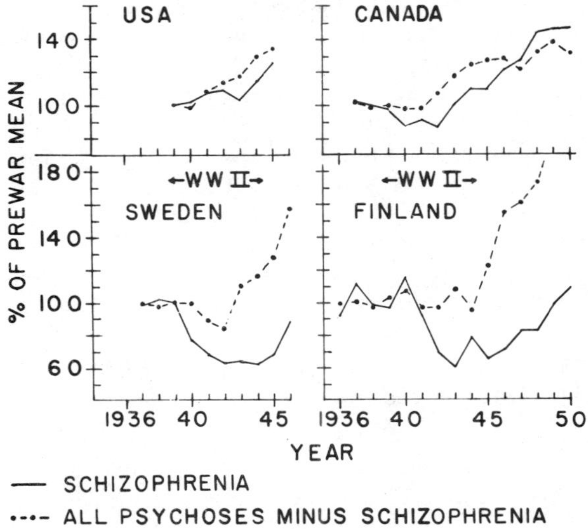

Figure 4 Changes during World War II in admissions of women to mental hospitals. Data for Finland are for first plus readmissions. Data for other countries are for first admissions only. First admissions of women for schizophrenia in Norway (not graphed) decreased 40% during World War II (see text)

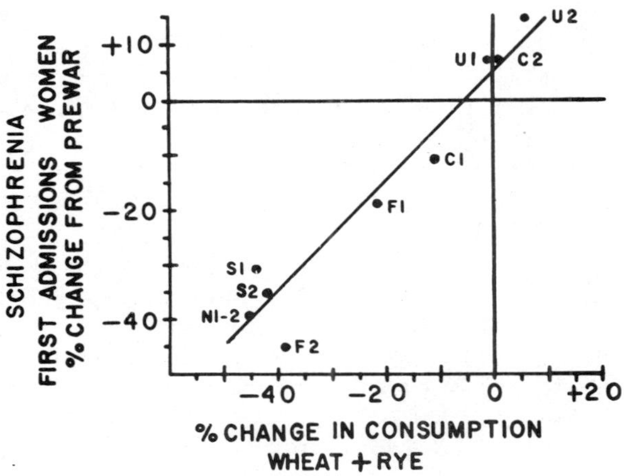

Figure 5 Percent changes from prewar values for first admissions of women for schizophrenia (ΔS) vs. weighted percent changes in wheat (ΔW) plus rye (ΔR) consumption. $\Delta S = 5\% + 1.04\,\Delta W + 0.48\,\Delta R$ (correlation coefficient$=0.96$, $p<0.01$). Letters indicate countries, e.g S=Sweden. The adjacent numbers indicate the first and second three-year periods of World War II, 1940–1945 inclusive. See Dohan (1966) for details and calculations of first admissions in Finland from first plus readmission data

marked changes in 'first admissions' for schizophrenia ($r=0.96$, $p<0.01$). Other factors such as admissions for each of the other psychoses, war status, number of doctors, number of beds available, consumption of alcohol, and employment were not correlated with these marked changes in admissions for schizophrenia (Dohan, 1966; 1969).

However, schizophrenia undoubtedly occurs among populations eating only grains other than wheat and rye; but it appears to do so with considerably lesser frequency (Dohan, 1966). Could this be due to a lesser content of the presumptively psychotoxic Glx Pro-rich polypeptides because of the lesser glutamine and proline content of the gluten proteins of the other cereal grains? I think this possibility is worth investigating.

ARE COELIAC DISEASE AND SCHIZOPHRENIA GENETICALLY RELATED?

There is circumstantial evidence that schizophrenia and coeliac disease (gluten enteropathy) may be genetically related disorders. Thus, clinical observations suggest that coeliac disease and schizophrenia have occurred sometime in the life of the same person more frequently than expected by chance alone (Graff and Handford, 1961; Dohan, 1970). Among other possibilities, this suggests that coeliac disease and schizophrenia, both apparently polygenic disorders (McCrae, 1970; Gottesmann and Shields, 1967) have one or more genes in common and that the differences in the phenotypes are determined by the dissimilar genes. Systematic family studies using proven coeliacs as probands are needed to test the validity of this hypothesis.

The main environmental factor producing symptoms in coeliacs is contained in the gluten of wheat and rye grains (Weijers, Van de Kamer and Dicke, 1957). Investigators in several countries are currently attempting to isolate the specific polypeptides from the gliadin fraction of wheat gluten which appear to be responsible for damaging the intestinal mucosa and for the other manifestations of coeliac disease (Kowlessar, Warren and Bronstein, 1970; Cornell and Townley, 1973; Dissanayake *et al.,* 1974). Recent evidence suggests that glycopeptides are the toxic agents (Phelan *et al.,* 1974).

The classical picture of coeliac disease, which may be episodic, is that of a child or adult with a characteristic gut lesion, who has lost considerable weight, has signs of vitamin deficiencies and is losing large amounts of fat in the stools. However, many patients do not show this classical picture (Brooks, Powell, and Cerda, 1966; Mann, Brown, and Kern, 1970). Intestinal biopsy studies of the relatives of coeliac probands and of 'treated' or spontaneously remitted coeliacs demonstrated that many individuals with the gut histology of coeliac disease admit to few or no symptoms.

Psychiatric symptoms of coeliacs

Coeliac disease may present with psychiatric symptoms, which, in association with other symptoms, may be of diagnostic help. The psychiatric symptoms often improve in a few days after starting a gluten-free diet (Townley and

Anderson, 1967). Käser (1961) described coeliac children as showing 'definite psychic symptoms in all cases. The children are conspicuously quiet, turned inward, often weepy, often discontented or surly and apparently lack all joy in living. They can take on negativistic and schizoid characteristics and may execute ceaseless stereotyped movements.' Paulley wrote in 1959: many (adult coeliacs) showed extreme obsessional neuroses, suffering delusions, frequently believing they had cancer. Paranoid ideas were also frequent and many were considered psychotic or near psychotic.'

The Glx Pro-rich polypeptides of wheat gluten or its subfraction, gliadin, resulting from digestion with pepsin, trypsin and other pancreatic enzymes have been fed to coeliac patients while on a gluten-free diet to test their effect on metabolism and on the histology of the intestine. In one such experiment Bayless and Cocco (1969) observed an acute psychotic reaction in a coeliac woman about three or four hours after the ingestion of a digestate from about 30 g of gluten. She was deluded, hallucinated, and was 'uncontrollable' for a few hours and then gradually became quieter and withdrawn. The psychosis disappeared in a few days. Her brother has schizophrenia. Acute severe psychiatric reactions in coeliac patients have also been observed by other investigators, such as Kowlessar (1968) and Cyrus Rubin (1973); under somewhat similar circumstances. Normal humans fed large amounts of gliadin do not develop psychiatric symptoms (Levine *et al.,* 1966).

The mechanisms accounting for the psychiatric symptoms produced by gluten ingestion in coeliacs (and schizophrenics) are unknown. I suggest that a 'direct' effect of specific Glx Pro-rich polypeptides deserves consideration. The important roles of glutamic acid and its decarboxylated derivative, γ-amino butyric acid, in neurotransmission, and the abundant evidence of the entrance into and modulation of brain function (Marx, 1975) by some polypeptides suggest a variety of speculations as to why Glx Pro-rich peptides might produce abnormal behaviour.

The gut

The evidence presented above provides only circumstantial evidence that Glx Pro-rich polypeptides from wheat gliadin (or other food proteins) pass the gut barrier of schizophrenics. However, in coeliac disease there is better evidence. Kowlessar *et al.* (1970) state that 'glutamine containing peptide is found in the plasma ultrafiltrate of coeliac patients after gliadin ingestion but not in normal subjects.' Coeliacs, but not normal humans, may have psychiatric symptoms after large doses of gliadin. In addition, using a more sensitive method, Hemmings *et al.* (1976) reported that some ^{125}I-labelled α-gliadin or its breakdown products pass the gut barrier of normal rats and bind to various tissues including the brain. Thus, in the future, studies on coeliacs, schizophrenics and normal subjects will be needed to determine (possibly by radioimmunoassay) the kinds and quantities of peptides passing the gut barrier and their disposition after absorption.

Gliadin (rich in glutamine and proline) is digested in the lumen of the gut to (glutamic acid, glutamine, proline-rich) polypeptides and amino acids. One or more of the polypeptides can damage the mucosa of the small intestine of coeliacs *in vivo* and *in vitro* by unknown mechanisms. A direct effect on gut mucosa of cytotoxic polypeptides which remain unhydrolysed because of genetic impairment of still undiscovered intestinal peptidases (Cornell and Townley, 1973) or immunological factors (Strober *et al.,* 1975) is thought to be primarily responsible also see Kowlessar, Warren, and Bronstein, 1970; and many articles in Hekkens and Peña, 1974). It has recently been proposed that incomplete oligosaccharide chains in cell surface-membrane glycoproteins allow gluten to act as a lectin (Weser and Douglas, 1976).

Immunological factors are undoubtedly important in the production of the characteristic changes in the gut mucosa, typically in the duodenum and upper jejunum, of coeliacs. The immunological response of the gut mucosa appears to be facilitiated (Strober *et al.,* 1975) by a gene or genes closely linked to that determining the HLA–B8 transplantation antigen. This cell surface antigen is much more common in coeliacs and, to a lesser extent, in patients with dermatitis herpetiformis – which is apparently genetically related to coeliac disease (Marks *et al.,* 1970) – than in the general population. However, it is not increased in schizophrenics (Cazzullo *et al.,* 1974; Zmijewski and Dohan, 1976).

Nevertheless, under certain circumstances, schizophrenics appear to have developed coeliac-like manifestations. Reports before World War II indicate that many schizophrenics had suggestive evidence of malabsorption and that at autopsy a significant proportion showed histologic changes in the gut which were similar to those now recognized as occurring in coeliac disease for discussion and references, see Dohan, 1969 and 1976, plus other information available from the author). The patchy and more extensive distribution and variability in severity of the mucosal lesions of the gut in schizophrenics, as compared to coeliacs, is similar to that reported during the past decade in patients with dermatitis herpetiformis (Marks *et al.,* 1970). However, post-mortem specimens (Dohan, 1969) and gut biopsy studies (Stevens *et al.,* 1975; Dean *et al.,* 1975) of present-day schizophrenics receiving anti-schizophrenic medication do not show the typical changes of coeliac disease. The effect of the generally higher consumption of cereal grains before World War II (Yates, 1960) on the dose-related responses of the gut mucosa to gluten (Weinstein, 1974) and the absence of chlorpromazine and other anti-schizophrenic medication may be related to this disparity.

Since chlorpromazine stabilizes lysosomal and other membranes (Guth *et al.,* 1965), I suggest its effect on symptomatic coeliac patients, who 'will not' follow a gluten-free diet, is worth investigating. If gut biopsy studies are done in schizophrenics I believe they should be done only after a high gluten diet (perhaps 30 g/d) for weeks or months in psychiatrically monitored patients not receiving anti-schizophrenia medication for at least a few weeks (Dohan and Grasberger, 1973).

The glutens

The cereal grain glutens generally accepted as pathogenic in coeliac disease are those from wheat, rye and barley. The toxicity is generally attributed to some component(s) of the prolamine fraction (e.g. gliadin, secalin, hordein) of these glutens. Gliadin is not toxic to the normal gut (Levine *et al.,* 1966). Furthermore, the peptides are rendered non-toxic to coeliacs by digestion with scrapings (containing peptidases) from hog intestine (Frazer, 1956). Duodenal mucosa from children without coeliac disease markedly reduced the lytic effect on lysosomes of certain gliadin peptides while mucosa from treated coeliacs did not do so (Townley *et al.,* 1973). Such studies of pathogenic mechanisms also suggest therapeutic possiblities.

The glutens in cereal grains (Gramineae) other than wheat, rye, and barley are generally regarded as innocuous for coeliacs. Yet, after initiation of a strict but conventional gluten-free diet the intestinal mucosa is usually not restored to normal for many months despite the often rapid disappearance of symptoms and the restoration to almost normal of the epithelium of gut biopsies from untreated coeliacs which had been cultured in the absence of gliadin peptides for 48 h (Jos *et al.,* 1975). These facts suggest that coeliacs on a strict gluten-free diet continue to eat other foods containing relatively small amounts of noxious substances.

The proteins of cereal grains other than those omitted in the usual 'gluten-free' diet are also Glx Pro-rich but less so than those of wheat, rye, and barley (Food and Agriculture Organization, 1970). Thus, cereal grain glutens may present a hierarchy of toxicity to coeliacs. Epidemiological evidence suggests this may also be true for schizophrenics.

ACKNOWLEDGMENTS

I thank the colleagues who have reviewed various drafts of this article and the many gastroenterologists, dermatologists, and psychiatrists who have shared their knowledge with me.

Figure 2 (slightly redrawn) and Figure 4 have been reproduced with the permission of the editor and publisher, from: 'Schizophrenia: Current Concepts and Research', edited by D. V. Siva Sankar, PhD., and published by PJD Publications, Hicksville, New York, 1969.

REFERENCES

Bayless, T. and Cocco, A. (1969). Personal communication

Brooks, F. P., Powell, K. C. and Cerda, J. J. (1966). Variable clinical course of adult celiac disease. *Arch. Intern. Med.*, **117,** 789

Cazzullo, C. L., Smeraldi, E. and Penati, G. (1974). The leukocyte antigenic system HL-A às a possible genetic marker of schizophrenia. *Br. J. Psychiatry*, **125,** 25

Cornell, H. J. and Townley, R. R. W. (1973). Investigation of possible intestinal peptidase deficiency in coeliac disease. *Clin. Chim. Acta*, **43,** 113

Dean, G., Hanniffy, L., Stevens, F., Temperley, I., O'Broin, J. D., Scott, J. and Cahalane, S. F. (1975). Schizophrenia and coeliac disease. *J. Irish Med. Assoc.*, **68,** 545

Dissanayake, A. S., Jerrome, D. W., Offord, R. E., Truelove, S. C. and Whitehead, R. (1974). Identifying toxic fractions of wheat gluten and their effect on the jejunal mucosa in coeliac disease. *Gut*, **15,** 931

Dohan, F. C., (1966). Cereals and schizophrenia – data and hypothesis. *Acta Psychiatr. Scand.* **42,** 125

Dohan, F. C. (1969) Schizophrenia: possible relationship to cereal grains and celiac disease. In S. Sankar (ed.) *Schizophrenia: Current Concepts and Research*, p. 539 (Hicksville, N.Y.: P. J. D. Publications, Ltd.)

Dohan, F. C. (1970). Coeliac disease and schizophrenia. (Letter) *Lancet*, **i,** 897

Dohan, F. C. (1973). Coeliac disease and schizophrenia. (Letter) *Am. J. Psychiatry*, **130,** 1400

Dohan, F. C. (1976). The possible pathogenic effect of cereal grains in schizophrenia – Celiac disease as a model. *Acta Neurol.* **31,** 195

Dohan, F. C., Grasberger, J., Lowell, F., Johnston, H. Jr. and Arbegast, A. (1969). Relapsed schizophrenics: More rapid improvement on a milk and cereal-free diet. *Br. J. Psychiatry*, **115,** 595

Dohan, F. C. and Grasberger, J. C. (1973). Relapsed schizophrenics: Earlier discharge from the hospital after cereal-free, milk-free diet. *Am. J. Psychiatry*, **130,** 685

Dohan, F. C., Levitt, D. and Kushnir, L. (1976). *Pavlov J. Biol. Sci.*, (In press)

Food and Agriculture Organization of the United Nations (1970). *Amino Acid Content of Foods and Biological Data on Proteins*. (Rome: FAO)

Frazer, A. C. (1956). Discussion on some problems of steatorrhea and reduced stature; on the growth defect in coeliac disease. *Proc. R. Soc. Med.*, **49,** 1009

Gottesman, I. and Shields, J. (1967). A polygenic theory of schizophrenia. *Proc. Nat. Acad. Sci. USA*, **58,** 199

Graff, H. and Handford, A. (1961). Celiac syndrome in the case history of five schizophrenics. *Psychiatr. Q.*, **35,** 306

Guth, P. S., Amaro, J., Sellinger, O. Z. and Lloyd, E. (1965). Studies *in vitro* and *in vivo* of the effects of chlorpromàzine on rat liver lysosomes. *Biochem. Pharmacol.*, **14,** 769

Hekkens, W. Th. J. M. and Peña, A. S. (1974). *Coeliac Disease*. Proceedings of the Second International Coeliac Symposium. (Leiden: H. E. Stenfert Kroese B. V.)

Hemmings, C., Hemmings, W. A. and Patey, A. L. (1976). The fate of the oral doses α-gliadin in suckling and adult rats. *IRCS Med. Sc.*, **4,** 39

Jos, J., Lenoir, G., de Ritis, G. and Rey, J. (1975). *In vitro* pathogenetic studies of coeliac disease. *Scand. J. Gastroenterol.*, **10,** 121

Käser, H. (1961). Diagnose und Klinik der Coeliake. *Ann. Paediatr.*, **197,** 320

Kowlessar, O. D. (1968). Personal communication.

Kowlessar, O. D., Warren, R. E. and Bronstein, H. D. (1970). Celiac disease: Enzyme defect or immune mechanism? In G. B. J. Glass (ed.). *Progress in Gastroenterology*, p. 409. (New York: Grune and Stratton)

Levine, R. A., Briggs, G. W., Harding, R. S. and Nolte, L. B. (1966). Prolonged gluten administration in normal subjects. *N. Engl. J. Med.*, **274,** 1109

McCrae, W. M. (1970). The inheritance of coeliac disease. In C. C. Booth and R. H. Dowling (eds.). *Coeliac Disease*, p. 55. (London: Churchill Livingstone)

Mann, J. G., Brown, W. R. and Kern, F. Jr. (1970). The subtle and variable clinical expressions of gluten-induced enteropathy (adult celiac disease, nontropical sprue). *Am. J. Med.*, **48,** 357

Marks, J., Burkett, D., Shuster, S. and Roberts, D. F. (1970). Small intestinal abnormalities in relatives of patients with dermatitis herpetiformis. *Gut*, **11,** 493

Marx, J. L. (1975). Learning and behaviour – I. Effects of pituitary hormones, II. The hypothalamic peptides. *Science*, **190,** 367 and 544

Paulley, J. W. (1959). Emotion and personality in the etiology of steatorrhea. *Am. J. Dig. Dis.*, **4**, 352

Phelan, J. J., McCarthy, C. F., Stevens, F. M., McNicholl, B. and Fottrell, P. F. (1974). The nature of gliadin toxicity in coeliac disease: A new concept. In W. Th. J. M. Hekkens and A. S. Peña. (eds.). *Coeliac Disease*, p. 60. (Leiden: Stenfert Kroese)

Rubin, C. (1973). Personal communication.

Singh, M. M. and Kay, S. R. (1976). Wheat gluten as a pathogenic factor in schizophrenia. *Science*, **191**, 401.

Stevens, F. M., Lloyd, R., Geraghty, S., Reynolds, M., Sarsfield, J., Wright, R. and McCarthy, C. F. (1975). Proceedings: Schizophrenia and coeliac disease: Is there a positive relationship? *Irish J. Med. Sci.*, **144**, 75.

Strober, W., Falchuk, Z. M., Rogentine, G. N., Nelson, D. L. and Klaeveman, H. L. (1975). The pathogenesis of gluten enteropathy. *Ann. Intern. Med.*, **83**, 242

Townley, R. R. and Anderson, C. M. (1967). Coeliac disease – A review. *Ergeb. Inn. Med. Kinderheilk.*, **26**, 1

Townley, R. R., Cornell, H. J., Bhathal, P. S. and Mitchell, J. D. (1973). Toxicity of wheat gliadin fractions in coeliac disease. *Lancet*, **i**, 1363.

Weijers, H. A., van de Kamer, J. H. and Dicke, W. K. (1957). Celiac disease. In S. Z. Levine (ed.). *Advances in Pediatrics*, p. 277. (Chicago: Year Book Publishers)

Weinstein, W. M. (1974). Latent celiac sprue. *Gastroenterology*, **66**, 489

Weser, M. M. and Douglas, A. P. (1976). An alternative mechanism for gluten toxicity in coeliac disease. *Lancet*, **i**, 567

Yates, P. L. (1960). *Food, Land and Manpower in Western Europe*. (London: MacMillan).

Zmijewski, C. and Dohan, F. C. (1976). Unpublished.

POSTSCRIPT

Klee and his co-workers have recently reported *that a peptide fraction (exorphins), produced by the digestion of wheat gluten (or gliadin) with pepsin alone, has naloxone-reversible endorphin-like activity in their *in vitro* test systems, while another fraction antagonizes these effects. The peptides in both fractions deserve careful study because of the well-known behavioural effects of endorphins and other brain peptides. The authors point out that the peptides in both fractions are very hydrophobic, and show a predominance of leucine and isoleucine and contain phenylalanine and tyrosine but almost no charged amino acids. They suggest that such peptides 'might be expected to traverse biological membranes, including the blood brain barrier with relative ease'. Thus, investigators of the psychotoxic effects of gluten and gliadin peptides and their passage across the gut barrier should direct their attention not only to the most common (glutamine, glutamic acid, proline-rich) peptides produced during digestion, but also to unusual peptides such as those described by Klee and his associates.

*Klee, W. A., Zioudrou, C. and Streaty, R. A. (1978). Exorphins – Peptides with opioid activity isolated from wheat gluten and their possible role in the etiology of schizophrenia. In: E. Usdin (ed.). *Endorphins in Mental Health Research.* (New York: Macmillan)

16

Some insights into the pathogenesis of schizophrenia

M. M. SINGH

INTRODUCTION

As has been usual throughout the history of human knowledge, numerous, often strongly held views tend to proliferate about the nature and causes of phenomena that are poorly understood but somehow seem imperative to 'know'. So it has been with schizophrenia – a profound and incapacitating disorder that usually afflicts youth, is world-wide in occurrence and involves about one per cent of any generation through its lifetime. There are many hypotheses but relatively few established facts about this condition, and some even argue its existence as a clinical entity. One could say with some surety that schizophrenic phenomena are mediated by the brain but that, like ordinary phenomena, they probably result from actions on the brain of stimuli from without or within, of ordinary or extraordinary kinds, for all behaviour is a product of interactions between the organism and its environment. Beyond that, the only hard facts about the syndrome called schizophrenia are: that genetic factors are aetiologically important (Kety, 1976) but operate in as-yet-unknown ways, and that several groups of chemicals – neuroleptics – act as relatively specific 'antischizophrenic' agents but are neither completely effective nor capable of 'curing' the illness forever (Cole and Davis, 1968; Singh and Smith, 1973a).

It was with an awareness of this kind that we began our researches in schizophrenia in the winter of 1969. The starting point was the use of neuroleptic treatment as a research tool to understand the nature of the processes or components that were drug-responsive and those which were drug-resistant. From the outset, we reminded ourselves of the need to take a broad, multifaceted approach to the problem in the hope that a synthesis might emerge from the small insights provided by different methods and viewpoints. Also, we proceeded with the belief that a longitudinal method of study, in which each patient served as his own control, was preferable to the usual cross-sectional test group versus control group method, because with the marked phenomenological, nosological, prognostic and possibly aetiological diversity of schizophrenia, it offered a greater promise of finding meaningful differences between patients that might be lost in the variabilities of samples in the cross-sectional approach (Singh, 1973).

METHODS

The essential method consisted of observing groups of schizophrenics, first drug-free and then with individually titrated dosages of neuroleptics for three months or more, within a therapeutically active, carefully organized ward programme which permitted control of environmental variables and an observation of patients within a variety of social, recreational and work situations (Singh, 1973). The patient selection required a clear-cut diagnosis of schizophrenia, age between 18 and 50 years, exclusion of epilepsy, organic brain diseases and other relevant somatic diseases, and a severity of illness that justified extended hospitalization. Periodically throughout the study, measurements were made for the clinical signs and symptoms of schizophrenia after at least an hour-long interview, for social functions within the context of various free-ranging and structured activities, and for certain biological functions such as sleep and resting pulse rate (Singh and Smith, 1973a; Singh, 1973; and Singh and Kay, 1975a). As work progressed, a number of special tests or rating scales were developed from the knowledge gained. These included a series of cognitive tests based on Piaget's developmental theory (Kay and Singh, 1975; Kay *et al.*, 1975), a temporal measure of attention or the ability to concentrate (Kay and Singh, 1974) and a number of ethologically-based measures of social behaviour (Singh and Gang, 1974). All the studies followed a longitudinal research design with each patient being compared with himself at different stages in the course of treatment.

ANTICHOLINERGIC–NEUROLEPTIC ANTAGONISM

The first finding of note from this work came from a chance observation, as do most scientific findings, suggesting that anticholinergic anti-Parkinsonism drugs, so frequently given to schizophrenics to counteract the extra-

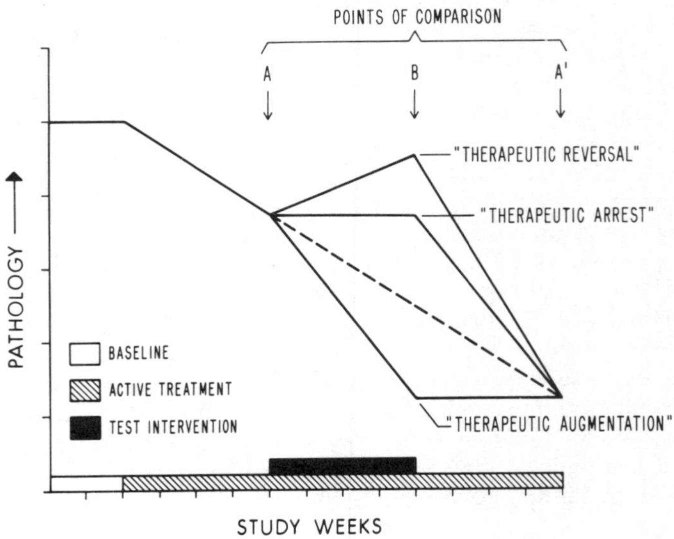

Deviation from the expected clinical course $= B - \frac{A+A'}{2}$

Figure 1 Research design. Downward curve indicates progressive decline in severity of psychopathology pyramidal side effects of medication, may have the more serious consequence of antagonizing the primary therapeutic effects of the neuroleptics. We systematically investigated this possibility in three studies (Singh and Kay, 1975a, Singh and Smith, 1973b; Singh and Kay, 1975b; Singh and Kay, 1975c; Singh and Kay, .in press) according to the method illustrated in Figure 1.

A predetermined dose of anti-Parkinsonism medication such as benztropine (two studies) or trihexyphenidyl (one study) was given non-blind (one study) or double-blind (two studies) for a specified period along the course of neuroleptic treatment, while holding the neuroleptic dosage factor constant. A period on neuroleptic alone both preceded (A) and followed (A′) the period on neuroleptic plus anti-Parkinsonism drug (B). If the test intervention had a countertherapeutic effect, the expected downward therapeutic curve would plateau or deflect upward with the intervention and then resume a downward course with the end of the intervention. The difference between B and an average of A+A′, using ratings at the end of each period, will give us the degree of deviation from the expected course. These differences calculated individually for each patient can then be subjected to statistical analysis with correlated *t* test. The data can also be analysed non-parametrically with a chi-square test comparing the number of patients showing therapeutic reversals, i.e. $B>(A+A')/2$, with those showing therapeutic augmentations, $B<(A+A')/2$.

Figure 2 illustrates the findings from the most detailed and the best controlled of the three studies (Singh and Kay, 1975a; Singh and Kay, 1975b and Singh and Kay, in press). It involved 18 schizophrenics, two prototypic neuroleptics – haloperidol and chlorpromazine – in a double-blind cross-over research design and three 2-week courses of benztropine, 4 mg per day, given 'double-blind' – one in the last two weeks of a 4-week baseline placebo period and one each in the middle two weeks of the two 6-week neuroleptic periods, which were separated by a 2-week placebo period for the cross-over. The relative dosages of haloperidol and chlorpromazine were 1 to 50. The solid line is for the nine patients who first received haloperidol and then crossed over to chlorpromazine, while the dotted line is for the nine who began with chlorpromazine and then switched over to haloperidol.

The following observations could be made: (1) Benztropine interventions were generally attended with upward deflections of the curves, that is, therapeutic reversals. (2) Benztropine alone worsened the clinical state and, when combined with neuroleptics, it reversed the therapeutic course. (3) In some instances, (e.g. thought disorganization; poor insight; poor rapport and blunting of affect) the clinical worsening with total neuroleptic withdrawal during the cross-over placebo weeks was less conspicuous than that with the addition of benztropine to neuroleptics. (4) Therapeutic changes with haloperidol were more dramatic than those with chlorpromazine (e.g. thought disorganization and social participation).

Statistical analyses of data from this study suggested that haloperidol was faster in action and more effective over a wide range of parameters than

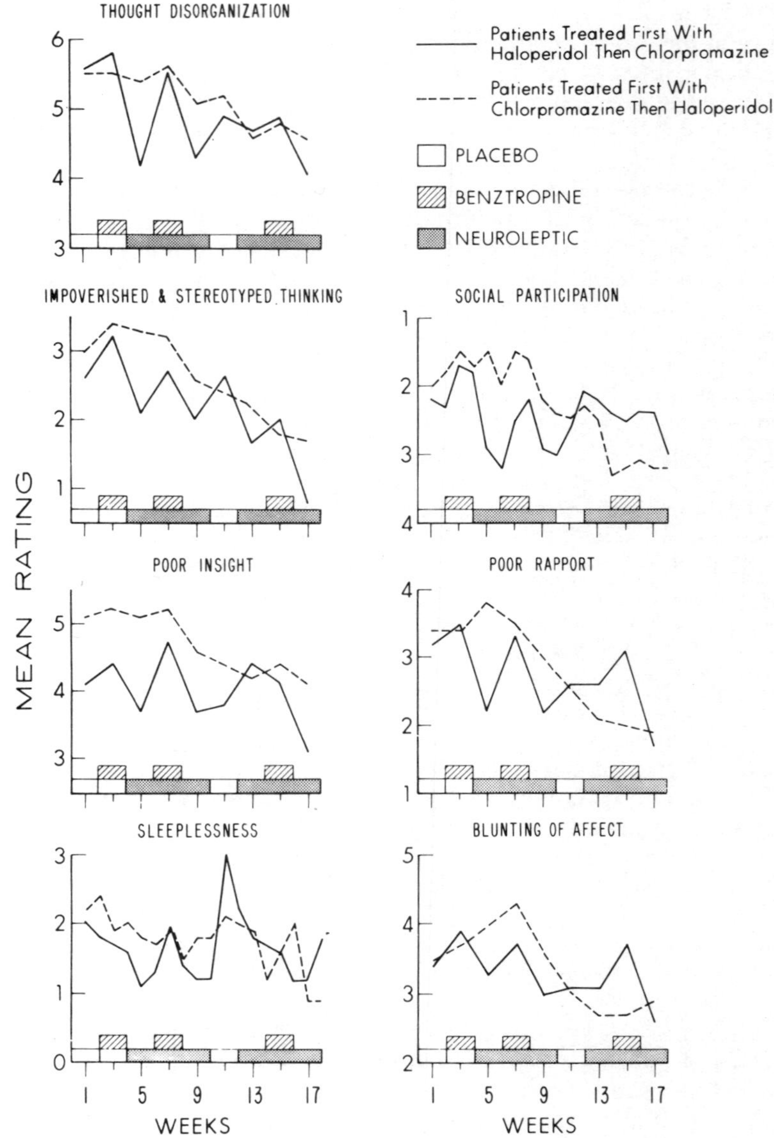

Figure 2 Countertherapeutic effects of benztropine when given alone under baseline placebo conditions and when added to ongoing treatment with haloperidol and chlorpromazine. Plateauing or upward deflections of the curves indicate a countertherapeutic change

chlorpromazine, and that treatment with chlorpromazine was much more susceptible to the countertherapeutic benztropine effect than that with haloperidol (Singh and Kay, 1975a). Data from a subsequent study, in which haloperidol and chlorpromazine, in a nearly 1 to 100 dosage ratio, were longitudinally compared over a 14-week treatment period in matched groups of 10 schizophrenics each, confirmed both these points (Singh and Kay, 1975c). Trihexyphenidyl, 6 mg per day, was the anticholinergic used in that study. These findings are of particular interest in that chlorpromazine, a low-potency, high-dose neuroleptic, has much more built-in anticholinergic activity than haloperidol, which is a high-potency, low-dose neuroleptic. This would suggest that inherent anticholinergic activity may be an important determinant of potency differences among the neuroleptics (Singh and Kay, 1975a; Singh and Kay, 1975c).

The data on anticholinergic–neuroleptic interactions from these two and an earlier study, with a combined sample of 47 subjects, could be analysed together because they had 28 clinical measures in common (Singh and Kay, in press). The significant results of correlated t tests (two-tailed) as well as the chi-square tests, are shown in Table 1.

Table 1 Countertherapeutic effects of anti-Parkinsonism drugs on the course of therapeutic changes in schizophrenia. Significant results of parametric (correlated t test) and nonparametric (chi-square) analyses are shown. n=47 (Combined sample from three studies)

Dimension	*Parametric analysis* t	p	*Non-parametric analysis* x^2	p
Social withdrawal	1.49	—	9.10	<0.01
Uncooperativeness	1.76	<0.10	11.56	<0.001
Hostility/belligerence	0.94	—	4.18	<0.05
Disorganized thinking	2.65	<0.05	6.00	<0.02
Bizarre and unusual thought content	2.88	<0.01	7.34	<0.01
Suspiciousness and paranoid ideas	2.08	<0.05	6.00	<0.02
Difficulty in abstract thinking	2.08	<0.05	2.58	—
Delusions	2.10	<0.05	1.32	—
Suicidal ideas and actions	.13*	—	4.46	<0.05
Disorientation	2.34	<0.05	8.04	<0.01
Disturbance of volition	1.35	—	6.54	<0.02
Sleeplessness	2.80	<0.01	12.46	<0.001
Pulse rate	2.43*	<0.05*	6.54*	<0.02*

Notes: (1) Tests performed on the differences between ratings in the period of anti-Parkinsonism drug intervention and an average of ratings in the periods before and after the intervention when patients received neuroleptic alone. Asterisked figures represent therapeutic augmentation in relation to the intervention
(2) Based on Singh and Kay (in press)

Apart from the pulse rate, which was significantly slowed during the anticholinergic interventions, the significant changes all indicated that anticholinergics antagonized the antipsychotic effects of neuroleptics. The clinical features most consistently worsened by them seemed to be those which characteristically and consistently show the therapeutic activity of neuroleptics (Cole and Davies, 1968; Singh and Smith 1973 a; Singh and Kay, 1975 a; Singh and Kay, 1975 c), thus suggesting a direct and rather specific antagonism between the two types of drugs. This was further brought into relief by the analyses of the data in terms of prognostic and therapeutic outcome subclassifications of patients (Singh and Kay, 1978).

The patients who were prospectively classified as schizophreniform according to Langfeldt's system and thus predicted to have favourable prognosis, and those who actually showed favourable treatment response, predominantly accounted for the significant therapeutic reversals with anti-Parkinsonism agents, thus suggesting that anticholinergics serve to increase the particular components of schizophrenic psychosis on which the neuroleptics have their specific therapeutic effects.

Table 2 Countertherapeutic effects of anti-Parkinsonism drugs in relation to prognostic classification and therapeutic outcome in schizophrenia

Dimension	*Prognostic classification*		*Therapeutic outcome*	
	Schizophreniform (*n*=19) *p*	*Nuclear* (*n*=28) *p*	*Favourable* (*n*=28) *p*	*Unfavourable* (*n*=19) *p*
Social withdrawal	<0.05	–	<0.02	–
Uncooperativeness	<0.02	–	<0.01	–
Disorganized thinking	<0.10	<0.10	<0.10	<0.10
Impoverishment and stereotypy of thought	<0.05	–	<0.02	–
Difficulty in abstract thinking	—	–	<0.05	–
Poor judgment and insight	<0.10	–	—	–
Delusions	—	<0.10	—	<0.05
Bizarre and unusual thought content	<0.02	–	<0.002	–
Suspiciousness and paranoid ideas	<0.05	–	<0.02	–
Disorientation	<0.05	–	<0.05	–
Disturbance of volition	<0.02	–	—	–
Blunting of affect	—	–	<0.01	–
Motor retardation	—	–	–	<0.10*
Sleeplessness	—	<0.002	–	<0.02
Pulse rate	<0.05*	–	–	<0.05*

Notes: (1) The results of correlated *t* test (two-tailed) analyses of the effects of anti-Parkinsonism drugs on the therapeutic course are shown. Asterisked figures represent therapeutic augmentation

(2) Based on Singh and Kay, (1978)

Consistent with this, of the three diagnostic types of schizophrenia, the catatonics, who are probably the most treatment-responsive schizophrenics, were those most involved in the countertherapeutic anticholinergic effects.

These studies of ours on the anticholinergic–neuroleptic antagonism in schizophrenics are supported by a number of studies in animals which show that almost all the behavioural pharmacological effects which predict antipsychotic activity are reversed by a variety of anticholinergics. These include conditioned avoidance response suppression (Hanson *et al.*, 1970), inhibition of amphetamine and apomorphine excitation and stereotypies (Scheel-Krüger, 1970; Fjalland and Møller-Nielsen, 1974), inhibition of amphetamine plus L-dopa induced mouse jumping (Colpaert *et al.*, 1975), and brain self-stimulation suppression (Wauquier *et al.*, 1975). It has further been reported that cholinomimetics potentiate the relevant behavioural effects of neuroleptics in animals (Scheel-Krüger, 1970) and tend to produce similar effects when given alone (Pfeiffer and Jenney, 1957). In schizophrenics, it has been observed that central muscarinic stimulation has effects resembling those seen with neuroleptics (Pfeiffer and Jenney, 1957) and can reverse the methylphenidate induced exacerbation of psychosis (Janowsky *et al.*, 1973).

So it seems that anticholinergics and neuroleptics act antagonistically in schizophrenia. Besides the obvious practical implications, this observation points to the involvement of some cholinergic brain mechanisms in the pathogenesis of the schizophrenic psychosis and its response to treatment.

A great deal of biochemical work in recent years has focussed attention on the actions of neuroleptics on the dopamine neuronal systems coursing between the midbrain, basal ganglia and limbic structures. In particular, it has been suggested that their receptor blocking actions on the mesolimbic dopamine pathways may be important for the antipsychotic activity of neuroleptics and that functionally the dopamine systems may be overactive in schizophrenia (Randrup and Munkvad, 1972; Snyder *et al.*, 1974; Stevens, 1973). The mesolimbic dopamine neurones are part of the medial forebrain bundle system which generally seems involved in the facilitation and repetition of behaviours (Stein, 1968). In a reciprocal relationship to this seems to be a cholinergic system, the so-called periventricular system, which acts, rather like the neuroleptics, to block the repetitious behaviour fostered by the medial forebrain bundle stimulation (Stein, 1968). Behavioural studies in animals suggest that anticholinergics interfere with the process of habituation or adaptation to repeated stimuli, and produce an intrusion of unrewarded responses into the behavioural repertoire (Carlton, 1968). Drugs such as amphetamines, which increase catecholaminergic activity, also have similar effects. At the same time, poor habituation, repetitiousness of behaviour and irrelevant responses are characteristics shown by schizophrenics (Shakow, 1971), so that it is very possible that actions on a reciprocal catecholaminergic –cholinergic system, such as the medial forebrain bundle and the periventricular system, are at the basis of the therapeutic actions of neuroleptics and the reversal of these effects by anticholinergics. The facility with which quite small amounts of anticholinergics were found in our studies to counteract the established therapeutic effects of fairly large amounts of neuroleptics may even indicate that primary neurobiological failures involve mechanisms which incorporate cholinergic pathways at some level and that the neuroleptics produce their therapeutic effects indirectly by acting on dopamine neurones that engage in a reciprocal relationship with these pathways. This may also mean that the hypothesized dopaminergic hyperactivity is relative rather than absolute – a conjecture that would be consistent with failure to find biochemical evidence of increased central dopamine activity in acute unmedicated schizophrenics (Bowers, 1974; van Praag and Korf, 1975).

However, it must be recognized that neuroleptics are only partially effective in schizophrenia, so that mechanisms involved in their actions can, at best, provide a partial explanation for schizophrenia. It may even be that an understanding of the drug-resistant components, which seem to predominate in the more seriously and fundamentally ill patients, will lead to more basic insights into the pathogenesis of this condition.

THE NATURE OF THE DRUG-RESISTANT COMPONENT OF SCHIZOPHRENIA

In looking for ways to characterize the drug-resistant aspects of schizophrenia, we were impressed by the fact that poor prognosis patients are often those with an early, slow and insidious onset of illness and a long history of premorbid failures (Gittelman-Klein and Klein, 1969), and that cognitive and social defects remaining after treatment in many ways resemble the premorbid styles of functioning in schizophrenics (Singh and Smith, 1973 a; Singh, 1973). This suggested that ontogenetic factors may be important in the pathogenesis of schizophrenia. Therefore, we devised a series of simple cognitive tests which could elicit responses related to various stages of intellectual development described by Piaget. These were repeatedly administered along the course of various studies mentioned earlier, and were also given to healthy volunteers (Kay and Singh, 1975, 1975; Kay *et al.*, 1975; Singh and Kay, 1976 a).

Table 3 Percentages of schizophrenics who, after 14 weeks of neuroleptic treatment, still scored abnormally on the three cognitive tests based on Piaget's developmental theory: Colour–Form Preference (CFP) test, Colour–Form Representation (CFR) test and Egocentricity of Thought (EOT) test

Test	*Diagnostic class*			*Prognostic class*		*Therapeutic outcome*		
	Heb. (%)	*Par.* (%)	*Cat.* (%)	*Nucl.* (%)	*Schizo.* (%)	*Poor* (%)	*Good* (%)	*Total* (%)
CFP *n*=31 Perseveration to Form 60–93%	79	11	38	75	20	75	20	48
CFR (*n*=50) 0–80%	79	47	57	55	57	64	48	56
EOT (*n*=50) 0–2	59	40	38	42	53	44	48	46

Notes: (1) Abbreviations: Heb.=Hebephrenic; Par.=Paranoid; Cat.=Catatonic; Nucl.=Nuclear schizophrenia; Schizo.=Schizophreniform psychosis
(2) Scores on test considered abnormal if below the norm determined on healthy individuals
(3) Based on Kay and Singh (1975), Kay *et al.* (1975) and Singh and Kay, (1976a)

The first of these tests, the *Colour–Form Preference* (CFP) test, requires matching one of three test cards with a standard card. One of the test cards matches for colour and another for the form of the standard, while the third is a no-match (Kay and Singh, 1975). This test depicts the earliest four stages of cognitive development: *purposeless perseveration* (up to 8 months), *random responding* (8 months to 1 year), classification by the single attribute of colour *(colour dominance)*, normally seen mainly in children of 2–4 years, and then by form *(form dominance)*, which becomes the preferential style between 4–7 years.

In schizophrenics, the first two types of responses, seen particularly in catatonics, seem to be mostly a function of the drug-responsive psychotic process. The colour dominance, that is the cognitive style of 2–4 year olds, is seen most typically and persistently in hebephrenics. Paranoids show very little abnormality on this test.

After 14 weeks of neuroleptic treatment, nearly 80% of hebephrenics and nuclear schizophrenics show some measure of abnormality on this test and account for most of the residual deficits among schizophrenics. In contrast, the paranoids seem to be largely free from cognitive deficits related to the preconceptual and preverbal cognitive stages depicted by the CFP.

The Colour–Form Representation (CFR) test measures the conceptualization by figural representation, which normally supersedes the classification by colour or form alone after about age 7 years (Kay *et al.*, 1975) and is the maturer style probably related to verbal language development, where a symbol comes to stand for the totality of a situation. The 'correct' responses on this test are those in which a test card is matched to the standard (a red circle with an embedded key) in terms of the representational cue (e.g., key, fish) rather than colour or form (Kay *et al.*, 1975).

This test provided the most effective discrimination between patients and healthy adults, with 90% of schizophrenics scoring abnormally before treatment and nearly 60% after treatment. Paranoids also were now abnormal both before and after treatment. However, hebephrenics still greatly outnumbered others in terms of residual deficits, but the deficits were about equally distributed between the prognostic and outcome subgroups.

Thus the results of the two tests (CFP and CFR) considered together indicated that whereas hebephrenics showed residual abnormalities related to both pre-verbal and verbal stages of development, those in paranoids were related mostly to the later verbal stages, and the catatonics probably were mixed in this respect. Nuclear, poor outcome patients resembled the hebephrenics, while others resembled the paranoids and catatonics.

The third test, the *Egocentricity of Thought* (EOT) test represents four stages of the maturation of right–left, subject–object positional concepts that normally develop between ages 5–11 years (Kay and Singh, 1975). Before treatment, 84% of schizophrenics scored either '0' (that is, unable to tell their own right from left). '1' (unable to tell another's right from left), or '2' (unable to tell positional relationships between various objects on a table) – that is, they corresponded in performance, respectively, to the stages of preconceptual thinking (less than 5 years), egocentric thinking (5–8 years) or socialized thinking (8–11 years) but were lacking in objective thinking that matures around 11 years (score 3=all three positional tests passed). After treatment, 46% had residual deficit which were distributed much in the same way as were those on CFR (Singh and Kay, 1976a).

So it seemed that hebephrenic and nuclear cases showed persistently primitive cognitive styles related to both early and later stages of development while the paranoid and schizophreniform cases had deficits related mainly to the later stages corresponding to language development. The catatonics mostly fell into the latter category but perhaps included some of the hebephrenic cases with catatonic features. This would suggest that the disease process probably begins much earlier in the hebephrenic and nuclear schizophrenics – perhaps as early as the first two years of life – than in others and is, therefore, associated with more profound developmental defects.

Testing in a group of 5–12 year old children (n=14) at *high risk for schizophrenia* has shown significantly lower levels of performance on the EOT test than seen in ordinary children at similar age periods. Indeed none of the high risk children scored beyond 1 on this test. They also scored quite poorly on a draw-a-person test, thus suggesting considerable problems in developing positional concepts, body image and subject–object differences.

Repeated behavioural measures of *sleeplessness* were taken every night in all our studies, and a *resting pulse rate* was recorded first thing each morning to provide indices of arousal or levels of excitation within the central nervous system. Before treatment, the catatonics showed the highest sleeplessness and pulse rate, the paranoids had moderate sleeplessness but near-normal pulse rate, while the hebephrenics had the least sleeplessness but moderately accelerated pulse rate. Calculating the post-treatment reduction in psychopathology as a percentage of the baseline scores showed that the catatonics had the highest percentage decrease in pathology, paranoids were next, while the hebephrenics had the lowest percentage decrease, and hence the largest residual deficit (Singh and Kay, 1976a). The treatment-responsive component thus seemed to correspond to the degree of over-arousal, especially as reflected in sleeplessness.

From findings such as these, it seems that the drug-responsive component in schizophrenia may be associated with an increased level of arousal or excitation within the central nervous system, particularly as it manifests in sleeplessness, and that this may be a relatively non-specific disorganizational or psychotic component, while the drug-resistant factor or factors may be largely of developmental origin and account for many of the differences between various forms of schizophrenia.

WHEAT GLUTEN AS A PATHOGENIC FACTOR

To be able to say that drug-resistant aspects of schizophrenia may be of developmental origin means that at least some rather incapacitating and perhaps more fundamental components of the disease evolve slowly during different stages of childhood growth. This does not, however, tell us what really causes the disease. Similarly, the knowledge that hereditary factors are important in this condition points to the possibility of a biochemical or metabolic abnormality as the basis of schizophrenia but it does not indicate the exact nature of such an abnormality.

To consider if a clue to these unknowns may be contained in Dr Dohan's hypothesis, which he has discussed in these proceedings, we performed the next study to be reviewed (Singh and Kay, 1976b). The research method was essentially the same as we had previously used in demonstrating the counter-therapeutic effects of anti-Parkinsonism medication (Figure 1). Fourteen schizophrenic subjects, selected as described before, were studied under carefully controlled conditions. From the day of admission to the research ward, the patients received a strict diet free of all cereal-grain and milk products, and throughout the period of study the patients were kept under close supervision. They were not studied all together; rather they entered the programme on a staggered schedule so that any results obtained could not be due to some coincidental factors or behavioural contagion affecting all patients at any time. For at least two weeks, each patient was observed drug-free and then he was placed on individually-titrated therapeutic dosages of haloperidol or occasionally a haloperidol and chlorpromazine combination for the next 12 weeks. During these 12 weeks, he received daily, in divided doses, a 'special drink'. Neither the patients, nor the raters knew the nature or composition of these drinks. In the first and last four weeks, i.e. periods A and A′, the drinks contained soy flour as a control substance, while in the middle four weeks, i.e. period B, the drinks contained 30 to 45 g a day of wheat gluten as the test substance. In other words, the patients were

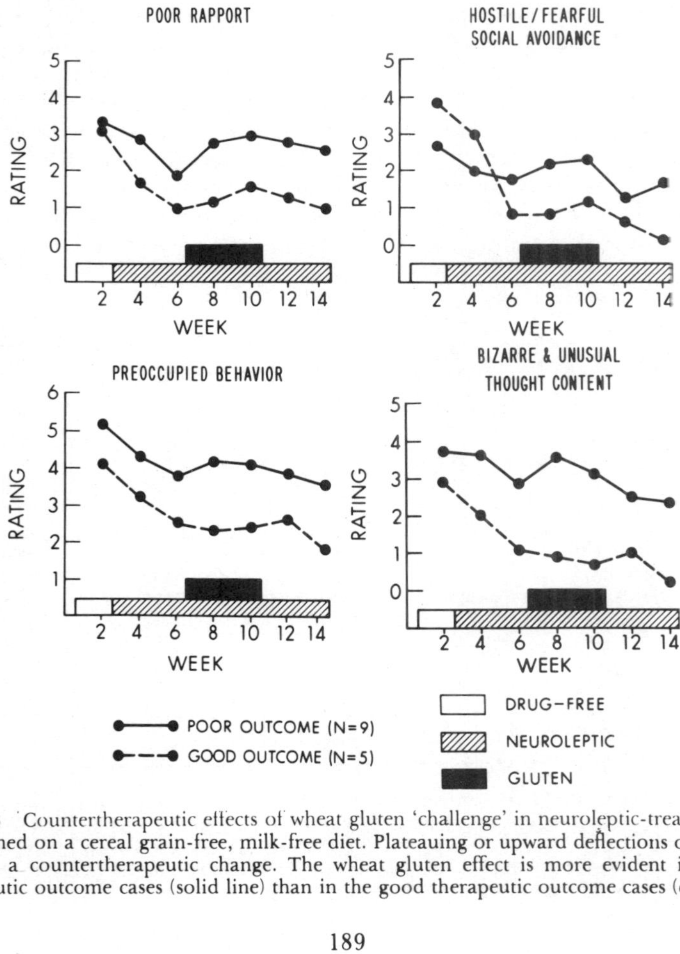

Figure 3 Countertherapeutic effects of wheat gluten 'challenge' in neuroleptic-treated patients maintained on a cereal grain-free, milk-free diet. Plateauing or upward deflections of the curves indicate a countertherapeutic change. The wheat gluten effect is more evident in the poor therapeutic outcome cases (solid line) than in the good therapeutic outcome cases (dotted line)

challenged with wheat gluten to determine if it would have an adverse effect on the therapeutic course. The results were analysed by comparing ratings at the end of the gluten period (B) with the combined average of ratings at the end of the pre-gluten (A) and post-gluten (A′) periods. Each patient served as his own control.

Every two weeks, the patients were rated on 33 dimensions of psychopathology after a 90 minute interview. Twice daily, five days a week, ratings were performed on five specially designed social avoidance behaviour scales on the basis of ongoing day-to-day social transactions of patients, and on a social participation scale on the basis of a structured programme of recreational activities. Before the study, each patient received a diagnostic and prognostic classification, while at the end of his stay on the research ward he was assessed for overall therapeutic outcome. In addition, I maintained detailed clinical notes independently of the ratings performed by various raters.

Ten out of 14 patients were clinically judged to have shown moderate to complete regression to the pre-treatment level of pathology, or worse, during the period of wheat gluten challenge. Statistical analyses suggested the same. Considering the data for each patient separately, the parameters in which B exceeded (A + A′)/2 were counted as 'therapeutic reversals' or hypothesized countertherapeutic effects and compared with others. In ten cases, the reversals outnumbered the other effects. However, the countertherapeutic gluten effects, unlike the anticholinergic effects described earlier, seemed much more in evidence in the poor therapeutic outcome cases. Eight out of nine poor therapeutic outcome patients belonged to the group in which therapeutic reversals outnumbered other ($p<0.02$) whereas only two out of

Table 4 Wheat gluten effects on psychopathology

Dimension	*t*	*p*
Preoccupied behaviour	2.72	<0.01
Hostile/fearful social avoidance	2.22	<0.02
Poor rapport	2.25	<0.02
Poor impulse control	1.38	<0.10
Poor judgment and insight	1.90	<0.05
Difficulty in abstract thinking	2.63	<0.02
Stereotyped thinking	1.35	<0.10
Bizarre and unusual thought content	1.45	<0.10
Tension state	2.19	<0.02
Anxiety	1.89	<0.05
Depression	1.40	<0.10
Elation	1.59	<0.10
Altered state of awareness	1.46	<0.10
Passive or apathetic withdrawal	1.71*	<0.10*

Notes: (1) Significant results of correlated *t* tests (one-tailed) on differences between end of gluten period ratings and an average of those at the end of pre-gluten and post-gluten periods are shown. All execpt one (marked with asterisk) of these supported the hypothesis that wheat gluten challenge exacerbated the schizophrenic process.
(2) Based on Singh and Kay, (1976b); (to be published)

five good outcome cases belonged to this group (Singh and Kay, to be published). Figure 3 illustrates this and, of course, the fact that wheat gluten challenge was attended with clinical worsening in neuroleptic-treated patients.

Table 4 shows the significant results of correlated *t* tests (one-tailed) on psychopathology ratings. These suggested that the most prominent changes with wheat gluten challenge consisted of an increase in autistic preoccupation, social avoidance, alienation from reality, impulsiveness, responsiveness to autistic experiences, vague, concrete and stereotyped thinking, bizarre ideas and a tense, fearful and unhappy state of being. Fundamental aspects of schizophrenia – aspects that would be particularly prominent in the nuclear or process type of schizophrenia – were thus enhanced by wheat gluten.

Since the social functions were very frequently rated, they could be subjected to Cox–Stuart tests of trend. The day and evening ratings were analysed separately for the three periods. There were no significant improvements during the gluten period, while nine out of the 12 measures showed improvement in the pre-gluten period and five did so in the post-gluten period. There was one significant trend towards deterioration in the gluten period and one in the post-gluten period. It could be concluded, therefore, that the wheat gluten challenge had had the effect of arresting therapeutic progress in terms of social parameters (Singh and Kay, to be published).

Thus it seemed that wheat gluten challenge had been countertherapeutic but that the wheat gluten effects contrasted with those we had earlier found with anticholinergic medication within a similar research framework. Using the previously discussed formulation, one could say that whereas anticholinergics increased the drug-responsive component of schizophrenia and directly antagonized the neuroleptic action, wheat gluten tended especially to increase the drug-resistant components and probably did not directly affect the neuroleptic activity. The latter was also suggested by the observation that the undesirable pharmacological effects of the medication were as frequent during the gluten period as they were during the gluten-free periods.

CONCLUDING REMARKS

We should be reminded at this point that the neuroleptics are only partially effective in schizophrenia. Also, it is well-known that if they are withdrawn, even after long periods, active manifestations of the disease tend to resurface, suggesting that the primary disease process remains active while the neuroleptics seem able to suppress or block some of its manifestations. The neuroleptics, therefore, probably act at a level removed from the primary site of origin of the disease process, and the mechanisms on which they act perhaps participate in only a part of what we see as the manifest condition. In terms of brain organization, this level will have to be on the distal or effector side of the disease site, so that without affecting the primary disease process, the neuroleptics can block or attenuate its manifestations.

On the other hand, the wheat gluten (and other cereal grain glutens), if proven to be pathogenic, will be expected to affect the primary site.

If one considers a reciprocal catecholaminergic–cholinergic neuronal system, such as that comprised of medial forebrain bundle and periventricular system within the brainstem, as the site where neuroleptics act to produce therapeutic effects and the anticholinergics to antagonize those effects, then the primary disturbance may be located in one or more of the limbic structures such as the hippocampus, septum and amygdala which seem to represent the next, and in terms of adaptive capability, very crucial level in the brain organization. Analysing the limbic functions within a three-level evolutionary brain model, Isaacson (1974) has recently suggested that these structures, comprising the middle or paleomammalian level, exercise a modulatory, essentially inhibitory control over the primitive or 'instinctual' mechanisms of the brainstem (the protoreptilian brain) which tend to respond to situations in immediate, automatic and inflexible ways acquired in the past from genetic programming or learning. Major cholinergic pathways are contained in them which may operate in part by enhancing the activity of the periventricular suppressor system (Stein *et al.,* 1972).

Many of the characteristic adaptational defects noted in schizophrenics (Shakow, 1971) bear close resemblance to what Isaacson (1974) has described as the consequences of the failure of paleomammalian functions. Included in these are: the tendency of such patients to react to recurrent or old situations as if they were new ones – failure to habituate, and to respond to new situations as if they were recent past ones – perseveration. They 'cling' to the old, according to Shakow (1971), and have marked 'neophobia' or difficulty in dealing with new situations or contingencies of life. They show considerable disturbance in the processes of arousal and attention, for irrelevancies from the recent and distant past, especially those emotionally charged, keep engaging them into various 'minor sets', segmentalizing the external and internal environments, and making it very difficult to achieve 'major sets' or a state of focussed alertness and preparedness needed for optimal response to any situation. The past forever keeps dominating and intruding on the present – a state of affairs much like what Isaacson (1974) believes happens with the failure of paleomammalian controls on the primitive protoreptilian systems.

According to Isaacson's model, paleomammalian failure will have two main consequences; a release of the primitive or instinctual mechanisms and an ability of the highest level in the mammalian brain organization – the neocortex or neomammalian brain – to perform its adaptive functions of thought and language, because for that it needs the paleomammalian control of protoreptilian mechanism. Elkes. (1961), over a decade ago, described these two factors – the emergence of primitive modes of behaviour and the failure of higher order functions of thought and language – to be the principal ingredients of the schizophrenic picture, and suggested that they both resulted from a failure of some crucial discriminative inhibitory mechanisms within the brain organization. It may well be, therefore, that the primary source of pathological process in schizophrenia is one or more of the paleomammalian structures which serve the crucial discriminative inhibitory functions in the brain. Some direct evidence for this has come from the work of Heath (1954) who has found abnormal electrical activity in the septal region in schizophrenics. Heath and Krupp (1967) have also reported immunoglobulin deposits in the same area in schizophrenic brains, but this finding has not been confirmed.

A disorder of paleomammalian functions beginning early in childhood could seriously interfere with the developing higher level cognitive and social functions leading to more or less permanent defects of the type that comprise the drug-resistant components of this disease. Wheat gluten and other cereal grain glutens would be plausible culprits for an exogenous pathogenic factor in genetically predisposed persons as they are part of our diet from early years. However, the main determinant of the onset and perhaps severity of the disease is likely to be the genetic susceptibility, as these proteins in themselves are quite harmless to a vast majority of humans even in large amounts.

With some optimism, therefore, it may be suggested that at least a faint outline of a neurobiological model that could explain the pathogenesis of schizophrenia is beginning to emerge. However, one must add a note of caution. Our findings on wheat gluten and to a lesser degree on anticholinergic–neuroleptic interactions are at this stage only preliminary observations. These findings, much less the hypotheses based on them, cannot be considered as proven until they have been confirmed by much more further work. What we can say is that they provide hopeful clues to the pathogenesis of schizophrenia.

ACKNOWLEDGEMENTS

The work described in this paper represents the combined effort of many persons who worked on the Clinical Psychopharmacology Unit, Bronx Psychiatric Center, 1500 Waters Place, Bronx, New York 10461. In particular, Stanley R. Kay, M.A., was an important partner in the studies. Special thanks are due to Barbara Mason for the manuscript preparation at very short notice.

REFERENCES

Bowers, M. B. (1974). Central dopamine turnover in schizophrenic syndromes. *Arch. Gen. Psychiatry,* **31,** 50

Carlton, P. L. (1968). Cholinergic mechanisms in the control of behaviour by the brain. In *Psychopharmacology—a Review of Progress 1957–1967.* D. H. Efron *et al.* (eds.) pp. 125–135 (Washington, D.C.: U. S. Government Printing Office)

Cole, J. O. and Davis, J. M. (1968). Clinical efficacy of the phenothiazines as antipsychotic drugs. In *Psychopharmacology—a Review of Progress 1957–1967.* D. H. Efron, *et al.* (eds.) pp. 1057–1063 (Washington, D.C.: U. S. Government Printing Office)

Colpaert, F. C., Wauquier, A., Niemegeers, C. J. E. and Lal, H (1975). Reversal by a central anticholinergic drug of pimozide-induced inhibition of mouse jumping in amphetamine dopa-treated mice. *J. Pharm. Pharmacol.* **27,** 536

Elkes, J. (1961). Schizophrenic disorder in relation to levels of neural organisation: The need for some conceptual points of reference. In *The Clinical Pathology of Nervous System.* J. Folch-Pi (ed.) pp. 648–665. (London: Pergamon Press)

Fjalland, B. and Møller-Nielsen, I. (1974). Methyl-phenidate antagonism of haloperidol: Interaction with cholinergic and anticholinergic drugs. *Psychopharmacologia (Berlin),* **34,** 111

Gittelman-Klein, R. and Klein, D. F. (1969). Premorbid asocial adjustment and prognosis in schizophrenia. *J. Psychiatr. Res.,* **7,** 35

Hanson, H. M., Stone, C. A. and Witoslawski, J. J. (1970). Antagonism of antiavoidance effects of various agents by anticholinergic drugs. *J. Pharmacol. Exp. Ther.,* **173,** 117

Heath, R. G. (1954). *Studies in Schizophrenia.* (Cambridge USA: Harvard University Press)

Heath, R. G. and Krupp, I. M. (1969). Schizophrenia as an immunological disorder. *Arch. Gen. Psychiatry,* **16,** 1

Isaacson, R. L. (1974). *The Limbic System.* (New York: Plenum Press)

physostigmine and methylphenidate in man. *Am. J. Psychiatry,* **130,** 1370

Kay, S. R. and Singh, M. M. (1974). A temporal measure of attention in schizophrenia and its clinical significance. *Br. J. Psychiatry,* **125,** 146

Kay, S. R. and Singh, M. M. (1975). A developmental approach to delineate components of cognitive dysfunction in schizophrenia. *Br. J. Social Clin. Psychol.,* **14,** 387

Kay, S. R., Singh, M. M. and Smith, J. M. (1975). Colour–form representation test: A developmental method for the study of cognition in schizophrenia. *Br. J. Social Clin. Psychol.,* **14,** 401

Kety, S. S. (1976). Genetic aspects of schizophrenia. *Psychiatric Ann.,* **6,** 11

Pfeiffer, C. C. and Jenney, E. H. (1957). The inhibition of the conditioned avoidance response and counteraction of schizophrenia by muscarinic stimulation of the brain. *Ann. NY Acad. Sci.,* **66,** 753

Randrup, A. and Munkvad, I. (1972). Evidence indicating an association between schizophrenia and dopaminergic hyperactivity in the brain. *Orthomolec. Psychiatry,* **1,** 2

Scheel-Krüger, J. (1970). Central effects of anticholinergic drugs measured by the apomorphine gnawing test in mice. *Acta Pharmacol. Toxicol.,* **28,** 1

Shakow, D. (1971). Some observations on the psychology (and some fewer, on the biology) of schizophrenia. *J. Nerv. Ment. Dis.,* **153,** 300

Singh, M. M. (1973). Psychopharmacological study of schizophrenia—Some ways out of an impasse. A case study with haloperidol, *Int. Pharmacopsychiatry,* **8,** 80

Singh, M. M. and Smith, J. M. (1973a). Kinetics and dynamics of response to haloperidol in acute schizophrenia: A longitudinal study of the therapeutic process. *Compr. Psychiatry,* **14,** 393

Singh, M. M. and Smith, J. M. (1973b). Reversal of some therapeutic effects of an antipsychotic agent by an anti-Parkinsonism agent. *J. Nerv. Ment. Dis.,* **157,** 50

Singh, M. M. and Gang, R. C. (1974). An ethological model of schizophrenia—A preliminary investigation. *Dis. Nerv. Syst.* **35,** 157

Singh, M. M. and Kay, S. R. (1975a). A comparative study of haloperidol and chlorpromazine in terms of clinical effects and therapeutic reversal with benztropine in schizophrenia. Theoretical implications for potency differences among neuroleptics. *Psychopharmacologia (Berlin),* **43,** 103

Singh, M. M. and Kay, S. R. (1975b). Therapeutic reversal with benztropine in schizophrenics: Practical and theoretical significance. *J. Nerv. Men. Dis.,* **160,** 258

Singh, M. M. and Kay, S. R. (1975c). A longitudinal therapeutic comparison between two prototypic neuroleptics (haloperidol and chlorpromazine) in matched groups of schizophrenics. Non-therapeutic interactions with trihexyphenidyl. Theoretical implications for potency differences. *Psychopharmacologia (Berlin),* **43,** 115

Singh, M. M. and Kay, S. R. (1976a). Cognitive and social dysfunctions in schizophrenia within an ethological developmental framework. Paper presented at the Annual Convention of Society of Biological Psychiatry, San Francisco, California, June 10–13, 1976

Singh, M. M. and Kay, S. R. (1976b). Wheat gluten as a pathogenic factor in schizophrenia. *Science*, **191**, 401

Singh, M. M. AND Kay, S. R. (1978). Nosological and prognostic classification of schizophrenia—Pharmacological validation in terms of therapeutic antagonism between anticholinergic anti-Parkinsonism agents and neuroleptics. *Neuropsychobiology*, **4**, 288

Singh, M. M. and Kay, S. R. (1978). Therapeutic antagonism between anticholinergic anti-Parkinsonism agents and neuroleptics in schizophrenia. Systematic evidence from three studies and implications for a neuropharmacological model. *Neuropsychobiology*, (In press)

Singh, M. M. and Kay, S. R. (to be published). Wheat gluten as an exogenous factor in the pathogenesis of schizophrenia.

Snyder, S. H., Banerjee, S. P., Yamamura, H. I. and Greenberg, D. (1974) Drugs, neurotransmitters and schizophrenia. *Science*, **184**, 1243

Stein, L. (1968). Chemistry of reward and punishment. In *Psychopharmacology—a Review of Progress 1957–1967*. D. H. Efron, *et al.* (eds.). pp. 105–123*a* (Washington, D. C.: U.S. Government Printing Office)

Stein, L., Wise, C. D. and Berger, B. D. (1972). Noradrenergic reward mechanisms, recovery of function and schizophrenia. In *The Chemistry of Mood, Motivation and Memory*, J. L. McGaugh, (ed.). pp. 81–103. (New York: Plenum Press)

Stevens, J. R. (1973). An anatomy of schizophrenia? *Arch. Gen. Psychiatry*, **29**, 177

Van Praag, H. M. and Korf, J. (1975). Neuroleptics, catecholamines, and psychoses: a study of their interrelations. *Am. J. Psychiatry*, **132**, 593

Wauquier, A., Niemegeers, C. J. E. and Lal, H. (1975). Differential antagonism by dexetimide of inhibitory effects of haloperidol and fentanyl on brain self-stimulation. *Psychopharmacologia (Berlin)*, **41**, 229

17

Nutrition and schizophrenia: Implications and problems

J. W. T. DICKERSON

INTRODUCTION

There is some truth in the old adage that 'we are what we eat', for the structural components of our bodies are derived from the building materials supplied in the diet. The energy to drive the complex mechanisms responsible for bodily function are likewise derived from the food that we eat. In the last decade or so there has been considerable interest in the relationship of nutrition to brain growth, development and function (Dickerson, 1978). It is now appreciated that nutrient deficiencies during the first 2 years or so of postnatal life may have their sequel in poor function later. But this is not the aspect of the problem of the inter-relationships of nutrition and the brain with which we are now concerned. In the present state of knowledge it is not possible to say that malnutrition in early life is an aetiological factor in any psychiatric disorder.

However, it has long been known that disturbed mental function is characteristic of certain vitamin deficiencies. Thus, a long-term deficiency of thiamin, accompanied by deficiencies of other nutrients, results in the Wernicke–Korsakoff syndrome in which there may be irreversible damage to the brain. Dementia is one of the characteristic three 'D's of the disease, pellagra, caused by a deficiency of niacin. Deficiencies of folic acid and vitamin B_{12} also result in damage to the central nervous system.

The genetically transmitted 'inborn errors of metabolism', of which phenylketonuria (PKU) and galactosaemia are possibly the best known examples, also result in brain damage and impaired mental function. Inborn errors of metabolism usually result from the deficiency of a particular enzyme that results in the inability to metabolize a dietary component which then causes damage by accumulation as in PKU, or in the inability to metabolize certain tissue components, as in the lipidoses. However, there are certain very rare inborn errors of metabolism in which it seems that the enzyme present has a much higher than normal requirement for a co-factor – these are the vitamin-responsive metabolic disorders (see Scriver and Rosenberg, 1973). The first example of this group of disorders to be described was a pyridoxine (vitamin B_6) dependency which results in intractable convulsions (Hunt *et al.*, 1954).

With this as a background I want now to discuss the possible relationships of nutrition and schizophrenia. The fundamental cause of these conditions is at present, I believe, unknown. As far as the involvement of nutrition is concerned, I would like to suggest somewhat of a parallel with coronary heart disease, for as in this disease, so too in schizophrenia, the involvement of nutrition is probably multifactorial.

FOOD ALLERGIES AND SCHIZOPHRENIA

Coeliac disease

It is now 30 years since Wallen (1948) described the presence of food aversion in behaviour disorders. However, the first clue that diet might be associated with schizophrenia came from the epidemiological studies of Dohan (1966). These seemed to indicate that the number of cases of schizophrenia admitted to psychiatric institutions fell during World War II in those countries in which bread was rationed, whereas there was no change in other countries with no rationing. He postulated that this association could be due to an association of a sensitivity to wheat gluten with schizophrenia. Sensitivity to this protein, or more specifically to a small fraction of it, causes coeliac disease, a disorder with a convincing familial tendency. In this disorder, the finger-like villi of the intestinal mucosa become flattened, and the symptoms of coeliac disease reflect a breakdown of the dual function of the intestine. The small intestine is the route of absorption of the products of digestion, and a major symptom of coeliac disease is malabsorption, but it also acts as a barrier to the entry into the body of unwanted materials and some of the symptoms of coeliac disease – anorexia, nausea, headaches are due to a breakdown of this barrier function.

Dohan and his colleagues (Dohan *et al.*, 1969) reported that patients with schizophrenia improved faster on a gluten-free, milk-free diet. This work has been repeated more recently by Singh and Kay (1976) in a double-blind cross-over study in New York. It does seem that some patients will benefit from such a dietary regime. Few patients with schizophrenia may show evidence of malabsorption like that demonstrated in coeliac disease by measurement of faecal fat or the xylose absorption test. It may well be that in those patients that respond to a gluten-free, milk-free regime, the intestinal mucosa is permeable to peptides, or indeed proteins, that are not normally absorbed. It is interesting in this connection to recall that at birth the intestine of a number of species of mammals is permeable to intact protein, and that this mechanism then shuts off after a few hours or days, depending on the species. Dr Hemmings, I know, is very interested in the continuance of some 'leak' in the intestine through into adult life. Here I return to my analogy with coronary heart disease, for workers in South Wales (Davies *et al.*, 1974) have demonstrated a raised titre of antibodies to milk protein in the blood of patients with myocardial infarction. The availability of a simple test for the identification of patients with a sensitivity to gluten would greatly assist in the identification of patients likely to respond to dietary therapy. Anand *et al.* (1977) have published a preliminary report of a skin test for coeliac disease using a sub-fraction of gluten which might be extremely useful in patients with schizophrenia.

For those patients whose mental condition is associated with an allergy to wheat gluten, the adoption of a gluten-free diet offers a means of keeping them well. There are a number of very helpful books of recipes for those on this diet (e.g. Hills, 1977), and it is a good practical suggestion for the whole family to adopt it. Catering is easier, and there is less chance of mistakes. Moreover, the patient is not made to feel 'odd' so that there is less risk of psychological upset.

Other allergies

It may well be, however, that only a few patients will respond to a gluten-free, or even to a gluten-free, milk-free diet. The work of Randolph (1974) and others in the United States, and of Mackarness (1976) in this country has, I believe, shown beyond reasonable doubt that some patients with psychiatric disorders may be allergic to other common foods, or to environmental pollutants (Randolph, 1970). The diagnosis of such allergies requires time, and a form of individualized medicine that may be beyond the resources of a National Health Service. Randolph's method is to hospitalize the patient in a ward in which he is carefully protected from possible allergens, fast for 5 days with magnesium sulphate to clear out the gut, and then to feed foods in sequence one at a time. The preliminary fasting period heightens the sensitivity of the gut and, from personal conversations with patients who have had psychiatric disorders, I can testify that there is no doubt about an allergic response when it occurs. Many cases of hyperactivity and other disorders could be cured if it was possible to identify the cause and omit the particular food, or foods, from the diet. It is possible that some patients with schizophrenia may have similar allergies. In Randolph's view, an allergy should certainly be suspected if there is any evidence of an addiction to a particular food.

Feingold (1973) has proposed that hyperkinesis in childhood is associated with the ingestion of salicylates, of compounds which cross-react with salicylates and of common food additives, i.e. artificial flavours and colours. A double-blind cross-over trial of this hypothesis in 15 hyperkinetic children (Conners *et al.*, 1976) has yielded encouraging results, though the authors stress the need for caution in the interpretation of their results, and to the need for further objective evaluation.

FASTING

It is perhaps worth mentioning in this review that there have been claims that controlled fasting is beneficial in the treatment of schizophrenia (Cott, 1974). This treatment is based on the experience of Russian psychiatrists and particularly of Professor Yuri Nikolaev of Moscow. The fast consists of total abstinence from food for a period of 25–30 days. Patients may drink as much water as they like but they must take a minimum of one litre each day. A fast of this severity cannot be undertaken without medical supervision and when feeding is started the patient remains in hospital for a period equal to the duration of the fast. Initially, the diet consists of salt-free fruit, vegetables and milk. Meat, eggs and fish are excluded from the diet, and bread is not taken until the sixth or seventh day. Reporting on his experience up to 1973, Cott said in his 1974 paper that of 35 cases of schizophrenia treated in the period July 1970 to April 1973, 24 patients remained well to date.

MINERALS

Schizophrenia is thought by some to be associated with abnormal levels of minerals in the body, and particularly of copper and zinc (Pfeiffer and Ilieu, 1972). Hair is being used as a biopsy material to identify these abnormalities, and to monitor the progress of treatment with supplements or chelating agents, as appropriate. It should be stressed that the inter-relationships of the trace elements are extremely complex, and it may be too early to assess the value of this treatment since data is only available on individual cases. Indeed the pattern of disturbances may be so complex that it may be impossible to draw general conclusions. There is, however, a fair amount of evidence, both human and experimental, that lead pollution can result in various mental abnormalities including hyperkinesis and aggression.

VITAMINS

The administration of vitamins in 'mega' quantities was the original cornerstone for Pauling's concept of 'orthomolecular psychiatry' (Pauling, 1968). The idea that large amounts of niacin might prove beneficial in the treatment of schizophrenia had been introduced by Osmond and Hoffer (1962), and megavitamin therapy is often taken to be almost synonymous with 'niacin therapy'. Indeed the APA Task Force Report *Megavitamin and Orthomolecular Therapy in Psychiatry* (1973), in discussing vitamins, addressed itself solely to the use of niacin. However, most of the psychiatrists who use this form of treatment today use large doses of other vitamins (including ascorbic acid, pyridoxine, pantothenic acid, riboflavin, thiamin, folic acid and cyanocobalamin) in various combinations. These combinations are sometimes tailored to suit the individual patient, or are given in standard doses according to the condition. It should be understood also that few orthomolecular psychiatrists claim that the vitamins totally replace drugs. In many cases, the use of vitamins allows drug dosage to be reduced and side-effects minimised. As with the effects of a gluten-free diet, it seems highly likely that the choice of patient is very important, and as yet it seems that there are no tests that can reliably help to distinguish those patients who are likely to benefit from megavitamin therapy and those who will not. This is not a cheap alternative therapy, for vitamins in the quantities usually administered are expensive, and cannot at present be supplied on prescription.

The biochemical basis for the use of these large quantities of vitamins is difficult to understand. It has been argued that there may be enzymes present in schizophrenic subjects somewhat like those in vitamin-responsive metabolic disorders. However, Rosenberg (1973) points out that there are a number of points of contrast and the only case of schizophrenia so far reported in which the condition responded to a single vitamin was a specific defect in folic acid metabolism (Freeman *et al.*, 1975). The existence of such a condition may, however, be an encouragement to think more about the possibility of specific vitamin abnormalities as a cause of the condition.

TRYPTOPHAN

It is, of course, well-known that nicotinic acid can be synthesized in the body from tryptophan, and this amino acid is known to play a key role in the metabolism and function of the brain, for it is the precursor of the neuro-transmitter, serotonin. The demonstration by Fernstrom and Wurtman that the entry of tryptophan into the brain can be facilitated by a high carbohydrate diet, or insulin, has opened up new avenues of thought and research for those interested in the relationship of nutrition to brain function. It is likely that tryptophan is involved in schizophrenia, but its exact role seems not to be known.

However, the work carried out over the past decade or so in Detroit by Frohman and his colleagues on the S-protein seems to be of considerable interest. It is claimed (Cladwell *et al.,* 1974) that there is circulating in the blood of schizophrenics an α_2-globulin which is predominantly in an α-helix conformation. This protein differs in conformation from that isolated with the same techniques from control subjects and furthermore, in contrast to that isolated from normal subjects, it facilitates the cellular uptake of trypto-phan and 5-hydroxytryptophan into cells. This high entry of tryptophan into brain cells in turn is said (Gottlieb and Frohman, 1974) to result in the synthesis of abnormal amounts of *N,N′*-dimethyltryptamine (DMT) and other powerful hallucinogens. Control of the conformation and activity of the α_2-globulin is exerted by means of an anti-S-protein which is deficient in the brains of schizophrenics. In other words, some schizophrenics have this deficiency as an inborn error of metabolism. This work has very attractive possibilities for it has been possible to synthesize the active part of the anti-S-protein and work is now in progress to find whether the administration of this peptide will control the condition of patients with schizophrenia (C. E. Frohman, personal communication). Again, this approach to the problem may offer hope to a proportion of those who suffer with the disease.

LIPIDS

It has recently been suggested that schizophrenia may be a prostaglandin deficiency disease (Horrobin, 1977). This could be another possible inborn error of metabolism. Prostaglandins are synthesized from the essential fatty acids which are liberated from membrane phospholipids by the enzyme phospholipase A. Horrobin visualizes the possibility that there may be defective enzyme systems for converting the essential fatty acids in the diet to arachidonic and dihomo-γ-linolenic acid, the immediate precursors of some of the prostaglandins. Alternatively a deficiency of prostaglandins could result from defective phospholipase. If this hypothesis is true then the administration of a single fatty acid, arachidonic acid, may help patients with schizophrenia.

CONCLUSIONS

There are a number of leads to the involvement of nutrition in the treatment of schizophrenia. One, or more likely a combination, of these may be useful in the treatment of individual patients. In the absence of precise means of determination, a combination of dietary, vitamin and mineral therapy would seem to offer the best hope of success. These various therapies, together with the newer work suggesting the presence of inborn errors of metabolism, seem to underline the multifactorial nature of the schizophrenias, at any rate as far as nutrition is concerned.

REFERENCES

Anand, H. S., Truelove, S. C. and Offord, R. F. (1977). Skin test for coeliac disease using a subfraction of gluten. *Lancet*, **i**, 118

APA Task Force Report 7 (1973). *Megavitamin and Orthomolecular Therapy in Psychiatry*. (Washington D.C.: American Psychiatric Association)

Caldwell, D. F., Frohman, C. E., Thomas, N., Zellers, R., Arthur, R. E. and Gottlieb, J. S. (1974). The effects of the S-protein on intracranial self-stimulation in the rat. *Biol. Psychiatry*, **8**, 235

Conners, C. K., Goyette, C. H., Southwick, D. A., Lees, J. M. and Andrulonis, P. A. (1976). Food additives and hyperkinesis: A controlled double-blind experiment. *Pediatrics*, **58**, 154

Cott, A. (1974). Controlled fasting treatment for schizophrenia. *Orthomolec. Psychiatry*, **3**, 301

Davies, D. F., Johnson, A. P., Rees, B. W. G., Elwood, P. C. and Abernethy, M. (1974). Food antibodies and myocardial infarction. *Lancet*, **i**, 1012

Dickerson, J. W. T., (1978). Nutrition and disorders of the nervous system. In J. W. T. Dickerson and H. A. Lee. *Nutrition in the Clinical Management of Disease* (eds.), Ch. 13 (London: Arnold)

Dohan, F. C. (1966). Cereals and schizophrenia: Data and hypothesis. *Acta Psychiatr. Scand.* **42**, 125

Dohan, F. C., Grasberger, J. C., Lowell, F. M., Johnston, H. T. and Arbegas, A. W. (1969). Relapsed schizophrenics: more rapid improvement on a milk- and cereal-free diet. *Br. J. Psychiatry*, **115**, 595

Feingold, B. B. (1973). *Introduction to Clinical Allergy* (Springfield, Ill: Thomas)

Freeman, J. M., Finkelstein, J. D. and Mudd, S. H. (1975). Folate responsive homocystinuria and 'Schizophrenia'. *N. Engl. J. Med.*, **292**, 491

Gottlieb, J. S. and Frohman, C. E. (1974). Towards a biologic mechanism in schizophrenia In H. Mitsuda and T. Fukuda (eds.). *Biological Mechanisms in Schizophrenia and Schizophrenia-like Psychoses*, pp. 156–166 (Tokyo: Igaku Shoin)

Hills, H. C. (1977). *Good Food: Grain-free, Milk-free* (London: Roberts Publications)

Horrobin, D. F. (1977). Schizophrenia as a prostaglandin deficiency disease. *Lancet*, **i**, 936

Hunt, A. D. Jr., Stokes, J. Jr., McCrory, W. W. and Stroud, H. H. (1954). Pyridoxine dependency: Report of a case of intractable convulsions in an infant controlled by pyridoxine. *Pediatrics*, **13**, 140

Mackarness, R. (1976). *Not all in the Mind* (London: Pan)

Osmond, H. and Hoffer, A. (1962). Massive niacin treatment in schizophrenia: review of a nine year study. *Lancet*, **i**, 316

Pauling, L. (1968). Orthomolecular psychiatry. *Science*, **160**, 265

Pfeiffer, C. C. and Ilieu, V. (1972). A study of zinc deficiency and copper excess in the schizophrenias. *Int. Rev. Neurobiol.*, (suppl.), **1**, 141

Randolph, T. G. (1970). Domiciliary chemical air pollution in the etiology of ecologic mental illness. *Int. J. Soc. Psychiatry*, **16,** 243

Randolph, T. G. (1974). Ecologic mental illness. In H. Mitsuda and T. Fukuda (eds.). *Biological Mechanisms of Schizophrenia-like Psychoses*. pp. 13–21 (Tokyo: Igaku Shoin)

Rosenberg, L. E. (1973). Contrasts between vitamin-responsive inherited diseases and vitamin use in schizophrenia. In *Nutrition and Mental Function*. G. Serban (ed.). pp 259–262 (New York: Plenum)

Scriver, C. R. and Rosenberg, L. E. (1973). *Amino Acid Metabolism and its Disorders*. (Philadelphia: Saunders)
(Philadelphia: Saunders)

Singh, M. M. and Kay, S. R. (1976). Wheat gluten as a pathogenic factor in schizophrenia. *Science*, **191,** 401

Wallen, R. (1948). Food aversions in behaviour disorders. *J. Consult. Psychol.*, **12,** 310

18

The cytotoxic properties of wheat proteins

D. A. HUDSON

Ingestion of wheat gluten by subjects with coeliac disease produces local tissue damage in the upper small intestine which leads to a number of characteristic clinical, metabolic and biochemical disturbances (*Coeliac Disease*, 1970, and *Coeliac Disease*, 1974). Light and electron microscopic examination of biopsy tissue taken within 3–6 h after the intake of gluten reveals villous epithelial cells with swollen mitochondria often with distorted cristae, dilated endoplasmic reticulum and increased numbers of lysosomal bodies (Dissanayake *et al.*, 1974, and Lancaster-Smith *et al.*, 1975). In untreated cases, there is complete mucosal atrophy with no distinguishable villous shape, elongated crypt regions in which increased mitotic figures are evident and a considerable infiltration of the mucosa by cells of the lympho-plasmacytic series. The specific activities of various epithelial cell enzymes, including those associated with the microvillous membrane, are considerably reduced upon exposure to gluten or certain of its constituent proteins and peptides. Withdrawal of gluten from the diet leads to an eventual recovery of the tissue to its normal structural and functional characteristics.

The epithelial tissue damage resulting from gluten ingestion can be reproduced in *in vitro* systems. Short-term culture of mucosal biopsy tissue from coeliac subjects in the presence of soluble gluten constituents induces both morphological and biochemical effects similar to those observed under normal conditions (Jose *et al.*, 1974, and Townley *et al.*, 1973).

Because of the dramatic increase in the numbers of mucosal lymphocytes and plasma cells consequent upon exposure to gluten, it is perhaps hardly surprising that a number of immunological mechanisms have been invoked as primary causes of the local tissue damage. Thus, Asquith (1974) and Ferguson (1975) and their co-workers have provided some experimental data to suggest that it is the cell-mediated reactions of a local immune response to gluten which causes the characteristic villous atrophy and crypt hyperplasia of this condition. The early infiltration of mucosal tissue by neutrophils and eosinophils, with oedema, endothelial swelling in lamina propria capillaries and the prominence of smooth muscle fibres in the lamina propria provides, according to Doe, Henry and Booth (1974), histological evidence consistent with complement activation in the lamina propria. The nature of timing of this acute inflammatory reaction suggests that complement activation, probably by an antigen-IgM antibody reaction, may be responsible for the initiation of the gluten-induced mucosal lesion. Shiner (1973) suggests that ultrastructural changes in the basement membranes and capillary endothelium are compatible with a complex-mediated minimal response of the Arthus type. Others (Ezeoke *et al.,* 1974) have investigated the possibility that epithelial cell damage results from the action of antibody-dependent K-cell activity.

However, in contrast to these hypotheses, the possibility of there being a direct cytotoxic effect of gluten on the epithelial cell was suggested at an early stage of investigative studies and has by no means been refuted (Knowlessar *et al.,* 1970). Recently, Weiser and Douglas (1976) have attempted to explain all the known facts in terms of a surface effect of gluten on susceptible enterocytes. They suggest that some component or components of this protein mixture initiate a cytotoxic effect in the enterocyte of coeliac subjects through reactions with surface glycoproteins which, it is envisaged, have incomplete oligosaccharide chains. This hypothesis does not exclude the possibility of there being a peptidase deficiency in these cells as was suggested by earlier work. If partially digested peptides were to gain access to the cytosol in large quantities it is not difficult to envisage a metabolic disturbance possibly through the release of lysosomal enzymes.

A third broad possibility in the explanation of the mode of action of toxic gluten constituents has been provided recently (Green and Freed, 1976). In this, the primary defect in coeliac disease is the production of intestinal anti-gluten antibodies of poor avidity which delays the intracellular proteolysis of the peptide or peptides. The low-avidity antibody-antigen complex when deposited in the tissue fixes complement and causes inflammation. Toxicity, according to this hypothesis, is caused by gluten itself and by the hypersensitivity reaction.

In view of the possibility that certain gluten proteins or peptides may indeed exert a direct cytotoxic effect on the enterocytes of coeliac patients, experiments are being undertaken in this laboratory to examine this in purified cell populations. There are few studies to date concerned with specificity of the cytotoxic effect of gluten.

Thus, Sikora and co-workers (1976) have shown that a particular group of gluten peptides is capable of stimulating peripheral lymphocytes (as expressed by increased DNA synthesis) of coeliac subjects. Other attempts to demonstrate such an effect by other workers have not been entirely successful (Holmes *et al.,* 1976). Incubation of fibroblasts from coeliac subjects with gluten causes severe fatty degeneration without there being a comparable effect on fibroblasts from a group of control subjects (Gordone *et al.,* 1975). The response of various human cell lines to specific gluten peptides has recently been investigated in this laboratory (Hudson *et al.,* 1976).

Chromatographically separated peptides were incubated over a 24 h period with human embryonic intestinal, lung, kidney, adrenal and HEp-2 cells. Toxicity, in this system, was assayed with a microtitre tissue-culture system and the observed effects scored according to the confluence of the cell monolayer sheets. It was found that a number of peptide fractions exhibited some effect on these cell lines over this period at relatively low concentrations. The most active of the peptide groups examined, both in terms of the time required and initial concentration necessary to produce an observable effect, was that which had previously been shown to affect the morphological and functional characteristics of the intestinal epithelium when fed to coeliac subjects. Casein, β -lactoglobulin and bovine serum albumin produced no observable effects in control experiments. These observations thus indicate that certain gluten peptides may well possess non-specific cytotoxic effects under certain conditions.

The mechanism by which toxic gluten peptides produce a direct effect upon certain cell types independently of the immune system is not yet known. Weiser and Douglas have presented, in their hypothesis of the mode of action of gluten, an amount of information which suggests that cell surface alterations may account for relative susceptibility to toxic effects. In the experiments described above, all the cell lines used were neoplastic or embryonic. It is known that such cells possess cell surface characteristics which are distinguishable from the normal adult cell. Additionally, if the presence or absence of genetically determined histocompatibility antigens reflects intrinsic differences in cell surface characteristics, the apparent linkage between coeliac disease, i.e. susceptibility to toxic gluten components, and related conditions with certain histocompatibility antigens may be of significance.

REFERENCES

Asquith, P. (1974). Cell-mediated immunity in Coeliac Disease. In *Coeliac Disease*, W. Th. J. M. Hekkens and A. S. Peña (eds.) (Stenfert-Kroese)

Coeliac Disease (1970). C. C. Booth and R. H. Dowling (eds.) (London: Churchill Livingston)

Coeliac Disease (1974). W. Th. J. M. Hekkens and A. S. Pena (eds.) (Leiden: H. E. Stenfert-Kroese, B. V.)

Dissanayake, A. S., Jerrome, D. W., Offord, R. E., Truelove, S. C. and Whitehead, R. (1974). Identifying toxic fractions of wheat gluten and their effect on the jejunal mucosa in coeliac disease. *Gut,* **15,** 931

Doe, W. F., Henry, K. and Booth, C. C. (1974). Complement in coeliac disease. In *Coeliac Disease,* W. Th. J. M. Hekkens and A. S. Peña (eds.) pp. 189. (Leiden: Stenfert-Kroese)

Ezeoke, A., Ferguson, N., Fakhri, O., Hekkens, W. Th. J. M. and Hobbs, J. R. (1974). Antibodies in the sera of coeliac patients which can co-opt K-cells to attack gluten-labelled targets. In *Coeliac Disease.* W. Th. J. M. Hekkens and A. S. Peña (eds.) p. 176. (Leiden Stenfert-Kroese)

Ferguson, A., MacDonald, T. T., McClure, J. P. and Holden, R. J. (1975). Cell-mediated immunity to gliadin with the small-intestinal mucosa in coeliac disease. *Lancet,* **i,** 895

Gordone, G., Gemme, G., Comelli, A., Vianello, M. G. and Caladni, S. (1975). Peptidase and coeliac disease. *Lancet,* **i,** 807

Green, F. H. Y. and Freed, D. L. J. (1976). Gluten toxicity in coeliac disease. *Lancet,* **i,** 749

Holmes, G. K. T., Asquith, P. and Cooke, W. T. (1976). Cell-mediated immunity to gluten fraction III in coeliac disease. *Clin. Exp. Immunol.,* **24,** 259

Hudson, D. A., Cornell, H. J., Purdham, D. R. and Rolles, C. J. (1976). Non-specific cytotoxicity of wheat gliadin components towards cultured human cells. *Lancet,* **i,** 339

Jose, J., Lenoir, G., de Titis, G. and Rey, J. (1974. *In vitro* pathogenic studies of coeliac disease. *Scand. J. Gastroenterol,* **10,** 121

Kowlessar, O. D., Warren, R. E. and Bromstein, H. D. (1970). Coeliac disease: Enzyme defect or immune mechanism. In *Progress in Gastroenterology,* G. B. Jerzy (ed.) p.409 (London: Grune and Stratton)

Lancaster-Smith, M., Kumar, P. J. and Dawson, A. M. (1975). The cellular infiltrate of the jejunum in adult coeliac disease and dermatitis herpetiformis following the reintroduction of dietary gluten. *Gut,* **16,** 683

Shiner, M. (1973). Ultrastructural changes suggestive of immune reactions in the jejunal mucosa of coeliac children following gluten challenge. *Gut,* **14,** 1

Sikora, K., Anand, B. S., Truelove, S. C., Cictitira, P. J. and Offord, R. E. (1976). Stimulation of lymphocytes from patients with coeliac disease by a subfraction of gluten. *Lancet,* **ii**, 389

Townley, R. R. W., Bhathal, P. S., Cornell, H. J. and Mitchell, J. D. (1973). Toxicity of wheat gliadin fractions in coeliac disease. *Lancet,* **i**, 1362

Weiser, M. M. and Douglas, A. P. (1976). An alternative mechanism for gluten toxicity in coeliac disease. *Lancet,* **i**, 749

19

5-Hydroxytryptamine metabolism in coeliac disease

D. N. CHALLACOMBE

Interest in 5-hydroxytryptamine (5-HT) metabolism in children with coeliac disease began with the finding of increased urinary excretion of 5-hydroxyindoleacetic acid (5-HIAA) in adults with this disorder (Haverback and Davidson, 1958; Kowlessar *et al.,* 1958). 5-HT is synthesized from dietary tryptophan by enterochromaffin (EC) cells in the gastrointestinal tract and is broken down by the enzyme monoamine oxidase (MAO) to 5-HIAA, which is excreted in the urine. Raised blood levels of 5-HT have been reported in patients with untreated coeliac disease (Pimparker *et al.,* 1961; Warner and Cohen, 1962), and both blood 5-HT and urinary 5-HIAA levels fell to normal after the introduction of a gluten-free diet (Sleisenger, 1961). Increased urinary excretion of 5-HIAA and diminished excretion following a gluten-free diet were confirmed in children with coeliac disease, in 24 and 8 hour urine collections (Challacombe *et al.,* 1972; Challacombe *et al.,* 1975), and measurement of 8 hour urinary 5-HIAA was proposed as an aid to diagnosis. The possible origins of these abnormalities of 5-HT metabolism in the small intestine of patients with coeliac disease were therefore studied.

EC cells in sections of the duodenal mucosa, obtained by peroral biopsy from children with coeliac disease, were stained with alkaline diazonium and were counted by inserting a grid into the eye piece of a light microscope (Challacombe and Robertson, 1976). A final image magnification of ×250 was used and EC cell counts in coeliacs were compared with similar counts in normal duodenal biopsies. Significantly greater EC cell counts were found in patients with coeliac disease (Figure 1). In a group of children with a clinical history suggestive of coeliac disease but with minor villous changes in the duodenum on light microscopy, gluten challenge over ten days resulted in more severe histopathological changes and raised EC cell counts. As EC cells in the duodenum are mainly found in the crypts, and crypt-cell hyperplasia is a feature of coeliac disease, our findings may be secondary to generalised crypt-cell proliferation. Concentrations of 5-HT were also measured in duodenal biopsies from adults and children with coeliac disease and from a group of controls with normal biopsies, and increased tissue concentrations of 5-HT were found in patients with coeliac disease (Challacombe *et al.,* 1976) (Figure 2). In three children with coeliac disease who initially showed equivocal changes in the duodenal mucosa, gluten challenge over ten days resulted in increased tissue concentrations of 5-HT. Although increased tissue concen-

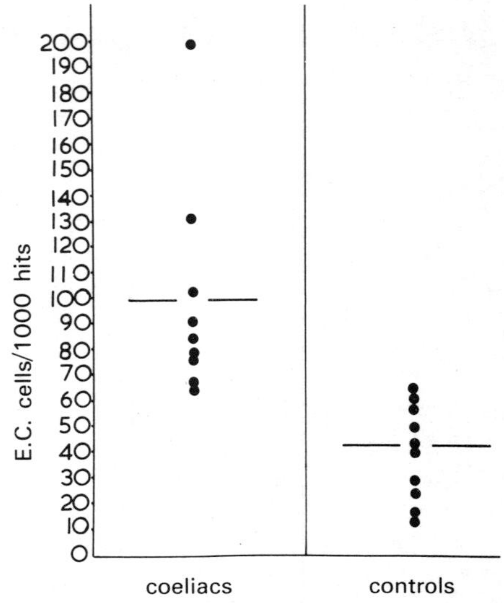

Figure 1 Elevated EC cell counts in coeliac disease patients

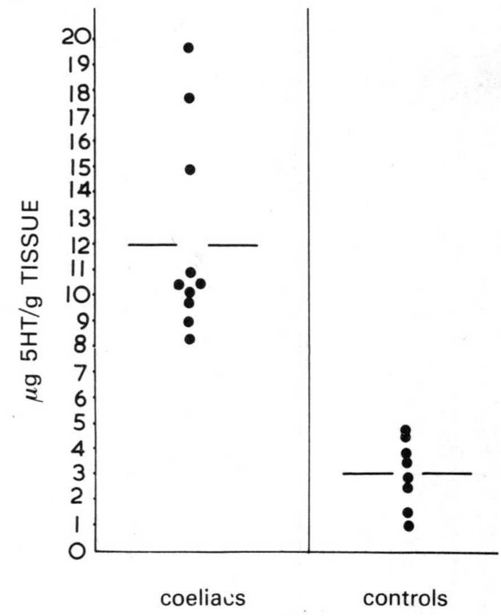

Figure 2 Elevated tissue concentrations of 5-HT in coeliac disease patients

trations may be secondary to EC cell hyperplasia, further studies will be necessary to exclude hyperactivity of individual EC cells.

Raised blood levels of 5-HT in patients with untreated coeliac disease may be caused by increased release of 5-HT from the small intestine into the

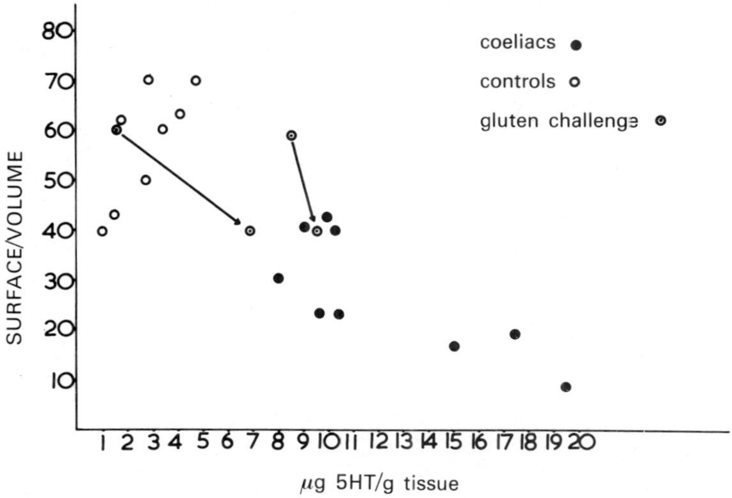

Figure 3 5-HT tissue concentration related to villous flattening using surface volume ratio

circulation, a finding which could also explain the finding of raised urinary excretion of 5-HIAA. Raised 5-HIAA levels however could also result from an increased rate of breakdown of 5-HT by monoamine oxidase. The activity of this enzyme has been studied and low concentrations were found in the duodenum of children with coeliac disease with normal levels in the platelets (Challacombe *et al.*, 1971). Increased monoamine oxidase activity is therefore unlikely to explain increased urinary excretion of 5-HIAA in coeliac disease.

Recent cell kinetic studies on the small intestine of rats (Tutton, 1974) have shown that 5-HT accelerates crypt-cell proliferation and shortens cell-cycle time. Similar abnormalities of cell kinetics have been reported in the duodenal mucosa of adults with coeliac disease (Wright *et al.*, 1973). While the cellular effects of 5-HT on the small intestine of rats may be species related, it is interesting to speculate whether increased local release of 5-HT in duodenal tissue in man is also responsible for villous flattening in coeliac disease. 5-HT concentrations in duodenal tissue have been related in our studies to the degree of villous flattening by the use of the surface : volume ratio (Dunnill and Whitehead, 1972). The lower the ratio (i.e. the flatter the villi) the higher the concentration of tissue 5-HT (Figure 3).

Although the findings of these studies may not have direct relevance to patients with schizophrenia, the depressed mood of children with untreated coeliac disease is an important diagnostic feature (Challacombe, 1971). Following withdrawal of gluten from the diet the mood improves during the first week and is often the first sign of recovery. If gluten is shown to be implicated in the aetiology of schizophrenia two possible mechanisms are suggested. Diminished activity of a surface epithelial enzyme in the small intestine, such as monoamine oxidase, could allow an overspill of potentially toxic amines from the intestinal lumen into the circulation, and lead to altered cerebral function (Challacombe, 1971). Alternatively, as published family studies of coeliac disease suggest that the incidence of this disease is greater among relatives of affected individuals than in the general population, and hereditary factors are also present in some patients with schizophrenia, an inborn error of amine metabolism may be present in the small intestinal mucosa, which is exacerbated by dietary gluten, leading to secondary abnormalities of cerebral metabolism.

REFERENCES

Challacombe, D. N. (1971). Coeliac disease and schizophrenia. *Lancet,* **i,** 89

Challacombe, D. N., Brown, G. A., Black, S. C. and Storrie, M. H. (1971). Increased excretion of 5-hydroxyindoleacetic acid in urine of children with untreated coeliac disease. *Arch. Dis. Child.,* **47,** 442

Challacombe, D. N., Dawkins, P. D. and Baker, P. (1976). Duodenal tissue concentrations of 5-hydroxytryptamine in coeliac disease. *Lancet,* **ii,** 522

Challacombe, D. N., Goodall, M., Gaze, H. and Brown, G. A. (1975). Urinary 5-hydroxyindoleacetic acid in 8 hour collections as an aid in diagnosis of coeliac disease. *Arch. Dis Child.,* **50,** 779

Challacombe, D. N. and Robertson, K. (1976). Enterochromaffin cells in the duodenal mucosa of children with coeliac disease. *Lancet,* **i,** 370

Challacombe, D. N., Sandler, M. and Southgate, J. (1971). Decreased duodenal monoamine oxidase activity in coeliac disease. *Arch. Dis. Child.,* **46,** 213

Dunnill, M. S. and Whitehead, R. (1972). A method for the quantitation of small intestinal biopsy specimens. *J. Clin. Pathol.,* **25,** 243

Haverback, B. J. and Davidson, J. D. (1958). Indole metabolism in the malabsorption syndrome. *Gastroenterology,* **35,** 570

Kowlessar, O. D., Williams, R. C., Law, D. H. and Sleisenger, M. H. (1958). Urinary excretion of 5-hydroxyindoleacetic acid in diarrheal states with special reference to nontropical sprue. *N. Engl. J. Med.,* **259,** 340

Pimparker, B. D., Senesky, D. and Kalser, M. H. (1961). Blood serotonin in nontropical sprue. *Gastroenterology,* **40,** 504

Sleisenger, M. H. (1961). Clinical and metabolic studies in nontropical sprue. *N. Engl. J. Med.,* **265,** 49

Tutton, P. J. M. (1974). The influence of serotonin on crypt cell proliferation in the jejunum of rat. *V. Arch. Abt. B. Zell. Pathol. (Berlin),* **16,** 79

Warner, R. R. P. and Cohen, N. (1962). Blood serotonin in malabsorption states. *Am. J. Dig. Dis.,* **7,** 553

Wright, N., Watson, A., Morley, A., Appleton, D., Marks, J. and Douglas, A. (1973). Cell-cycle time in the flat mucosa (avillous) of the human small intestine. *Gut,* **14,** 603

20

A preliminary investigation of dietary constituents and amphetamine-induced abnormal behaviour

M. TAYLOR

The influence of diet on brain metabolism has attracted great interest over recent years. In particular, investigators have concentrated on the relationship between dietary tryptophan intake and consequent changes in brain trypto-phan and 5-hydroxytryptamine levels (Wurtman and Fernstrom, 1975). Although dietary manipulation of tryptophan intake results in profound central changes in the rat, there is little evidence of corresponding behavioural effects in normal animals (Taylor, 1976). Recent evidence, however, has suggested that diet may act as a pathogenic factor in *abnormal* behaviour states in humans (Singh and Kay, 1976). Although there are no parallel abnormal behaviour states in animals, the stereotyped behaviour produced by high doses of amphetamine is thought to have features in common with some psychotic states (Randrup and Munkvad, 1967; Taylor *et al.*, 1974). As such, it offers a means of experimental investigation of the action of dietary constituents on abnormal behaviour in animals.

The preliminary experiments reported here investigate the effects of the essential amino acids tryptophan and methionine, and the gluten protein fraction γ -gliadin, on amphetamine-induced abnormal behaviour. All these agents have been implicated in the aetiology of abnormal behaviour states in humans.

Subjects were adult male Wistar rats weighing approximately 300–350 g, housed individually under normal lighting conditions with water available *ad lib.* Experimental groups consisted of seven rats. After 24 h food depriv-ation, three groups of animals were individually given access to 4 g of food in their home cage for an hour; the food was powdered standard diet (Purina Lab Chow) mixed with a 10 ml solution containing 120 mg L-tryptophan, 150 mg L-methionine or water. This was repeated a second day. A further group was given an injection (i.p.) of 0.1 mg/kg γ -gliadin, in a volume equivalent to 2 ml/kg body weight, which was followed half an hour later by access to 4 g of powdered food mixed with water. This was also repeated a second day. Ninety minutes after access to food on the second day, all animals received an injection of 10 mg/kg D-amphetamine (i.p.) in a volume equivalent to 2 ml/kg body weight.

Immediately after amphetamine injection, each rat was individually placed in an evenly illuminated open field (45 cm × 45 cm) where its behaviour was observed and recorded for one minute intervals every 5 min until 70 min after injection. A time-sampling 'all-or-nothing' system of recording was used, with the incidence of the following behaviour categories being noted: rearing, walking, sniffing, grooming, immobility, head movements, circling and backward walking (Taylor *et al.,* 1974). Frequency of occurrence of the behaviours within the one minute interval was not recorded. Summation of the categories rearing and walking was defined as 'active behaviour'.

The effects of the various pretreatment conditions on the amphetamine stereotyped behaviour are presented in Figure 1. All the conditions produced a significant reduction in the amount of active behaviour ($p < 0.05$) and a significant increase in the incidence of head movements ($p < 0.05$). No differences in the form of the stereotyped behaviour was apparent, but its latency of onset was much shorter after pretreatment with γ-gliadin, followed by methionine, and then tryptophan. No occurrence of circling or backward walking were noted. Replication of the above conditions without amphetamine injections revealed no effects on behaviour.

These results demonstrate that dietary constituents can have substantial effects on drug-induced behaviour. The experimental conditions served to increase the occurrence of stereotyped behaviour, both in terms of latency of onset and incidence of the 'abnormal' behaviour category of head

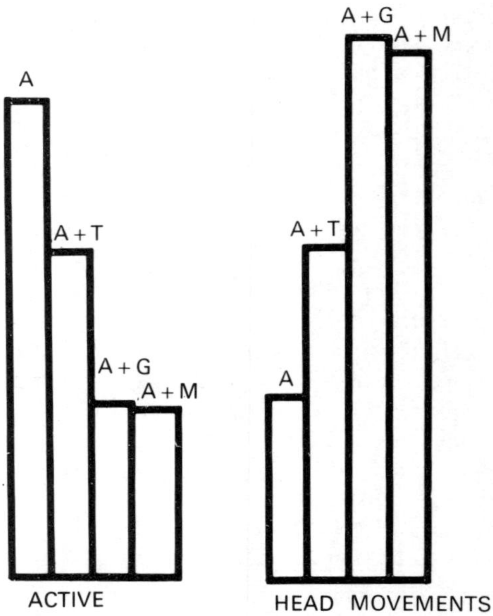

Figure 1 The incidence of amphetamine-induced-active behaviours and stereotyped head movements after the various pretreatment conditions. A=Amphetamine control. A+T=Amphetamine plus 120 mg L-tryptophan. A+G=Amphetamine plus 0.1 mg/kg γ-gliadin. A+M=Amphetamine plus 150 mg L-methionine

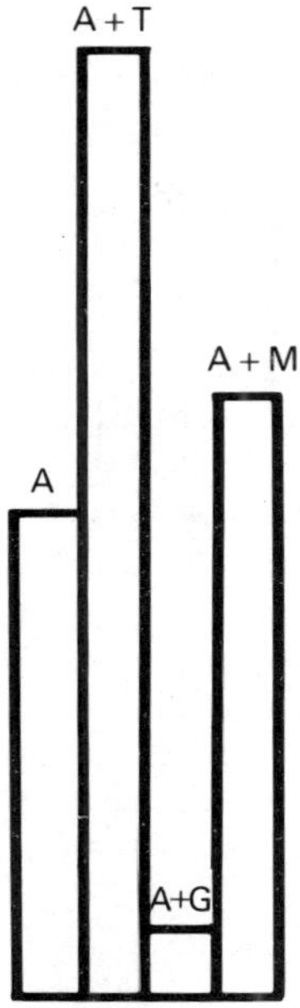

Figure 2 The incidence of amphetamine-induced active behaviour after the various dietary pretreatment conditions and after pretreatment with 0.5 mg/kg pimozide. A=Amphetamine control. A+T=Amphetamine plus 120 mg L-tryptophan. A+G=Amphetamine plus 0.1 mg/kg γ-gliadin. A+M=Amphetamine plus 150 mg L-methionine

movements. It is tempting to suggest this may result from some central interaction between the experimental conditions and the action of amphetamine. Other workers have drawn attention to the possible central actions of tryptophan and methionine, and some presumed central action may also be suggested for γ-gliadin. This view is supported by Hemmings *et al* (1976) who has reported the presence of large molecular breakdown products of orally ingested α-gliadin in brain tissue.

The occurrence of amphetamine stereotypy is dependent upon functional central dopaminergic systems (Creese and Iverson, 1975). Blockade of dopamine receptors might be expected to throw further light on the nature of the behavioural action of the above and therefore the initial experimental conditions were replicated, with pretreatment on the second experimental day, four hours before amphetamine injection, with a single dose of 0.5 mg/kg of the dopamine receptor blocker pimozide. The results of this are presented in Figure 2. The action of pimozide on amphetamine stereotypy was to completely eliminate stereotyped behaviour and to reduce the level of active behaviour. None of the experimental groups showed any evidence of stereotyped behaviour but considerable differences in active behaviours were apparent. No significant difference between control conditions and methionine treatment was evident, but tryptophan treatment resulted in a significant increase in active behaviour ($p<0.05$), wheras γ-gliadin resulted in a significant decrease in active behaviour ($p<0.05$). The γ-gliadin animals in particular showed very slow movements, holding positions for long periods.

The above suggests some distinctive interaction between the various treatment conditions and the action of amphetamine. It is particularly worthy of note that this interaction can take place with a very low dose of γ-gliadin.

Singh and Kay (1976). have demonstrated that diet may be an important factor in the pathogenesis of abnormal behaviour. The preliminary experiments outlined above show that drug-induced abnormal behaviour can be greatly influenced by dietary constituents, and it is suggested that this technique may be of great value in further investigations of the role of diet in abnormal behaviour.

ACKNOWLEDGEMENTS

This work was supported by grants from The Schizophrenia Association of Great Britain and The National Research Council, Canada.

REFERENCES

Creese, I. and Iverson, S. D. (1975). The pharmacological and anatomical substrates of the amphetamine response in the rat. *Brain Res*, **83**, 419

Hemmings, C., Hemmings, W. A. and Patey, A. L. (1976). The fate of oral doses of α-gliadin in suckling and adult rats. *IRCS Med. Sci.*, **4**, 38

Randrup, A. and Munkvad, J. (1967). Stereotyped activities produced by amphetamine in several animal species and man. *Psychopharmacologia (Berlin)*, **11**, 300

Singh, M. M. and Kay, S. R. (1976). Wheat gluten as a pathogenic factor in schizophrenia. *Science*, **191**, 401

Taylor, M. (1976). Effects of L-tryptophan and L-methionine on activity in the rat. *Br. J. Pharmacol.*, **58**, 117

Taylor, M. Dietary modification of Amphetamine stereotyped behaviour: the action of tryptophan, methionine and lysine. *Psychopharmacology*, (1978), in press

Taylor, M., Goudie, A. J., Mortimore, S. and Wheeler, T. J. (1974). Comparisons between behaviours elicited by high doses of amphetamine and fenfluramine: implications for the concept of stereotypy. *Psychopharmacologia (Berlin)*, **40**, 249

Wurtman, R. J. and Fernstrom, J. D. (1975). Control of brain monoamine synthesis by diet and plasma amino acids. *Am. J. Clin. Nutr.*, **28**, 638

Postscript –

'A PRELIMINARY INVESTIGATION OF DIETARY CONSTITUENTS AND AMPHETAMINE-INDUCED ABNORMAL BEHAVIOUR'

Subsequent experiments (Taylor, 1978) have confirmed the effects noted above, and extended them to include as a control condition, the addition of Lysine to the diet. Lysine failed to have any effect on amphetamine-induced stereotyped behaviour, in contrast to the effects of both tryptophan and methionine which are reported here. A further control condition explored the effects of administering tryptophan plus methionine to the diet. As reported in Taylor (1976), the effects of this condition are intermediary to both tryptophan and methionine administered singly. This effect extended to whole brain dopamine and 5-hydroxytryptamine levels.

SECTION 6:
Immunological Factors

21

Immunological approaches to the study of gut function

W. P. FAULK

THE IMMUNOLOGICAL SYSTEM

Cells that ultimately constitute the immune system initially arise as stem cells in the yolk-sac and migrate through the embryonic liver. They differentiate into two populations of lymphocytes (Figure 1). One population matures in

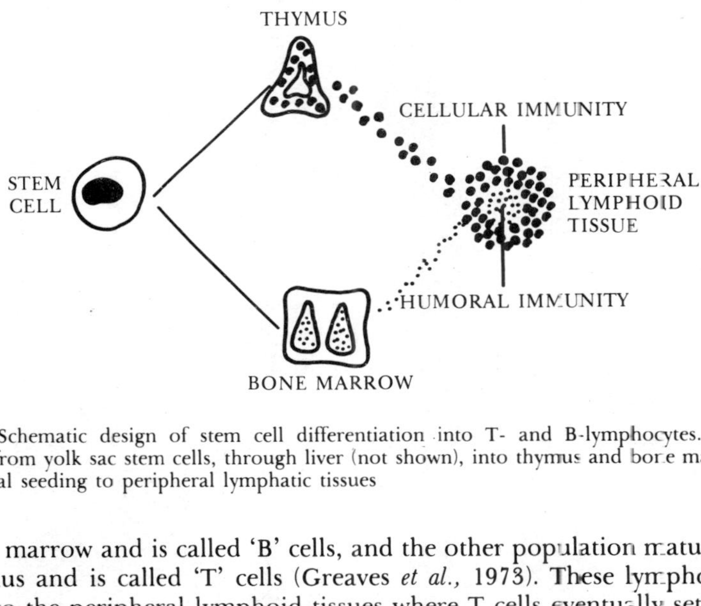

Figure 1 Schematic design of stem cell differentiation into T- and B-lymphocytes. Note migration from yolk sac stem cells, through liver (not shown), into thymus and bone marrow, and eventual seeding to peripheral lymphatic tissues

the bone marrow and is called 'B' cells, and the other population matures in the thymus and is called 'T' cells (Greaves *et al.*, 1973). These lymphocytes migrate to the peripheral lymphoid tissues where T cells eventually settle in the paracortical areas of lymphoid structures such as tonsils, spleen, and lymph nodes, and B cells settle in the medulla and cortex of lymphoid tissues and eventually constitute the well-known germinal centers (White, 1975). Plasma cells (Figure 2) are also found in germinal centers, and the job of both B cells and plasma cells is to produce immunoglobulins (Ig). There are five classes of Ig, and these are designated IgG, IgM, IgA, IgD, and IgE. Plasma cells and B cells normally produce only one class and subclass of Ig and antibody (Fudenberg *et al.*, 1972).

T and B cells and their products, along with macrophages, complement, and certain non-specific factors of resistance, are responsible for the bulk of

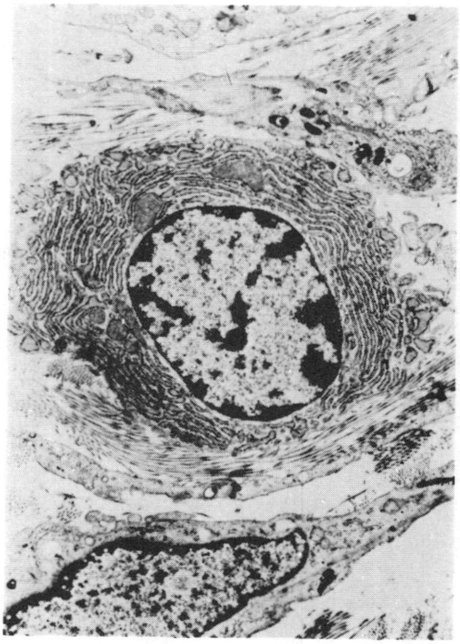

Figure 2 Electron-photomicrograph of Ig-producing plasma cell with rough endoplasmic reticulum. Cell in lower aspect of photograph is a fibroblast

host defences. The T and B cells work together in healthy persons to produce an adequate immune response to most infections, but some infections, such as pneumococcal pneumonia, are relatively more dependent on adequate B-cell function, and other infections, such as tuberculosis, are relatively

Figure 3 Some distinguishing features of B- and T-lymphocytes. Note membrane-bound Ig on B cells. This can be detected by immunofluorescence using fluorochrome-labelled anti-Ig sera. T cell on right forms spontaneous rosettes with untreated sheep red blood cells (diagrammatically indicated by black circles)

dependent on T-cell function. This division of labour within the immune system has been revealed largely as a result of extensive studies on patients suffering from primary immunodeficiency diseases (Good *et al.*, 1970). T cells can be quantified according to their ability to form rosettes with sheep erythrocytes, and one aspect of their function can be measured by their proliferative response to phytohaemagglutinin (PHA), a plant glycoprotein that has a non-specific nitogenic effect on T cells. The B cells can be quantified according to their ability to form rosettes with either antibody-coated or antibody- and complement-coated sheep erythrocytes. They can also be measured by membrane immunofluorescence (Figure 3), because they bear Ig on their cell membranes, and the type of Ig can be determined by using fluoresceinated class-specific antisera (Faulk and Hijmans, 1972). Since B cells produce antibodies and all antibodies are Ig, one of the most commonly used measurements of B-cell function is simply to estimate serum Ig levels, or to measure the production of antibody subsequent to antigenic stimulation.

Since T cells are responsible for cell-mediated immunity (CMI) it is important to know more about these cells. T cells in mice are distinguished by characteristic membrane markers, and human T cells are identified by several rosetting and mitogenic tests. Human T cells form rosettes with sheep erythrocytes. These rosettes form spontaneously and do not require antibody or complement as do the B-cell rosettes mentioned earlier. This test simply provides information about the number of T cells. It neither measures the capacity of T cells to respond to an environmental stimulus nor does it measure T-cell function. Diminished numbers of T-cell rosettes have been reported both in chronic infections and in certain immunodeficiency states (Cooper *et al.*, 1974). The capacity of T cells to respond to an environmental stimulus can be measured either with a non-specific T-cell mitogen such as PHA or with specific antigens. In both instances a proliferative response is generated, and the number of cells responding can be measured either by counting cells in metaphase or by pulsing the culture with a labelled DNA precursor such as tritiated thymidine. Antigen of course stimulates only a small clone of committed T cells, but the proportion of cells responding to PHA should be roughly the same as the proportion of cells forming spontaneous rosettes. Furthermore, the sum of the percentage of T-cell rosettes in a normal blood sample plus the percentage of B-cell rosettes in the same sample should theoretically equal about 100%.

The most reproducible measure of T-cell function in humans is the skin test response to antigens, such as purified protein derivative (PPD) following BCG immunization for tuberculosis, that is characterized by delayed-hypersensitivity reactions (Turk, 1975). Another aspect of T-cell function can be measured by the capacity of stimulated cells to release soluble factors that inhibit the outward migration of macrophages from a capillary reservoir. One such factor, popularly known as macrophage inhibitory factor (MIF), is only one of a heterogeneous group of substances that are released from activated T cells and are known as lymphokines. It might be borne in mind that most of these assays are specific for T cells only within the context of the test system employed. For example, cells other than T cells will form spontaneous rosettes with sheep cells (Papamichail *et al.,* 1975), many cells have PHA receptors and some of these will actually incorporate tritiated thymidine when stimulated with PHA (Faulk and Temple, 1975), and MIF is found in several types of cells. Nevertheless, tests for T-cell numbers, T-cell responses, and T-cell function are reliable and accurate tools if carefully used and controlled, and they have produced useful information about human immunobiology (Faulk and Chandra, 1976).

Another important mechanism of resistance is that of phagocytosis and intracellular digestion. This mechanism is found in animals which lack a well-organized immunological system, and in mammals it is more specialized and integrated with a protease-containing system of lysosomes. Organisms are recognized and bound by phagocytic cells either by virtue of membrane receptors or by the presence of cytophilic antibodies. Bound organisms are then endocytosed into a phagosome, and the phagosome fuses with lysosomes to form a phagolysosome. Acid proteases are released from the lysosome into the phagolysosome, and the phagocytosed organism is degraded and killed. Defects can occur in each of these steps, and several diseases in man are associated with increased infections due to faulty phagocytosis and killing (Douglas and Faulk, 1976).

Host defences thus rely upon non-specific factors of resistance as well as upon specific immunological responses. The non-specific factors include a complex of seemingly unrelated phenomena such as endocrine functions, serum iron, adequate nutrition, and the ability to mount appropriate febrile and leukocytosis responses. On the other hand, the immunological system is a well-defined series of lymphoid tissues that are responsible for the production of antibodies and CMI. Immune responses are also amplified through the mediation of several other systems such as blood complement, and both specific and non-specific factors participate in the generation of adequate inflammatory responses (Notkins and Lodmell, 1975).

IMMUNOLOGICAL SYSTEM IN THE GUT

The gastrointestinal (GI) tract contains large numbers of lymphocytes. Indeed, some structures in the gut, such as Peyer's patches, are specialized aggregates of lymphoid follicles (Faulk *et al.,* 1971). Other aggregates of lymphocytes are scattered through the GI tract from stomach to rectum, and they are generally referred to as solitary lymphoid nodules (Yoffey and Courtice, 1970). Some lymphocytes in these areas are able to migrate to different areas in the gut (Gowans and Knight, 1964), and a unique sequestration of lymphocytes is often noticed within the mucosal epithelium which overlays the gut-associated lymphoid tissues (GALT). These lymphocytes are separated from the lumen of the gut by the intervening epithelial cell membranes. The epithelium is pinocytotically active and is capable of taking up antigens from the gut lumen and transferring them to these lymphocytes as well as to the GALT. It is possible to remove lymphocytes from the GALT and to study them for several immunological properties such as rosette formation, the presence of Ig on the cell membrane, lymphokine release, etc. It is also possible to study the metabolism of these cells using various *in vitro* and *in vivo* systems. For instance, when lymphocytes of the GI tract are labelled *in vitro* and studied by radioautography for their capacity to incorporate radiolabelled DNA precursor (Meuwissen *et al.*, 1969), a larger proportion of lymphocytes from the appendix are labelled than are lymphocytes prepared from other lymphoid structures such as lymph nodes and spleen (Table 1). This can be confirmed by *in vivo* studies using tritiated

Table 1 ***In vitro*** **labelling of rabbit lymphocytes from different lymphoid tissues**

	Origin of cells					
	Appendix	*Sacculus*	*Thymus*	*Peyer's patch*	*Mesenteric node*	*Spleen*
Cells labelled (%)	17	14	7	7	4	2

9×10^6 rabbit lymphocytes from each organ in complete growth medium were exposed to 4 μCi of tritiated thymidine for 1 h, washed, and radioautographs prepared

thymidine, and gut lymphocytes from other organs in the same animal (Table 2). In other words, the rate of turnover as measured by the incorporation of DNA precursors is much higher in GALT than in other lymphoid tissues such as spleen and lymph nodes (Faulk *et al.*, 1971).

In view of the anatomical proximity of GALT cells to the gut lumen and their impressively active metabolic state, it is important to learn if GALT cells are capable of entering into immune reactions when they are exposed to various antigens. This problem has been studied by means of co-culturing

Table 2 ***In vivo*** **labelling of rabbit lymphocytes from different lymphoid tissues**

	Origin of cells				
	Appendix	*Sacculus*	*Peyer's patch*	*Lymph nodes*	*Spleen*
Cell labelled (%)	24.1	16.7	10.4	4.9	3.3

Data from 10 healthy, non-immune rabbits injected i.v. 7 h before sacrifice with 2 μCi/g body weight of tritiated thymadine (sp. act. 11 Ci/μmol), animals were then killed and cells removed from lymphoid centers under study for radioautography

lymphocytes prepared from different lymphoid aggregates in the gut (Henry *et al.*, 1970), and other lymphoid organs such as spleen, lymph nodes and thymus, with a standardized antigen (sheep red blood cells). Following co-culture with antigen, the lymphocytes are assayed for antibody to sheep erythrocytes using the Jerne haemolytic plaque test in agar with guinea pig complement. The results of this type of experiment show that lymphoid cells from the GI tract are capable of mounting an immune response that compares favourably with that produced by lymphocytes from lymph nodes and spleen (Table 3). This type of experimental model is equally applicable to antigens other than erythrocytes, and gluten or gluten fractions could probably be used. Interpretation of such experiments to the human situation requires rigid experimental design and control, partly due to the complex

Table 3 Generation of immune responses *in vitro* by co-culturing rabbit lymphocytes with sheep erythrocytes

Source of cells	*Control cultures*	*Test cultures*
Peyer's patch	3.7(1–17)	62(22–134)
Spleen	18.0(4–58)	140(28–475)
Thymus	0.1	0.1

Results are given as plaque forming cells per million lymphocytes recovered on the 5th day of culture. These data represent the mean of 12 experiments. The range of responses obtained is given in parentheses

patterns of lymphocyte migration. For instance, lymphocytes from different organs tend to migrate within a certain axis of lymphocyte traffic as well as moving in the physiological traffic which carries lymphoid cells throughout the body. In this regard it is relevant that some GALT cells migrate away from the gut, and Goldblum *et al.* (1975) have recently shown that human mothers orally immunized with *E. coli* produce immunized lymphocytes in their breast milk.

As has been discussed above, B lymphocytes are responsible for the production and secretion of immunoglobulins G, M, A, E, and D, and T lymphocytes are responsible for CMI. These two populations of lymphocytes co-operate with each other as well as with macrophages to produce an immune response, and immune responses are amplified through the mediation of complement and other amplification systems (Faulk and Greenwood, 1976). The immune response together with non-specific factors of resistance and inflammatory responses constitute the bulk of host defences (Faulk, 1975). However, different parts of the body are subjected to different environmental stresses and infections, and the above general comments must be tailored to meet these varying needs. This is represented by the necessity of HCl secretion in the maintenance of gastric function and by the need for mechanical flushing in the maintenance of normal emptying in the GI tract. In the gut, as well as in other mucosal surfaces, there is a specialized system called secretory immunity (Hanson and Brandtzaeg, 1972). IgA present in secretions is a dimer composed of IgA monomers connected by a joining-chain (J-chain) that is coupled to another molecule of molecular weight 58 000 called secretory component (S-C) produced by epithelial cells (Figure 4). This secretory IgA (S-IgA) is resistant to enzymatic breakdown and is thus ideally suited to survive in the gut (Lamm, 1976). As a general rule, serum IgA is monomeric and does not contain either J-chain of S-C, and IgA

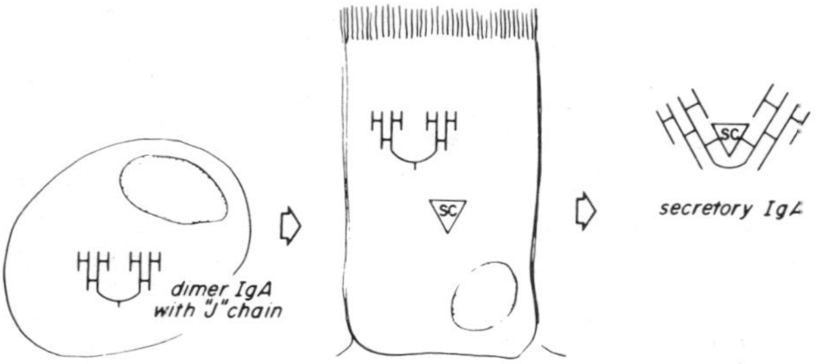

Figure 4 The two-component cell system of secretory immunity. Note two molecules of IgA bound together into dimer by J-chain within IgA-producing B lymphocytes. The dimer then passes to an intestinal epithelical cell where it acquires secretory component and ultimately is secreted in gut (From Walker, W. Allan and Hong, Richard (1973). Immunology of the gastro-intestinal tract: Part I, *J. Pediatr.*, **83**, 517)

identified in secretions is S-IgA (Figure 5). In some diseases, such as vaginal candidiasis, a great deal of S-IgA is identified in serum (Mathur *et al.*, 1976), and, in those uncommon circumstances where persons lack the capacity to make IgA, there is a compensatory mechanism whereby IgM couples with S-C and mucosal surfaces are protected by secreted IgM (Ogra *et al.*, 1974).

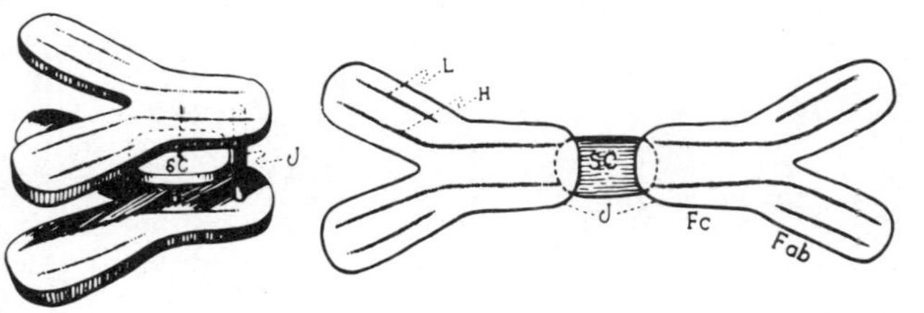

Figure 5 Secretory IgA. Note two molecules of IgA coupled together by J-chain with secretory component inserted between (left). The unfolded dimer is to the right. Abbreviations are: J for joining-chain, S-C for secretory component, L for light-chain, H for heavy-chain. Fc and Fab are fragments (F) produced for study in the laboratory. L, H, Fc, and Fab are designations used for all Ig. and J and S-C are usually limited to S-IgA. (From Walker, W. Allan and Hong, Richard (1973). Immunology of the gastrointestinal tract: Part I, *J. Pediatr*, **83**, 517)

The function of S-IgA seems to be principally concerned with selectively impeding the absorption of certain substances from the gut lumen by a process called antigen trapping (Walker and Hong, 1973a). In the case of a normally functioning gut, S-IgA with specificity for dietary proteins such as gluten, egg albumin or milk proteins is secreted into the gut lumen. This binds to the antigen in question and inhibits its absorption (Figure 6). If a person is unable to mount an adequate S-IgA response and the antigen is not trapped into the gut lumen by antibody, the protein is then available for pinocytosis across mucosal epithelium into GALT where it is likely to generate a sensitized population of lymphocytes which are substantially able to initiate immunopathology locally or at distant sites following migration. In other

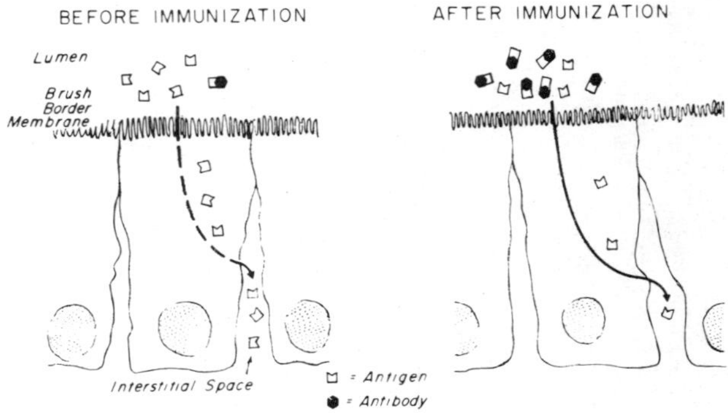

Figure 6 Antigen-trapping mechanism of S-IgA. Note on left deficient S-IgA to trap antigen in gut lumen and consequent entrance of large amounts of antigen through gut cells and into interstitial space. Adequate S-IgA on right traps antigen in lumen and prevents it from entering into interstitial spaces. (From Walker, W. Allan and Hong, Richard (1973). Immunology of the gastrointestinal tract: Part I, *J. Pediatr*, **83**, 517)

words, if the S-IgA mechanism of antigen trapping is not operative, dietary antigens in the gut lumen have an increased possibility of absorption and thus of initiating either local or distant hypersensitivity reactions with either the same or cross-reacting antigens. This is clinically manifest by the increased serum antibody titres to several bacteria in individuals who lack IgA (Brown and Lee, 1974) as well as in the observations of antibodies to dietary proteins reported in the sera of malnourished children who lack S-IgA (Chandra, 1975).

GUT IMMUNOPATHOLOGY

The normal immune system in the gastrointestinal tract manifests several different types of responses or reactions to disease. Indeed, there is some evidence that certain forms of pathology occur as a result of immunologically mediated damage to the bowel. Generally, there are four types of immunopathology that occur in the body (Figure 7), and each of these has been identified in the gastrointestinal tract. The types of immunopathology that can be generated by humoral or cellular immune reactions can be grouped into the following four types according to Gell, Coombs and Lachmann (Coombs and Gell, 1975). The first type involves the release of pharmacologically active substances such as histamine from most cells subsequent to the binding of antigen by antibody on the cell's membrane. Type I reactions can apparently occur in the gut inasmuch as Dr Shiner and her colleagues at Northwick Park have presented evidence for mast cell degranulation in the bowel of children with clinical allergy to milk proteins (Shiner *et al.,* 1975). The second type of immunopathological reaction involves the binding of antibodies to basement or cell membranes either with or without the participation of complement. Regarding complement, although IgA and S-IgA cannot fix complement through the classical pathway of activation, the alternative pathway of complement fixation can be activated

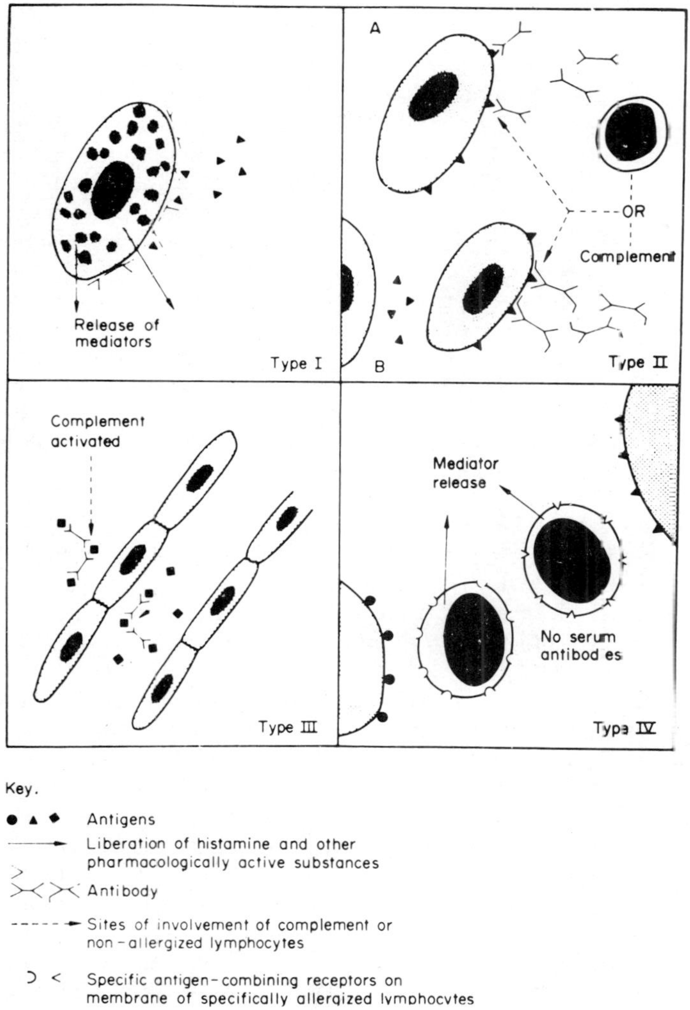

Figure 7 The four types of immunopathological damage. (With kind permission of Blackwell Scientific publications)

by both IgA and S-IgA (Colten and Bienenstock, 1974). Auto-antibodies which react directly with colonic epithelial cells have been found in the sera of some patients with ulcerative colitis (Wright and Truelove, 1966). In Crohn's disease, there is less evidence for Type II reactions, but auto-antibodies to reticulin have been reported in the sera of some of these patients (Alp and Wright, 1971). Reticulin is a type of collagen that is found on fibroblast cell membranes as well as basement membranes (Beard *et al.*, 1976). Another example of a Type II reaction in the gut is the identification of

S-IgA antibodies to intrinsic factor in the gastric juices of patients with pernicious anaemia (Goldberg *et al.,* 1968). The third type of immunopathological reaction involves damage caused by immune complexes. There are several conditions in the gut that could result in immune-complex formation. For instance, patients lacking S-IgA who form IgG or IgM antibodies to absorbed food antigen would tend to form antigen–antibody complexes in the gut, and these same patients often have gastrointestinal infections which could also result in immune-complex mediated tissue damage (Lamm, 1976). Certain strains of *E. coli* produce immunogenic glycoproteins which cross-react with bowel tissues, and it has been speculated that immunity to these could result in inflammatory conditions possibly on the basis of Type III reactions (Lyampert and Danilova, 1975). It has also been shown that antigen–antibody complexes are present in the sera of patients with ulcerative colitis, and their presence in serum can be correlated with the severity of the bowel disease as judged clinically and by sigmoidoscopy (Jewell and MacLennan, 1973). The fourth type of immunopathological reaction involves cell-mediated immunity (CMI). type IV reactions have been demonstrated in ulcerative colitis inasmuch as lymphocytes from these patients have been shown to be cytotoxic for colonic epithelial cells growing in tissue culture (Ansell, 1976). An antibody-dependent modification of CMI has also been shown to be operative in ulcerative colitis; cytotoxicity for colonic epithelial cells can be conferred on normal lymphocytes by sera from these patients, and the cytotoxic property is lost following colectomy (Shorter *et al.,* 1971).

Although most immunopathology can be accounted for according to the above four types of reactions, there are, of course, other mechanisms of damage which are not so readily apparent. For instance, certain diseases of the bowel are more manifest in individuals who have a genetic propensity for the disease. This is demonstrated by the predominance of HLA-B8 among patients with gluten-sensitive enteropathy (Strober *et al.,* 1975) as well as by the high incidence of gastrointestinal diseases in patients with primary immunodeficiency syndromes and disorders of granulocyte function (Ochs *et al.,* 1975).

Another interesting genetic correlate of gastrointestinal diseases is the association of ulcerative colitis with ankylosing spondylitis. This disease is about 25 times more common in patients with ulcerative colitis than in the general population (Brewerton, 1976), and the diagnosis of ankylosing spondylitis sometimes precedes the clinical onset of ulcerative colitis by 10–20 years (Brewerton, 1976, and Jayson *et al.,* 1970). Furthermore, patients who have ulcerative colitis and no evidence of rheumatic disease have an increased prevalence of ankylosing spondylitis in their first-degree relatives (Macrae and Wright, 1973). Patients with ankylosing spondylitis almost always possess HLA-B27 whereas this antigen is uncommon in patients with ulcerative colitis and no ankylosing spondylitis, suggesting that other unknown variables are important in the pathophysiology and pathogenesis of these diseases (Walker and Hong, 1973b). Immunological approaches have been of great assistance in helping to build a more intelligent understanding of gastrointestinal diseases, and similar approaches should be useful in broadening present concepts of mental illness. Indeed, the relationship between schizophrenia and dietary gluten suggests that existing immunological technology might profitably be applied to this important and hitherto poorly understood disease.

ACKNOWLEDGEMENTS

This work was supported in part by USPHA grants AI-13484 and HD-09938. Dr R. Galbraith provided useful suggestions and criticism.

REFERENCES

Alp, M. H. and Wright, R. (1971). Autoantibodies to reticulin in patients with idiopathic steatorrhoea, coeliac disease, and Crohn's disease, and their relation to immunoglobulins and dietary antibodies. *Lancet,* **ii,** 682

Ansell, B. M. (1976). Arthritis in gastrointestinal disease; In *Infection and Immunology in the Rheumatic Diseases* (D. C. Dumonde, ed.) p. 129. (London: Blackwell Scientific Publications)

Beard, H. K., Faulk, W. P., Conochie, L. B. and Glynn, L. E. (1976). Some immunological aspects of collagen. *Progr. Allergy,* **22,** 45

Brewerton, D. A. (1976). HL-A antigens in ankylosing spondylitis and related diseases; In *Infection and Immunology in the Rheumatic Diseases* (D. C. Dumonde, ed.) p. 333 (London: Blackwell Scientific Publications)

Brown, W. R. and Lee, E. (1974). Radioimmunological measurements of bacterial antibodies. II. Human serum antibodies reactive with Bacteroides fragilis and Enterococcus in gastrointestinal and immunological disorders. *Gastroenterology,* **66,** 1145

Chandra, R. K. (1975). Food antibodies in malnutrition. *Arch. Dis. Childh.,* **50,** 532

Colten, H. R. and Bienenstock, J. (1974). Lack of C3 activation through classical or alternate pathways by human secretory IgA anti blood group A antibody. *Adv. Exp. Med. Biol.,* **45,** 305

Coombs, R. R. A. and Gell, P. G. H. (1975). Classification of allergic reactions responsible for clinical hypersensitivity and disease. In *Clinical Aspects of Immunology.* (P. G. H. Gell, R. R. A. Coombs and P. J. Lachmann, eds.) p. 761 –London: Blackwell Scientific Publications)

Cooper, M. D., Faulk, W. P., Fudenberg, H. H., Good, R. A., Hitzig, W., Kunkel, H. G., Rosen, F. S., Seligmann, M., Soothill, J. and Wedgewood, R. J. (1974). Primary immunodeficiency diseases in man. *Clin. Immunol. Immunopathol.,* **2,** 416

Douglas, S. D. and Faulk, W. P. (1976). Immunologic aspects of protein-calorie malnutrition. In *Advances in Clinical Immunology,* Vol. 1 (London: Churchill Livingstone)

Faulk, W. P., McCormick, J. N., Goodman, J. R., Yoffey, J. M. and Fudenberg, H. H. (1971). Peyer's patches: morphologic studies. *Cell. Immunol.,* **1,** 500

Faulk, W. P. and Hijmans, W. (1972). Recent developments in immunofluorescence. *Prog. Allergy,* **16,** 9

Faulk, W. P. (1975). Immunity and infection. *Medicine,* **2 (1),** 13

Faulk, W. P. and Chandra, R. K. (1977). In *CRC Handbook of Nutrition and Food* (Cleveland: CRC Press) (In press)

Faulk, W. P. and Temple, A. (1975). Fibroblast immunobiology. In *Regulation of Growth and Differentiated Function in Eukaryote Cells* (G. P. Talwar, ed.) pp. 295–306 (New York: Raven Press)

Faulk, W. P. and Greenwood, B. M. (1977). Clinical immunology of infectious diseases. In *Medical Immunology* (E. J. Holborow and G. Reeves, eds.) pp. 433–472 (London: Academic Press)

Fudenberg, H. H., Pink, J. R. L., Stites, D. P. and Wang, A. C., (eds.) (1972) *Basic Immunogenetics* (London: Oxford University Press)

Goldberg, L. S., Shuster, J., Stuckley, M. and Fudenberg, H. H. (1968). Secretory IgA: Autoantibody activity in gastric juice. *Science,* **160,** 1240

Goldblum, R. M., Ahlstedt, S., Carlsson, B., Hanson, L. A., Jodal, U., Lidin-Janson, G. and Sohl, A. (1975). Antibody forming cells in human colostrum after oral immunization. *Nature,* **257,** 797

Good, R. A., Finstad, J. and Gatti, R. A. (1970). In: *Infectious Agents and Host Resistance* (S. Mudd, ed.) p. 76 (Philadelphia: W. B. Saunders)

Gowans, J. L. and Knight, E. J. (1964). The route of re-circulation of lymphocytes in the rat. *Proc. R. Soc., Ser. B,* **159,** 257

Greaves, M. F., Owen, J. T. and Raff, M. C. (1973). *T and B Lymphocytes: Their Origin, Properties, and Roles in Immune Responses* (Amsterdam: Excerpta Medica)

Hanson, L. A. and Brandtzaeg, P. (1972). Secretory antibody systems; In: *Immunologic Disorders in Infants and Children* (E. R. Stiehm and V. A. Fulginiti, eds.) p. 107 (Philadelphia: Saunders)

Henry, C., Faulk, W. P., Kuhn, L., Yoffey, J. M. and Fundenberg, H. H. (1970). Peyer's patches: immunological studies. *J. Exp. Med.,* **131,** 1200

Jayson, M. I. V., Salmon, P. R. and Harrison, W. J. (1970). Inflammatory bowel disease in ankylosing spondylitis. *Gut,* **11,** 506

Jewell, D. P. and MacLennan, K. C. M. (1973). Circulating immune complexes in inflammatory bowel disease. *Clin. Immunol.,* **14,** 219

Lamm, M. E. (1976). Cellular aspects of immunoglobulin A. *Adv. Immunol.,* **22,** 223

Lyampert, I. M. and Danilova, T. A. (1975). Immunological phenomena associated with cross-reactive antigens of micro-organisms and mammalian tissues. *Progr. Allergy,* **18,** 423

Macrae, I. and Wright, V. (1973). A family study of ulcerative colitis, with particular reference to ankylosing spondylitis and sacro-ilitis. *Ann. Rheumat. Dis.,* **32,** 16

Mathur, S., Virella, G., Koistinen, J., Mahvi, T., Horger, E. and Fudenberg, H. H. (1976). Humoral immunity in vaginal candidiasis. *Infect. Immun.*

Meuwissen, H. J., Kaplan, G. T., Perey, D. Y. and Good, R. A. (1969). Role of rabbit gut-associated lymphoid tissue in cell replication. *Proc. Soc. Exp. Biol. Med.,* **130,** 300

Notkins, A. L. and Lodmell, D. L. (1975). Cellular immune response in viral infections. In *Perspectives in Virology* (M. Pollard, ed.) p. 115 (New York: Academic Press)

Ochs, H. D., Ament, M. E. and Davis, D. D. (1975). Structure and function of the gastro-intestinal tract in primary immunodeficiency syndromes (IDA) and in granulocyte dysfunction. In *Immunodeficiency in Man and Animals* D. Bergsma, R. A. Good and J. Finstead, eds.) p. 199 (Sunderland, Mass.: Sinaver Asso., Inc.)

Ogra, P. L., Coppola, P. R., MacGillivray, M. H. and Dzierba, J. L. (1974). Mechanisms of mucosal immunity to viral infections in gammaA immunoglobulin-deficiency syndromes. *Proc. Soc. Exp. Biol. Med.,* **145,** 811

Papamichail, M., Gutierrez, C., Temple, A. and Faulk, W. P. (1975). Spontaneous rosette formation by mouse L-cells. *Immunology,* **30,** 129

Shiner, M. *et al.* (1975). Intestinal biopsy in the diagnosis of cow's milk protein intolerance without acute symptoms. *Lancet,* **ii,** 1060

Shorter, R. G., Huigenga, K. A., Spencer, R. J., Aas, J. and Guy, S. K. (1971). Inflammatory bowel disease. Cytophilic antibody and the cytotoxicity of lymphocytes for colonic cells *in vitro. Am. J. Digest. Dis.,* **16,** 673

Strober, W., Falchuk, Z. M. and Gebhard, R. L. (1975). Gluten-sensitive enteropathy. In *Immunodeficiency in Man and Animals* (D. Bergsma, R. A. Good and J. Finstead, eds.) p. 208 (Sunderland, Mass: Sinaver Assoc.)

Turk, J. L. (1975). *Delayed Hypersensitivity* 2nd Ed. (Amsterdam: North Holland Publishing Co.) lishing Co.)

Walker, W. A. and Hong, R. (1973a). Immunology of the gastrointestinal tract. Part I. *J. Pediatr.,* **83,** 517

Walker, W. A. and Hong, R. (1973b). Immunology of the gastrointestinal tract. Part II. *J. Pediatr.,* **83**

White, R. G. (1975). Immunological functions of lymphoreticular tissues. In *Clinical Aspects of Immunology* (P. G. H. Crell, R. R. A. Coombs and P. J. Lachman, eds.) p. 411 3rd Ed. (London: Blackwell Scientific Publications)

Wright, R. and Truelove, S. C. (1966). Autoimmune reactions in ulcerative colitis. *Gut,* **7,** 32

Yoffrey, J. M. and Courtice, F. C. (1970). *Lymphocytes, Lymph and the Lymphomyeloid Complex,* p. 686 (London: Academic Press)

22

Nutrition and immunity: possible new approaches to research in schizophrenia

W. P. FAULK AND J. R. COCKRELL

INTRODUCTION

Host resistance depends upon specific immunological responses and non-specific factors of resistance. The immunological system consists of two lymphoid components, and both components apparently arise from the same stem-cell series. Lymphocytes arising in the thymus are called T cells, ('T' indicating thymus), and lymphocytes arising from bone marrow are called B cells ('B' indicating bone marrow). T cells are responsible for cell-mediated immunity reactions such as graft rejection and delayed hypersensitivity, and B cells are responsible for the production of immunoglobulins and antibody. T and B cells and their products, along with macrophages, complement, and certain non-specific factors of resistance co-operate to provide the bulwark of host defences (Good *et al.*, 1970). Non-specific factors of resistance include phenomena such as certain endocrine functions, serum iron, and the ability to mount appropriate febrile and leukocytosis reactions. The effect of certain hormones on the immune system can be particularly striking (Braun and Unger, 1973). Both specific and non-specific factors participate in the generation of adequate inflammatory responses.

Just as there is increased incidence of infection in patients with immunodeficiency diseases, so also there appears to be a relationship between malnutrition and infection. Indeed, Richter (1976) has pointed out that the existence in some populations of a sub-group of encephalitis-induced schizophrenia suggests that an infectious aetiology should be given careful consideration in schizophrenia research. Nutritional factors can interact with infections in at least two ways: (1) by malnutrition increasing host susceptibility to infection, and (2) by infection precipitating malnutrition. The relationship is cyclic insofar as one pathophysiological condition is capable of accentuating the other (Faulk *et al.*, 1974). In the nutrition studies which we will cite, the major dietary deficiency is protein. Information has recently been collected from several quarters which suggests that dietary factors may participate in the pathophysiology of schizophrenia. This comes mainly from reports of schizophrenics with allergic reactions to certain food proteins such as wheat flour, eggs, or milk, who improve when these items are removed from the diet. For instance, Dohan *et al.*, (1969) reported that the substitution of a gluten-free diet reduced the time that schizophrenics remained in the hospital, and that the effect was no longer evident when gluten was added to the gluten-free diet. Much of these data are reviewed in this volume. In the first part of this paper we will briefly describe the immune system and review examples showing the effects of diet on immune tissues as well as on the immune response.

It should be stressed at the onset that the immune system functions in other areas than host defense. For instance, immunoglobulins can carry out certain hormone-like functions, such as that caused by the long-acting thyroid stimulator (LATS), which is a non-species specific IgG found in 20–40% of thyrotoxic sera. Although one is usually taught that antibodies destroy their targets, such as the classical examples of sheep red cells or bacteria, it is now well accepted that certain antibodies can either protect, as represented by blocking antibodies, or stimulate, as represented by the above LATS example. Some populations of lymphocytes also seem to contribute a non-cytotoxic or physiological function. For instance, some T cells enhance or suppress the function of other cells, although the extent to which these reactions occur *in vivo* is not yet clear.

HISTOPATHOLOGY OF IMMUNE SYSTEM IN MALNUTRITION

T and B lymphocytes are seeded from the thymus and bone marrow to peripheral lymphoid organs such as lymph nodes, spleen, tonsils, Peyer's patches, and other lymphoid aggregates in the gastrointestinal tract. Histopathological examination of these tissues in conditions of poor nutrition reveals morphological abnormalities of both central and peripheral lymphoid tissues (Faulk *et al.,* 1976). These findings are particularly striking in young children. For example, thymus glands from healthy 4-month-old children weigh about 25 g, but thymuses from children of comparable age with malnutrition weigh less than 10 g, frequently 1 g or less. Thymuses from healthy neonates during the first several days of life weigh about 20 g, but those from neonates who sustain intrauterine malnutrition also reveal morphological alterations and reduction in weight. The histology of the thymus of a normal child is that of lobules well demarcated by thin connective tissue septa; each lobule is differentiated into medullary and cortical regions. The medulla contains large lymphocytes and the cortex gives rise to T lymphocytes. Thymus histology varies according to the degree of malnutrition; in the initial or intermediate stages of malnutrition there is seen a progressive loss of cortico-medullary differentiation and lymphocyte depletion, and severe stages of malnutrition can show complete loss of normal thymus architecture with lymphocyte depletion and interstitial fibrosis.

The peripheral lymphoid organs of the immune system also show gross and microscopic evidence of damage in malnutrition. The spleen is small and contains fewer and smaller germinal centres, and the amount of fibrous connective tissue increases. The palatine tonsils are also small, and Peyer's patches as well as other lymphoid aggregates in the gut are hypoplastic. It is not clear, however, whether these morphological changes in the thymus and peripheral lymphoid tissues are primarily the result of malnutrition or the secondary effects of infection or stress. Histopathological findings in thymuses from intra-uterine malnourished neonates might suggest that the changes are primarily due to malnutrition, but the possibility of transplacental transport of maternal stress hormones, endotoxin, or viruses as possible augmenting factors has not been excluded. Whatever the cause, it is clear that both the central and peripheral components of the immune system undergo drastic changes during malnutrition, and these alterations are clinically associated with a compromised ability of the host to deal effectively with infections (Douglas and Faulk, 1977).

LYMPHOCYTE POPULATIONS IN MALNUTRITION

B lymphocytes

B lymphocytes produce antibodies, all of which are immunoglobulins (Ig) and of which five classes are known: IgG, IgA, IgM, IgD, and IgE. Nutritional deprivation is usually not associated with a significant change in the proportion or absolute number of B lymphocytes, suggesting a selective sparing of this population of cells in conditions of sub-optimal nutrition (Stiehm *et al.,* 1977). Indeed, in occasional patients with prolonged infection, these cells may be slightly increased. An estimate of the capacity of the B cells to synthesize antibodies can be obtained by quantitative measurements of immunoglobulins. The serum concentrations of all Ig classes are usually elevated in malnutrition (Neumann *et al.,* 1975), and in some subjects IgA is increased more than other immunoglobulins, perhaps as a consequence of gastrointestinal and respiratory infections (Mata and Faulk, 1973). Serum IgE is also often elevated, particularly in patients with certain parasitic infestations. In severe and seriously ill undernourished infants, low levels of IgG, IgA and IgM are sometimes seen. Studies of antibody responses following immunization in malnutrition seem to indicate that one might expect either a decreased or relatively normal antibody response, dependent on the type of antigen and other technicalities relevant to the method of immunization (Faulk *et al.,* 1975).

Mucosal immune responses are largely independent of systemic immunity. These are achieved by locally produced secretory IgA, and it is important in this regard that malnourished children have decreased concentrations of secretory IgA in secretions from their mucosal surfaces. Mucosal immune responses are thus impaired, and this is thought to contribute to the increased frequency and severity of gut and pulmonary infections associated with nutritional deficiency. Also, with mucosal immunity impaired, systemic spread of infection can more easily occur from gastrointestinal and respiratory surfaces. Due to the failure of secretory IgA and mucosal immunity, certain potential food antigens from the diet can also cross the gut wall and result in the formation of antibodies to food products (Chandra, 1977).

T LYMPHOCYTES

The capacity of T cells to proliferate in response to an environmental stimulus can be measured with substances which either non-specifically or specifically stimulate T-cell proliferation. Antigen of course stimulates only a small clone of committed or primed T cells, but the proportion of T cells responding to a non-specific mitogen such as the plant glycoprotein phytohaemagglutinin (PHA) should be roughly the same as the proportion of T cells present. Furthermore, the sum of the percentage of T cells in a normal blood sample and the percentage of B cells in the same sample should approximately equal 100%. This is normally about 70% T cells, 20% B cells, and 10% cells which cannot be classified as either T or B cells (these are referred to as null cells, and their proportion increases in certain conditions of chronic inflammation such as rheumatoid arthritis).

Studies indicate that lymphocytes from malnourished individuals do not respond normally to mitogenic stimulation with PHA. Original studies from South Africa reported a significantly depressed response (Smythe *et al.*, 1971), and these results have been confirmed by several other laboratories. Other investigators have, however, reported either normal or elevated responses to PHA, and a report from Gambia has suggested that sera from children with protein-calorie malnutrition may contain factors that inhibit lymphocyte responses to PHA (Moore *et al.*, 1974). Factors involved in diminished response could include some alteration in the lymphocytes themselves, the presence of circulating inhibitors (Heyworth *et al.*, 1975), and the action of suppressor cells.

A simple and useful measure of T-cell function in malnutrition is the skin test response to antigens, such as purified protein derivative (PPD) following BCG immunization for tuberculosis, that are characterized by delayed hypersensitivity reactions. Many different antigens have uniformly failed to elicit normal delayed hypersensitivity reactions in malnourished individuals (Edelman *et al.*, 1973). One assumes that the skin test for delayed hypersensitivity is an accurate measure of cell-mediated immunity, but non-immune factors such as hormones or biochemical alterations in the skin can presumably depress the skin test. Many virus infections can also depress delayed hypersensitivity reactions in the skin, and the role of either superimposed virus infections or the activation of latent viruses in malnutrition has not been adequately explored.

COMPLEMENT

The complement system is a complex set of sequentially interacting proteins (C1, C4, C2, C3, C5, C6, C7, C8 and C9), which are present in the serum and which can be activated by a variety of agents such as antibodies, microbial products, and enzymes. In addition to the classical pathway of complement activation, the early reacting components can be by-passed through the mediation of another system which is initiated by substances such as endotoxin. The end result of the activated complement system is membrane damage and cell death by lysis. In addition, several of the components involved in either the classical or by-pass reactions play contributory roles in chemotaxis, blood clotting, anaphylaxis, and other systems that amplify the immune response.

Total haemolytic complement activity and levels of almost all complement components except C4 are reduced in malnourished patients (Sirisinha *et al.*, 1973). In severe malnutrition all the serum complement components are at significantly lower levels than in normal controls. Moreover, sera from malnourished individuals have been reported to contain electrophoretically altered complement components (Chandra, 1975), suggesting *in vivo* activation of the complement sequence. Such activation could be triggered by immune complexes or endotoxin which result from superimposed infections. Impaired complement activity in nutritional deficiency could also be the consequence of reduced protein synthesis by liver, gut and lymphocytes. Also, loss of complement proteins may occur through protein-losing gastroenteropathy associated with malnutrition. Nutritional recovery is associated with a return of complement levels and function to normal, athough the long-term effect of nutritional deprivation on the complement system is not known.

PHAGOCYTOSIS

Phagocytosis and intracellular digestion of micro-organisms is accomplished by fixed-tissue phagocytes as well as by phagocytic cells in the peripheral circulation such as neutrophils and monocytes. The mechanism is integrated with a protease-containing system of lysosomes. Organisms are recognized and bound by phagocytic cells either by virtue of membrane receptors or by the presence of cytophilic antibodies. The organism is then endocytosed into a phagosome, and the phagosome fuses with lysosomes to form phagolysosomes. Acid proteases are released from the lysosome into the phagolysosome, and the phagocytosed organism is degraded. Studies done on phagocytic cells, mostly neutrophils, from malnourished children have shown that recognition and endocytosis of bacteria are normal, but that these cells have a delayed chemotactic response, particularly in the presence of infection (Douglas and Schopfer, 1976). There is no characteristic abnormality in the enzymes from leukocytes of malnourished individuals, but the time required for intracellular killing of phagocytosed micro-organisms is increased (Douglas and Schopfer, 1974).

NON-SPECIFIC FACTORS

Non-specific factors of resistance include many different mediators such as C-reactive protein, lysozyme, B lysins, serum iron, and hormones (Braun and Unger, 1973). Many of these factors are affected by alterations in the status of particular nutrients. Some attention has focused on the transferrins. These are iron-binding proteins that reportedly indicate a poor prognosis if depressed in the serum of malnourished children (McFarlane *et al.*, 1977). It is not altogether clear why depressed serum transferrin values should herald a poor prognosis, but this is thought to be related to their iron-binding capacity. Iron is important in the killing of endocytosed bacteria by phagocytes (Bullen *et al.,* 1972), and certain bacteria require iron to manifest their pathogenicity (Elin and Wolf, 1974).

Breast milk contains many substances which are important as non-specific factors of resistance (Goldman and Smith, 1973), and breast-fed infants seem to thrive better than do bottle-fed infants even if they are living under very deficient environmental sanitation (Mata and Urrutia, 1971). Certain indigenous microflora which form a protective barrier in the gut against pathogenic organisms appear to be important in this as well as other mechanisms such as the elaboration of vitamin K used in the establishment of homeostasis and blood clotting. The diets of many malnourished persons also lack adequate vitamins, and several vitamins have been shown to be important in mounting an adequate immune response (Scrimshaw *et al.,* 1968). More relevant to the aims of this symposium is the observation that a diet low in nicotinic acid can cause the schizophrenia-like psychoses of pellagra, but there is little evidence that schizophrenics derive benefit from treatment with even megavitamin doses of nicotinic acid or nicotinamide (Wyatt *et al.,* 1971).

POSSIBLE INTER-RELATIONSHIPS OF NUTRITION AND IMMUNITY WITH RESEARCH IN SCHIZOPHRENIA

Several years ago one would not have been able to anticipate that nutritionists and immunologists would be working closely together to solve problems of inadequate host defence, but today one of the most rapidly expanding areas of immunology has to do with nutritional–immunological interactions. A good example of this is contemporary interest in the failure of gastrointestinal secretory immunity in conditions of sub-optimal nutrition (Chandra, 1975a). One of the most important functions of the secretory immunity system is its capacity to bind antigen in the gut lumen and thereby inhibit the antigen's capability to cross the gut wall and enter circulation. A vigorous mucosal immunity to a protein antigen such as gluten could block or trap dietary gluten in the gut lumen and protect potentially sensitive individuals from this protein. By the same token, failure of secretory immunity for genetic or environmental (e.g. nutritional) reasons would allow entrance, exposure, and hypersensitivity. The form of hypersensitivity would also be of more than academic interest. Coombs (1975) has defined four basic types of hypersensitivity reactions, each with different immunopathology. The type I reaction involves histamine release from mast cells by reagenic or IgE antibody, and chronic exposure to this reaction could tend to promote a condition of histamine tolerance. It is interesting in this regard that schizophrenics are unusually resistant to injected histamine, and that tolerance to histamine is said to increase with increased chronicity of illness (Smythies, 1975). The other types of immunopathology could also be relevant in schizophrenia research, but to our knowledge no such studies have been done. However, as the hiatus has closed between nutritionists and immunologists, one trusts that a similar welding of talents will occur between immunology and research in schizophrenia.

Malnutrition is not the only circumstance in which gluten seems to be central in the interplay between the gastrointestinal tract and the immune system. Coeliac disease, whose pathophysiology is related to dietary gluten, has many immunopathological manifestations. For instance, serum IgA levels in coeliac disease are elevated, sometimes with values increased up to ten-fold (Visakorpi, 1977). Some patients show anti-gluten antibodies in their sera, and many of the patients have anti-reticulin antibodies. Following a challenge with gluten, patients show deposition of IgM, fibrinogen and C3 in the gut lamina propria basement membranes. Contemporary genetic evidence suggests that HLA markers may also be important in building an understanding of the pathophysiology and immunopathology of coeliac disease (Strober, 1974). Dermatitis herpetiformis also has intestinal mucosal lesions and immunological findings which are similar to those seen in coeliac disease, and which similarly normalize on a gluten-free diet (Weinstein, 1974). These experimental approaches, particularly the acquisition of more immunogenetic data as has been begun by Cazzullo *et al.*, 1974), could obtain information which would help immunologists think more intelligently about possible new approaches through immunology to research in schizophrenia.

The effects of diet on brain function have been poetically expressed for centuries. In the Nun's Priest's tale, during Chanticleer's dreams, Chaucer (Morrison, 1949) has Dame Portlet report that 'Dreams are produced by such unseemly capers as overeating; they come from stomach vapours when a man's humours aren't behaving right.' Even though the relationship of brain function and diet still isn't clear, some of the effects of diet on immune function are beginning to be understood. The emerging model of the immune system is a confirmation and a refinement of its traditionally accepted role as a network for the storage and retrieval of information vital for the health of the host. Current understanding emphasizes the intricacies of the system and its interplay with other processes taking place in the body, and within this context an analogy can be drawn between the immune and central nervous systems. Both of these systems are superbly and uniquely qualified for the computer-like functions of data storage and retrieval. Observations of nutritional effects upon the immune system carry even further this analogy with the nervous system, as in the example of gluten enteropathy and schizophrenia, which in fact combines nutritional, immune, and central nervous system manifestations. As more is learned about these three different diciplines, it might be expected that their interactions will be more intelligently perceived, and thereby offer new understandings of the pathophysiology of schizophrenia.

REFERENCES

Braun, W. and Ungar, J. (1973). *Non-specific Factors Influencing Host Resistance*, (Basel: Karger)

Bullen, J. J., Rogers, H. and Leigh, L. (1972). Iron-binding proteins in milk and resistance to Escherichia coli infection in infants. *Br. Med. J.*, **1**, 69

Cazzulo, L. L., Smeraldi, E. and Peuato, G. (1974). *Br. J. Psychiatry*, **125**, 25

Chandra, R. K. (1975a). Reduced secretory antibody response to live attenuated measles and poliovirus vaccines in malnourished children. *Br. Med. J.*, **2**, 583

Chandra, R. K. (1976). Serum complement and immunoconglutinin in malnutrition. *Arch. Dis. Child.*, **50,** 225

Chandra, R. K. (1977). In *Food and Immunology (1977)* p. 58 (L. Hambraeus, L. A. Hanson and H. McFarlane, eds.) (Stockholm: Almqvist & Wiksell)

Cooms, R. R. A. (1975). In *Clinical Aspects of Immunology* (P. G. H. Gell, R. R. A. Coombs, and P. Lachmann, eds.) 3rd edn. pp. 761–781. (Oxford: Blackwell Scientific Publications)

Dohan, F. C., Grasberger, J. C., Lowell, F. M., Johnstone, H. T. and Abergast, A. W. (1969). *Br. J. Psychiatry,* **115,** 595

Douglas, S. D. and Schopfer, K. (1974). Phagocyte function in protein-calorie malnutrition. *Clin. Exp. Immunol.,* **17,** 121

Douglas, S. D. and Schopfer, K. (1976). Host defence mechanisms in protein-energy malnutrition. *Clin. Immunol. Immunopathol.,* **5,** 1

Douglas, S. D. and Faulk, W. P. (1977). In *Advanced Clinical Immunology* (R. A. Thompson, ed.) (London: Churchill-Livingstone)

Edelman, R., Suskin, R. M., Olson, R. E. and Sirisinha, S. (1973). Mechanisms of defective delayed cutaneous hypersensitivity in children with protein-calorie malnutrition. *Lancet,* **i,** 506

Elin, R. J. and Wolff, S. M. (1974). The role of iron in non-specific resistance to infection induced by endotoxin. *J. Immunol.,* **112,** 737

Faulk, W. P., Mata, L. J. and Edsall, G. (1975). The effects of malnutrition on the immune response in humans: A review. *Trop. Dis. Bull.,* **27,** 89

Faulk, W. P., Pinto-Paes, R. and Marigo, C. (1976). The immunological system in health and malnutrition. *Proc. Nut. Soc.,* **35,** 253

Goldman, A. S. and Smith, C. W. (1973). Host resistance factors in human milk. *J. Pediatr.,* **82,** 1082

Good, R. A., Finstad, J. and Gatti, R. A. (1970). In *Infectious Agents and Host Reistance.* (S. Mudd, ed.) pp. 76–114. (Philadelphia: Saunders)

Heyworth, B. Moore, D. L. and Brown, J. (1975). Depression of lymphocyte response to phytohaemagglutinin in the presence of plasma from children with acute protein-energy malnutrition. *Clin. Exp. Immunol.,* **22,** 72

Mata, L. and Faulk, W. P. (1973). The immune response of malnourished subjects with special reference to measles. *Arch. Latinoam. Nutr.,* **23,** 345

McFarlane, H., Olusi, S. O., Adeshina, H. A., Ade-Serrano, M. A. and Osunkoya, B. O. (1970). In *Food and Immunology* (L. Hambraeus, L. A. and H. McFarlane, eds.) pp. 23–41 (Stockholm: Almqvist and Wiksell)

Moore, D. L., Heyworth, B. and Brown, J. (1974). PHA-induced lymphocytic transformation in leucocyte cultures from malarious malnourished and control Gambian children. *Clin. Exp. Immunol.,* **17,** 651

Morrison, T. (1949) *The Portable Chaucer.* p. 203. (New York: The Viking Press)

Neuman, C. G., Lawlor, G. J., Stiehm, E. R., Swedseid, M. E., Newton, C., Herbert, J., Ammann, A. J. and Jacob, M. (1975). Immunologic responses in malnourished children. *Am. J. Clin. Nutr.,* **28,** 89

Richter, D. (1976). In *Schizophrenia Today* (D. Kemali, G. Bartholini and D. Richter, eds.). p. 71. (Oxford: Pergamon Press)

Scrimshaw, N. S., Taylor, C. E. and Gordon, J. E. (1968). Interactions of nutrition and infection. *WHO Monogr. Ser.,* **57**

Sirisinha, S., Edelman, R., Suskin, R., Charupatana, C. and Olsen, R. E. (1973). Complement and C3-proactivator levels in children with protein-calorie malnutrition and effect of dietary therapy. *Lancet,* **i,** 1016

Smythe, P. M., Brereton-Stiles, G. G., Grace, H. J., Mafoyane, A., Schonland, M., Coovadia, H. M., Loening, W. E. K., Parent, M. A. and Vos, G. H. (1971). Thymolymphatic deficiency and depression of cell-mediated immunity in protein-calorie malnutrition. *Lancet,* **ii,** 939

Smythies, J. R. (1975). In *New Prospectives in Schizophrenia.* (A. Forrest and J. Affleck, eds.) pp. 51–68 (London: Churchill Livingstone)

Stiehm, E. R., Neumann, C. G., Swendserd, M. E., Lawlor, G. E. and Ferguson, A. C. (1977). In *Food and Immunology* (L. Hambraeus, C. A. Hanson and H. McFarlane, eds.) pp. 69–85. (Stockholm: Almqvist and Wiksell)

Strober, W. (1974). In *Coeliac Disease.* (Leiden: Stenfert Kroese)

Visakorpi, J. K. (1977). In *Food and Immunology.* (L. Hambraeus, L. A. Hanson and H. McFarlane, eds.) pp. 92–98 (Stockholm: Almqvist and Wiksell)

Weinstein, W. M. (1974). *Castroenterology,* **66,** 489

Wyatt, R. J., Termini, B. A. and Davis, J. (1971). *Schizophrenia Bull.,* **4,** 11

23

The absorption of large breakdown products of dietary proteins into the body tissues including brain

W. A. HEMMINGS

INTRODUCTION

For many decades it has been accepted doctrine that dietary protein is broken down to amino acids in the gut lumen, before absorption of these amino acids by the gut wall. Thus Bayliss (1918), Hammarsten-Mendel (1909) and Fisher (1954) held to this view. Only recently has it been accepted that small peptides may be absorbed through the gut wall faster than amino acids (Matthews, 1975). Yet since the first decade of this century it has been known that immunologically significant amounts of protein evade this mechanism and reach the circulation as intact native protein. This finding has lain in the literature and has been rediscovered anew in each decade, but has had little effect on our thought on the digestive process. Recently from my laboratory has come evidence that certain proteins seem to be absorbed in very high degree in almost intact form, or at least in the form of large cleavage products. These products pass the gut wall, permeate the body and enter the cells, and, what is particularly relevant to the present topic, they enter the brain and its cells apparently passing freely across the blood–brain barrier, whatever that is (Brightman and Reese, 1969).

Immunization by uptake of the antigen from the gastro-intestinal tract was first demonstrated by Uhlenhuth (1900) who fed hen's egg white to rabbits and showed that they developed circulating precipitins to that protein. Later Ascoli (1902) used the method of detecting the antigen directly by precipitin tests against specific antiserum raised in the normal manner, to show the presence of egg albumin in blood and urine after a test oral dose of that antigen, in rabbits. It appeared in demonstrable amounts in blood one or two hours after the feed. In healthy men it was demonstrated in the blood $1\frac{3}{4}$ hours after eating raw egg white. Various other workers soon confirmed these findings. In the light of modern findings this is especially remarkable as it is now known that the albumins are more subject to gastric degradation than some other proteins. Wells and Osborne (1911) carried out experiments with a variety of quite well characterized plant proteins such as edestin from hemp seed, vetch legumin and pea vicilin, wheat gliadin, barley hordein and others.

These authors also, for the first time, employed the very sensitive method of anaphylaxis in guinea pigs, first immunizing the animal parenterally with the antigen, and then demonstrating anaphylaxis as the result of a test dose of antigen. They observed positive anaphylactic reactions with the whole range of vegetable proteins described, but noticed that the globulins of squash seed, vignin, excelsin and castor bean globulin were effective in lower doses than others, edestin being least harmful. Since a major effect in anaphylaxis is 'intoxication' and was often the only symptom shown with such a protein as edestin, one might record that these authors were for the first time investigating the cerebral effects of diet

Most of the work on antigen absorption in the first decades of the century was carried out using immunological techniques, especially anaphylaxis. The use of horse serum as antigen was common. Thus Hettwer and Kriz-Hettwer (1926) record that it is virtually impossible to give an oral dose of sufficient magnitude to kill the test animal, and that if a dose was placed in an isolated intestinal loop, it had to be larger than that given intraperitoneally to induce symptoms of shock. They concluded that anaphylactic intoxication followed intermittent ingestion of a food stuff.

An entirely novel and independent technique of assaying intestinal transport of intact proteins was used by Mills, Dorst, Mynchenberg and Nakayama (1922). They fed fibrinogen to human volunteers and assayed the clotting time of the blood thereafter: they demonstrated that an oral dose of 75 mg of fibrinogen taken in a pint of water after fasting was followed within an hour by a dramatic fall in the clotting time, for example from 2½ min to 1 min in one volunteer. A haemophiliac patient showed a reduction of clotting time from 14 min to 4½ min. The fibrinogen was shown to pass into urine also. Similar experiments were carried out using rats and dogs.

The next major technical advance was that of Walzer (1927) who took advantage of the ability of certain rare sera from food-sensitive individuals to give passive cutaneous anaphylaxis (PCA) reaction, the Prausnitz–Kustner reaction. Using this very elegant test system in large numbers of normal individuals Walzer showed the transport of intact fish antigen and egg albumin across the GI tract. He fully appreciated that the phenomenon he was demonstrating was a normal physiological process from its universality, and that it implied the transport of substantial amounts of protein from the test dose, although he made no attempt to quantitate the process of transport. He did however demonstrate uptake from rectal doses, thus confirming Croftan's (1908) experiments.

Yet despite these excellent papers, scepticism seems at that time to have been dominant. Subsequently Ratner and Gruehl (1934) were primarily concerned to ensure that their technique of feeding guinea pigs should be as natural as possible so as to be above the criticism of forced feeding possibly causing distension or other damage to the gut. These authors however successfully confirmed the older work and reviewed it at considerable length.

Winter (1944) made a further technical innovation, in that he employed the guinea pig uterus and the Schultze–Dale technique for demonstrating sensitivity and desensitization, and he showed by this means that oral doses would desensitize an immune animal: this of course requires a much larger influx of antigen than that needed merely to induce acute shock.

In relatively modern times, Cooper's school of workers have been concerned with immunity to the normal flora of the gut which is presumably induced by the uptake of metabolites by the gut wall. Thus Lee (1975) reviews this aspect of the work and reports on the occurrence of natural antibodies to the gut flora. Husband and Lascelles (1974) report that the response of sheep to egg albumin and ferritin administered into isolated intestinal loops is largely one of specific IgA production.

The Brussels group of workers had demonstrated the dynamics of oral immunization (Bazin, André and Heremans 1973), for example to red cells, showing that there appeared not to be a secondary response to repeated antigen administration, but rather that the primary response of circulating IgA production was repeated after a suitable resting phase. Wells and Osborne (1911) had shown that guinea pigs might be innoculated successfully with plant antigens while occasionally receiving these per os, but when the antigen was fed continuously, the guinea pigs could not be immunized. This was perhaps the first demonstration of what we know as immunological tolerance. The mechanism by which it comes about is suggested by recent work (André and Vaerman, 1978) on the tolerogenic capacity of complexes of antigen with IgA antibody. It is clear that this effect must be influential in the setting up of pathological conditions such as sensitivity to dietary protein, but much work remains to be done to elucidate the conditions under which immunity/tolerance for the various classes of immunoglobulins exist. At first sight, tolerance in the IgG class would seem to be a disadvantage, in that it leads to a lack of blocking antibody, yet it would seem to be a common condition. Circulating antibodies to common foodstuffs, such as gliadin and bovine milk protein, are of frequent occurrence in man (Mascord *et al.*, 1978).

Clearly, such antibodies must influence how readily BDPs of these dietary proteins reach the tissues, including the brain. The idea that immunological defences should be mobilized first as secretory antibody, IgA, in the gut lumen and mucosa, perhaps influencing the course of digestion, and secondly as blocking IgG antibody in the circulation to 'mop up' such protein as escapes the first line of defence, seems to be altogether too naive to fit the facts as we know them even at present.

Oral immunization seems to have an effect on the subsequent uptake of the antigen, during the period of IgA production. Thus André *et al.* (1974) show that a preliminary oral dose of human serum albumin depresses subsequent uptake of the labelled antigen. Walker, Isselbacher and Bloch (1974) suggest that immunization and the presence of secretory IgA in the gut lumen lead to enhanced breakdown of the antigen. In gut sacs from immunized rats there is apparently enhanced localization of the antigen on the mucosal surface, and enhanced breakdown of the antigen there. It may be that the antibody is located in the glycocalyx, and that the antigen–antibody complex may be less rapidly absorbed into the epithelial cell and would therefore be longer exposed to lumenal enzymes. Green and Freed (1978) discuss the implications of such interactions for human medicine.

Despite the long history of the knowledge of passage of immunologically significant amounts of intact protein across the gut, apparently little effort has been made to determine the quantities involved in this process. Such work as that of Mills *et al.* (1922) on the passage of fibrinogen, though strictly qualitative, implied a substantial passage of the antigen to bring about the effect demonstrated. Again, the work of Walzer (1927) demonstrated not only the universality of the passage as a qualitative demonstration, but also implied the passage of substantial amounts of protein into the circulation to bring about the effect described. The same can be said of Winter's (1944) work on desensitization of immunized animals by the oral route.

The first serious attempt to quantitate the uptake of a defined antigen seems to be the work of Warshaw, Walker and Isselbacher (1974) who followed the entry of tritium-labelled bovine serum albumin into blood and lymph after oral administration, and found that 2% of the dose could be demonstrated in those fluids in immunologically intact form. They did not look at any tissues nor look for breakdown products of the antigen. Work in our laboratory on the passage of ferritin and its breakdown products across the gut of the suckling rat used a technique of assaying the content of the whole carcase and presenting a balance sheet of the whole process of assimilation, and it was demonstrated that the circulating concentrations of the antigen or its BDPs was a poor guide to estimating the total absorption (Hemmings and Williams, 1974). This is presumably due to a short half-life of the material in the circulation, a thesis confirmed by Morris and Morris (1976) also in the suckling rat. The extension of this work to the adult is a simple step.

Passage of protein across the blood–brain barrier, except in injury, is far less well documented. The basic experiment is the exclusion of vital dyes, such as T1824, which link to the serum proteins and were historically regarded as efficient protein markers. These, when injected into the circulation, permeate the tissues with the exception of the brain, and this first gave rise to the concept of a blood–brain barrier to the entry of proteins (Ehrlich, 1885; Tschirgi, 1950). Modern work at the electron microscope level employing peroxidase as the protein tracer had demonstrated that the tracer is confined to the lumen of capillaries in the parenchyma of the brain. These capillaries have tight intercellular junctions (Reese and Karnovsky, 1967) except in certain circumscribed regions like the choroid plexus. However, albumin and IgG in the CSF originate from the plasma (Frick and Schied-Seydel, 1958), and material present in the CSF is available to brain cells in the parenchyma (Brightman and Reese, 1969). It is not however clear how the rapid entry of BDPs of dietary protein reported herein might take place.

In Bangor we have long been interested in the massive passage of protein, especially the passage of IgG, which occurs across the gut of the suckling rat and mouse during the first weeks of life (Brambell, 1970). This mainly is a duodenal process, it would appear, and it is subject in the rat to cessation abruptly at the age of 21 d, following a sharp decline from day 18. There is however a second process of absorption in the suckling which seems to be characteristic of the ileum, where the protein is absorbed after some degree of proteolysis has occurred, as large cleavage fragments (Hemmings 1975a). This process of absorption of BDPs continues after 'cut off' at 21 d and persists in the adult (Hemmings, 1975b,c). It reaches a maximum at about 100 d p.p. (C. Hemmings *et al.,* 1977) with bovine IgG. The proteins tested so far which give rise to BDPs in large amount in the tissues include horse spleen ferritin (Hemmings, 1975a), bovine and rat IgG (Hemmings, 1975c), α, β, γ gliadins (C. Hemmings *et al.,* 1976a,b), and porcine haemoglobin (Hemmings, 1976).

RESULTS

Uptake of horse spleen ferritin from the gut

Horse spleen ferritin has been widely employed as a tracer for macromolecular transport processes because it is electron dense so long as it retains its native configuration. It is also a good immunizing agent and specific antisera are easily raised for its immunological estimation. It can be easily labelled *in vitro* with radioiodine. It has been shown by all these methods to penetrate the enterocyte, and has been found in the cytoplasm of both duodenal and ileal cells of the adult rat given it intestinally (Williams, 1976). It is also demonstrable as an antigen in such organs as spleen and liver after oral administration to adult rats, implying a substantial transmission of intact protein, and this has been confirmed by quantitative studies (Hemmings and Williams, 1974, 1975a) which show that a very large part of the dose can be recovered in protein-bound form from the tissues after feeding a dose of labelled ferritin. Entry of ferritin to the brain from an oral dose has however not yet been studied. Figures 1 and 2 show ferritin entering and leaving the ileal cells of rat intestine.

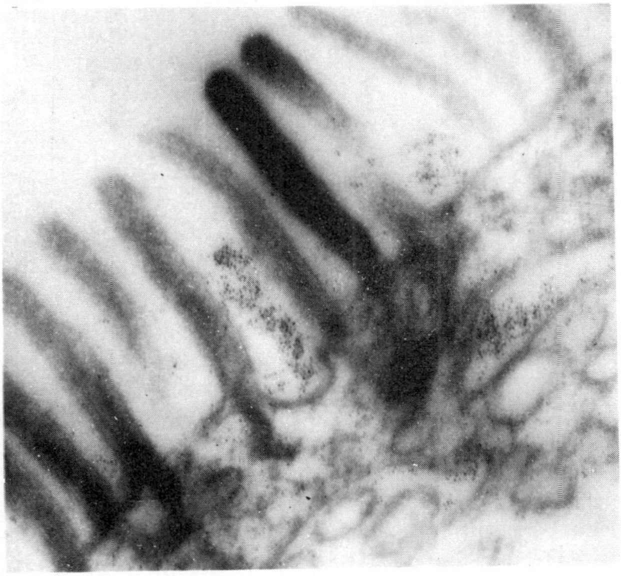

Figure 1 Section of the apical cytoplasm of an ileal cell of a 14 d old rat, after feeding horse-spleen ferritin (×19 500). (By permission of Cambridge University Press)

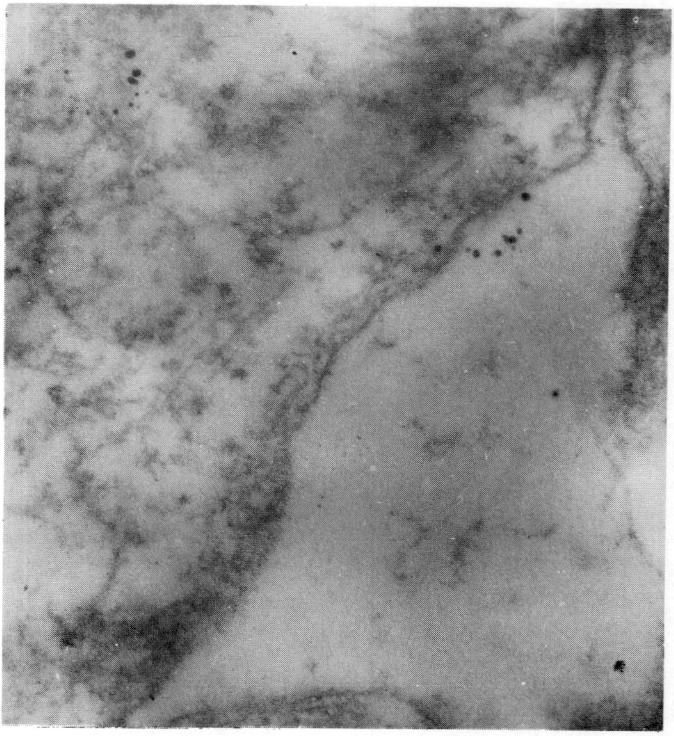

Figure 2 Intercellular space of the same tissue as Figure 1. Note the two groups of ferritin molecules, one in process of passing the bounding membrane, one approaching through the cytoplasm, but not enclosed in a vacuolar membrane (×45 000). (By permission of Cambridge University Press)

Similar experiments have been carried out with IgG, using, instead of the electron dense marker at EM level, the technique of direct deposition autoradiography to localize the protein in the cells, and preliminary results (Hemmings and Williams, 1976b) show the protein in the cytoplasm of epithelial cells of the intestine of adult rats.

The quantitative studies described in the present paper confirm that, as with ferritin, a large part of the dose of labelled bovine or rat IgG is present in the carcase as protein bound activity a few hours after feeding (Table 1). In fact in the case of bovine IgG fed to 300 g rats approximately 60% of the absorbed dose is present in that form.

Table 1 gives the distribution of radioactivity in the carcase after feeding bovine and rat IgG. Figure 3 illustrates the profile of BDPs in the carcase of an adult rat after feeding bovine IgG, as demonstrated by sucrose gradient ultracentrifugation. It can be seen that there is very little material present of the size of the initial IgG, but a large peak of material sedimenting with the albumin and pepsin markers. Figure 4 presents similar data for the brain

Table 1 Percentage of the dose fed in various body fractions after feeding ^{131}I-labelled bovine IgG and ^{125}I labelled rat IgG to adult rats. Exposure time 8 h, means of five animals±SD

Fraction	*Bovine IgG*		*Rat IgG*	
Gut wash	5.58	0.31	11.42	1.68
Stomach	27.4	8.3	29.0	17.5
Gut, protein	2.77	0.36	1.66	0.48
Gut, non-protein	1.59	0.19	2.56	0.58
Liver, protein	0.96	0.18	0.48	0.057
Liver, non-protein	0.56	0.26	0.76	0.092
Carcase, protein	43.7	7.98	34.1	5.84
Carcase, non-protein	17.5	3.0	20.0	2.56

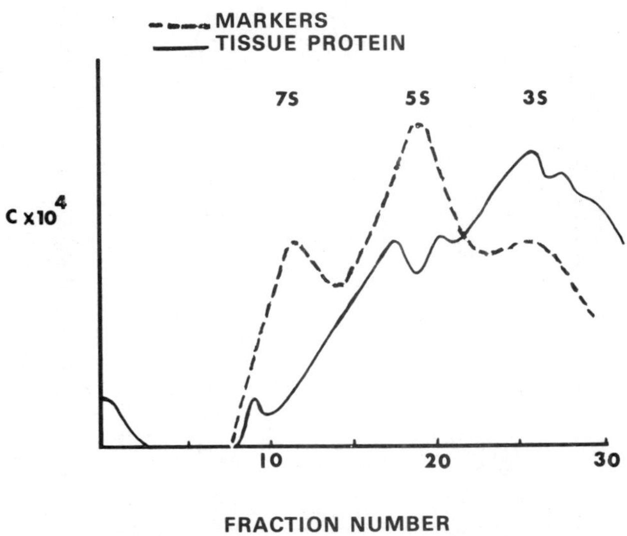

Figure 3 Sugar gradient ultracentrifugation profile of radioactivity of clarified carcase macerate after feeding ^{125}I-labelled bovine IgG to adult rats. ^{131}I-labelled markers are incorporated of IgG (7S), bovine serum albumin (5.5S) and hog stomach pepsin (3S)

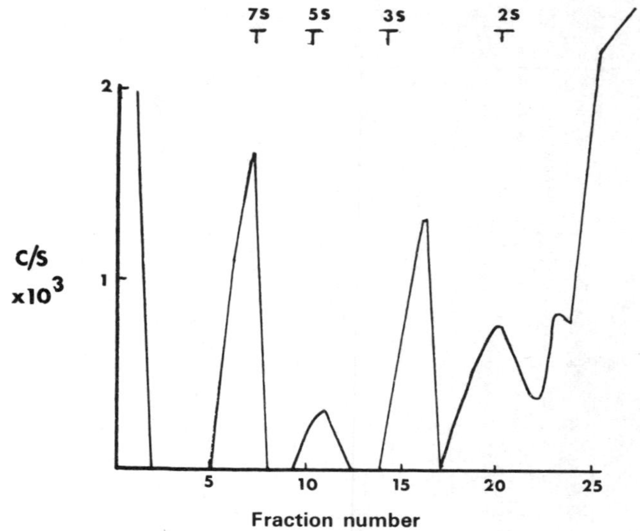

Figure 4 Sugar gradient ultracentrifugation pattern of clarified brain macerate from the same experiment as Figure 3

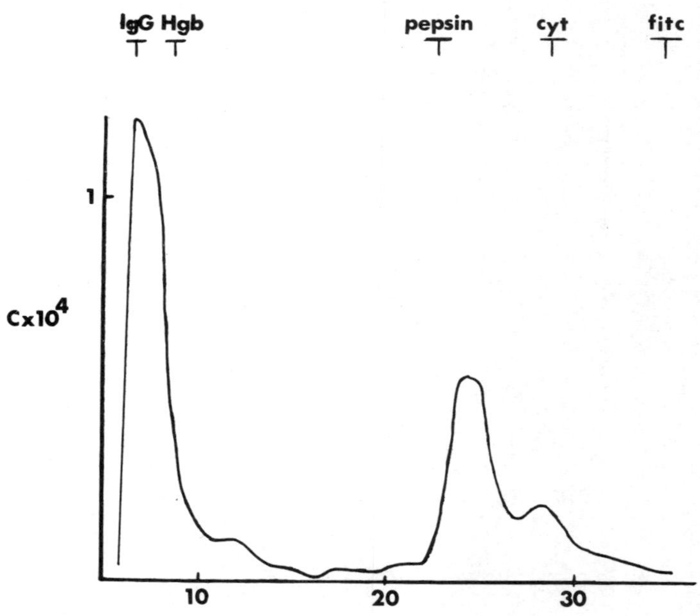

Figure 5 Gel filtration elution profile of radioactivity of the same material as Figure 4. Run on a column of Sephadex G-75, 1 cm ×50 cm, elution rate with PBS 26 ml/h

macerate after feeding bovine IgG: the macerate had been centrifuged for 30 min at 100 000 *g* to clarify it before being layered on the sugar gradient, so that it contained no organelles but represented the cell sap. Yet there is a predominant peak sedimenting at the bottom of the gradient, indicating an association of the labelled BDPs with native material to form a macromolecular complex of a high S number. Unfortunately this cannot be specified because no marker of sufficient size was included in the run, as this result was unexpected. Figure 5 presents the gel filtration profile of the same material, using Sephadex G-75, and illustrates that there are two peaks, one eluting with the exclusion volume, the other coming off close to the pepsin marker. Thus, the two techniques essentially agree with each other: the three left-hand peaks of the ultracentrifuge pattern would be combined in the exclusion volume peak of the chromatographic pattern, and the major right-hand peak is indicated by both techniques to be of slightly smaller size than the pepsin marker, with a smaller peak approximating to the cytochrome marker. There is clear evidence therefore of the presence of material of the same molecular size as the original molecule in the cell sap fraction of the brain, as well as material of greater and smaller size ranges. Whether this, or any of it, is unaltered protein remains to be tested.

In attempts to elucidate this we carried out antigen determinations with the use of a serum specific for bovine IgG. Labelled bovine IgG was fed to adult rats and serum and clarified brain macerate collected 8 h later were set up in precipitation tests at the equivalence points. Unlabelled antigen and an equivalent quantity of antiserum were added, with the intention of co-precipitating any fragments that retained their antigenic activity. The results of this experiment are given in Table 2. It can be seen that while the

Table 2 **Percentage of the total radioactivity of serum and brain macerate of adult rats, which had been fed ^{125}I-labelled bovine IgG 24 h before killing, which is perceptible with specific rabbit antiserum to bovine IgG. Means of five animals ±SD**

Sample	*Percentage precipitated*	*SD*
Serum	6.74	2.84
Brain	57.2	10.6

reaction of the serum is low, that of the brain is over half of the radioactive content of that organ, including the tungstic acid-soluble fraction. Hence it would appear that virtually all the tungstic acid-insoluble fraction of the cell sap of the brain retains antigenicity in this test. This would seem to show that the peaks of radioactivity seen in the ultracentrifuge pattern are indeed of intact bovine IgG or large cleavage fragments of the molecule.

Immunofluorescent demonstration of bovine IgG in the tissues

IgG was prepared from rabbit antiserum to bovine IgG, and labelled with fluorescein isothiocyanate (FITC). This antibody, FITC-antibovine IgG, was used as staining reagent in the classical Coon's technique (Coons *et al.*, 1941) and the sections examined in the UV microscope. Figure 6 shows a section of the ileum of an adult rat after feeding bovine IgG, developed for fluorescence: it can be seen that there are many light spots running down the centre of the villi, indicating the presence of bovine IgG in the lymphatic drainage of the villus. The larger lacteal vessels are also uniformly stained.

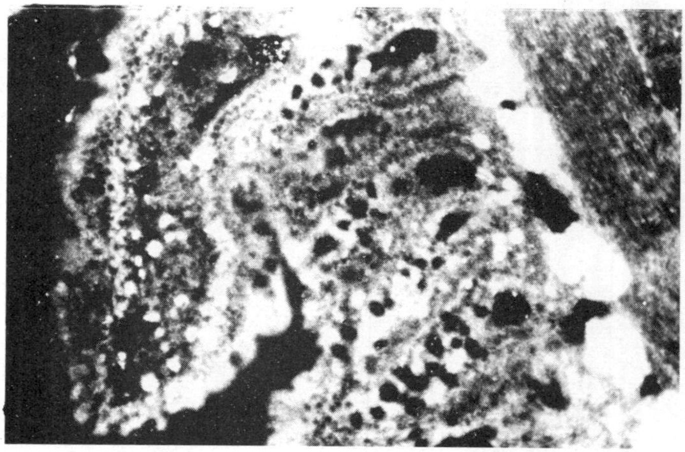

Figure 6 Fluorescent micrograph of the intestine of an adult rat which had been fed bovine IgG, developed with FITC-antibovine IgG (×125)

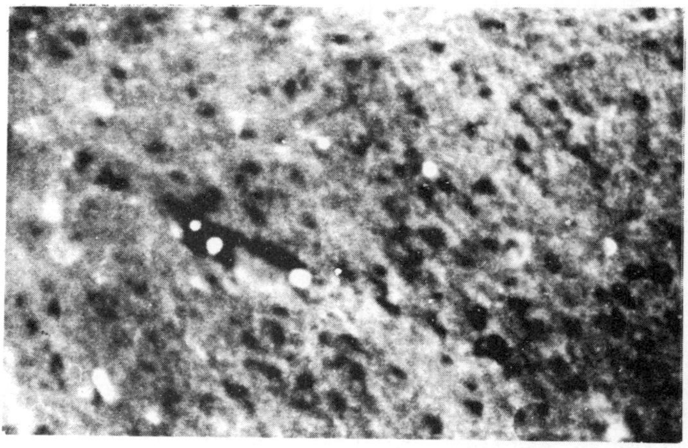

Figure 7 Fluorescent micrograph of the serebrum of the same rat as Figure 6 developed with FITC-antibovine IgG (×125)

A large amount of bovine IgG must therefore be passing the epithelium and mucosa, although these tissues are not themselves significantly fluorescent. Tests on the antiserum have shown that it does not react significantly with BDPs, so that these positive staining reactions must be taken as indicating the presence of substantially unaltered bovine IgG. Figure 7 is a section through the cerebrum of the same rat as Figure 6, developed in the same way, and clearly shows a number of discrete fluorescent foci here deep in the brain. It is very hard to interpret this appearance, but it does not seem that these foci indicate capillaries. Further work is in progress along these lines.

The uptake of wheat gliadins from the gut

Certain further experiments were carried out with gliadin fractions derived from Kolibri wheat flour. This work was undertaken after the initial findings were made on the entrance of BDPs to the tissues, because of the importance especially of α-gliadin in the causation of coeliac disease (Hekkens *et al.*, 1970) and because of the association of gluten, of which the gliadins are components, with the aetiology of schizophrenia (Dohan, 1966).

Table 3 Percentage of remaining dose in body fractions after feeding ^{125}I-labelled α-gliadin to rats. Ten suckling rats were exposed for three hours, six adult rats for 24 h. Means±SD

Sample	*Suckling rats*		*Adult rats*	
Stomach			2.94	0.67
Intestinal washing			27.89	5.46
Hind gut			9.18	1.72
Washed intestine	34.75	1.016	2.98	0.57
Carcase, tungstic ppt	15.8	0.576	46.34	6.91
Carcase, tungstic sol	45.99	0.683	9.71	1.70
Brain	0.656	0.072	0.145	0.0199
Blood (1 ml serum)	3.49	0.107	0.135	0.017

^{125}I-labelled α-gliadin was fed to groups of adult and suckling rats, which at autopsy some hours later were fractionated to reveal how much of the dose had been absorbed, and what its distribution was in the body. Table 3 represents the results of these experiments. It can be seen that there is a very large part of the dose in the fraction of the 'carcase' precipitable with tungstic acid. This represents protein-bound activity in the skeletal muscle primarily, the animals having been skinned before maceration. There is also a small but quite significant portion in the brains. As can be seen, the specific activity of the brain, which weighs approximately 1 g, is not very dissimilar from the specific activity of the serum. Since the contamination level of brain with blood, as measured by haemoglobin assay of the extracts, is of the order of 1% it is impossible that the radioactivity of the brain could arise by contamination with blood.

Table 4 **Specific activities of brain fractions analysed by differential centrifugation after feeding ^{125}I-labelled α-gliadin to rats. Means of six animals (%total activity of brain±SD)**

Sample	*Content*	*Suckling rats*		*Adult rats*	
P1	Nuclei, cell membranes ets	38.0	4.50	30.8	4.24
P2	Mitochondria and lysosomes	3.15	0.268	5.9	1.14
P3	Microsomes				
P4	Tungstic acid ppt of supernatant 3	12.88	3.23	29.8	6.19
S4	Tungstic acid supernatant of supernatant 3	42.28	1.96	29.2	2.85

Table 4 shows the result of differential centrifugation of the brain macerate, showing the distribution of radioactivity in the sub-cellular fractions. It can be seen that while about one-third of the total activity is associated with sample P1, which includes nuclei and larger fragments of cell membrane (so the activity may be inside or on the surface of the cell) there are low but significant counts on the organelle fractions, and a considerable amount,

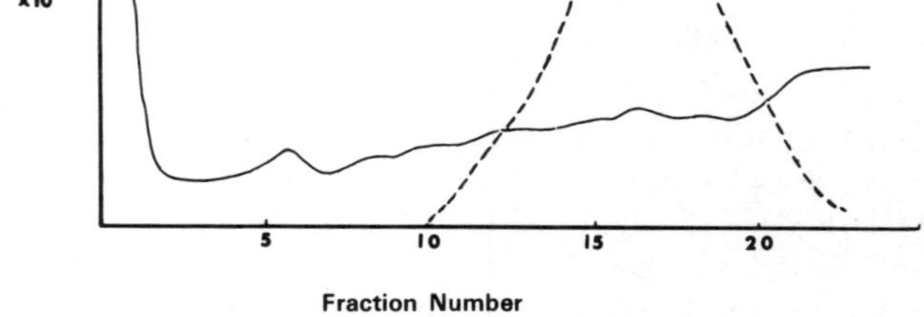

Figure 8 Sugar gradient ultracentrifugation profile of brain macerate of adult rats after feeding ^{125}I-labelled α-gliadin. The superimposed dotted line is the profile of the α-gliadin fed

another one-third in the adult, in the protein-bound portion of the cell sap. Thus this is clearly protein-bound activity from within the cell.

Figure 8 shows the result of sugar gradient ultracentrifugation of the clarified brain macerate in these experiments. The dotted line shows the distribution of activity in the control tube containing the original preparation of α-gliadin fed, the continuous line is the profile of activity of the brain macerate. It can be seen that, as in the case of bovine IgG, there is a large peak right at the bottom of the tube, but here there is little differentiation in the rest of the profile. There is no large peak of BDPs to the right of α-gliadin as might be expected. But it is clear that a large part of the activity in the brain is bound up in the rapidly sedimenting material at the left of the profile. The profile of the serum of this experiment is shown in Figure 9.

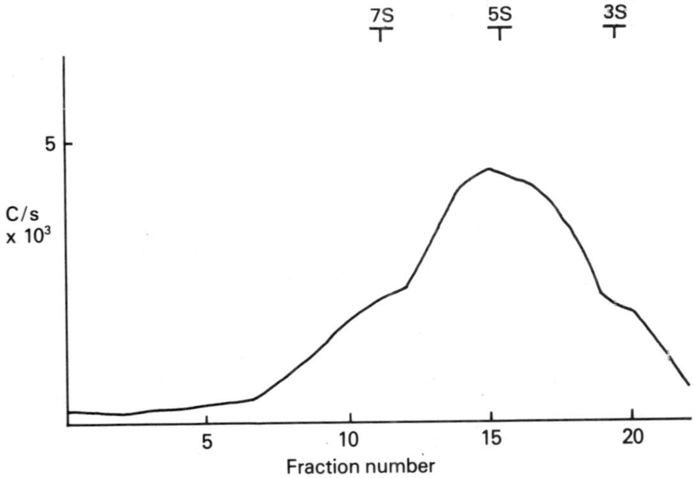

Figure 9 Sugar gradient ultracentrifugation profile of the serum of the experiment of Figure 8

Uptake of porcine haemoglobin from the gut

Adult rats were fed porcine haemoglobin labelled with ^{125}I, and their bodies analysed in the same way as with α-gliadin. The results are presented in Table 5. It can be seen again that there is a large part of the absorbed dose in the protein-bound activity of the carcase: and again there is a small but significant activity in the brain. The clarified brain macerate was therefore placed on sugar-gradient ultracentrifugation, and the profile is shown in Figure 10. Here the run was kept deliberately short in the expectation that there might be resolution of heavy material thereby: the peak of haemoglobin would be under the 5.5S marker. There are three major peaks to the left of this marker, and yet there is still an unresolved peak of ultra-heavy material sedimented to the bottom of the tube. The pattern with haemoglobin is thus very complex.

Table 5 **Distribution of radioactivity through the organs of adults rats fed ^{125}I–swine haemoglobin eight hours previously. Means of five animals ± SE**

Sample	*Dose* (%)	± *SE*
% of dose absorbed	45.82	12.34
Intestine	17.85	5.04
Liver, tungstic ppt	5.92	6.50
Liver, tungstic soluble	4.74	1.84
Brain, tungstic ppt	0.151	0.196
Brain, tungstic soluble	0.326	0.476
Carcase, tungstic ppt	24.82	9.89
Carcase, tungstic soluble	40.10	10.58

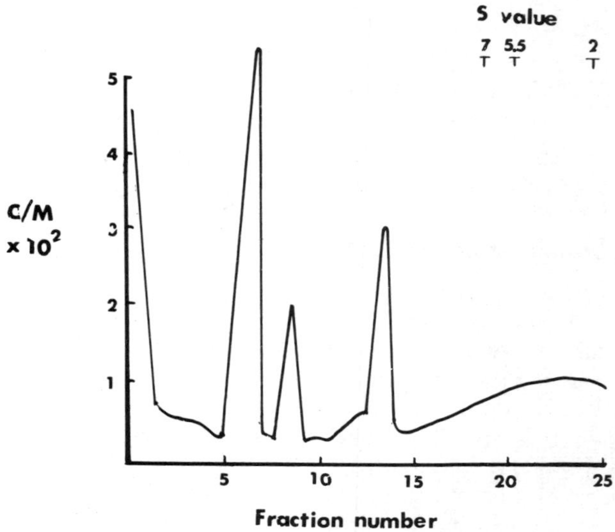

Figure 10 Sugar gradient ultracentrifugation profile of the clarified brain macerate from rats fed porcine haemoglobin labelled with ^{125}I

DISCUSSION

The choice of proteins studied to date must inevitably influence our present view of this new phenomenon, and serendipity may have played a part in that the choice has been suggested in the case of ferritin by its utility as a tracer, in the case of the IgGs because they were the standard study of this laboratory, and in the case of the gliadins because they were of pathological significance in man. Haemoglobin has some significance in the husbandry of piglets. These are all proteins which appear to be resistant to proteolytic assault in the gut lumen of the rat. It does not necessarily follow that the same list of proteins would be resistant in another species, and trials of this point are clearly a matter of some urgency. Are there exceptions to this rule of resistance to proteolysis? Clearly yes. Serum albumin is relatively readily broken down in the stomach (Jones, 1974) and gives rise to very low concentrations in the circulation, even of suckling rats after gastric digestion becomes overt about 7 d after birth (Jordan and Morgan, 1968). Despite this suscepti-bility to proteolysis, Warshaw *et al.* (1974) have succeeded in demonstrating the presence of no less than 2% of bovine serum albumin (BSA) in blood and lymph of adult rats a few hours after feeding tritium-labelled BSA. Never-theless serum albumin is clearly an unfortunate choice of protein to demon-strate the passage of undegraded material. Ovalbumin might be far better, because Sussman *et al.* (1928) and his colleagues demonstrated absorption of sufficient amounts of this protein from oral doses to give PCA reactions in normal humans. Our knowledge of this field is as yet very limited, and clearly another matter of great urgency is the need for trials of a great variety of normal dietary proteins to test their susceptibility to enzymatic degradation in the normal gut.

Is this phenomenon what it seems? The quantitative studies with isotope show the presence of considerable amounts of protein-bound material in the tissues, including brain, and the ultracentrifuge studies show that the isotope is bound to high molecular weight complexes or degradation products. The word complex is chosen because in some cases the radioactivity is associated with component peaks sedimenting faster than the original material fed. Since complexing is being considered, may it not be that quite small degrada-tion products are becoming bound to carriers in the recipients' serum and lymph or tissues, and so appearing in the tungstic precipitation in the centrifuge, and as material of much higher molecular weight in the gel filtration? This is a possibility not easily tested. One approach is to look for the immunological properties of the foreign BDPs in the tissues, either as an immunogen or as an antigen reactive with specific antiserum to the original molecule. In fact when the latter test is made with bovine IgG, as Table 1 shows, virtually all the protein-bound activity of the cell sap of the brain turns out to be specifically precipitable. A similar test of the same fraction after feeding α-gliadin (Hemmings *et al.*, 1976) also showed a high proportion of the protein-bound content to be precipitable with specific antiserum. Hence it would seem that the material in the brain does retain its antigenic structure to a very large extent, and so must be considered to be indeed large molecular forms of the original material, rather than small peptides associated with carrier molecules as was suggested in the alternative hypothesis above. The other serological test, of the potency of the BDPs in tissue as immunogen is also in hand, but necessarily requires a longer period of experiment. It is also qualitative only.

A further point of great interest, referred to briefly above, is the formation of ultra-heavy complexes by the BDPs in brain cell sap. α-Gliadin especially might be suspected of forming complexes with itself: such aggregates though would be expected to occur universally if they were prone to be formed, and this does not occur. α-Gliadin run on sugar gradient by itself forms a nearly symmetrical sedimentation peak at about 4S, as would be expected for the unaggregated molecule. In the serum of fed animals the situation is somewhat different, and the protein appears (Figure 9) predominantly in a 5S peak, with a minor 7S component. This certainly indicates complexing of some sort, but it is evidently not common to the undigested α-gliadin and its BDPs. The situation in brain is different again, with the formation of the ultra-heavy component at the bottom of the tube, and no sign of especial peaks at any of the above positions. If it were self-aggregation that was occurring, the picture should be constant. It therefore appears far more probable that the BDPs are combining with a variety of different native proteins according to the milieu in which they occur.

Clearly such ability to combine with native tissue components needs much more proof, and investigation. But it suggests a potential mechanism of cytotoxicity of the molecule, in that its capacity to combine, perhaps specifically, with native cell components, leading probably to the inactivation of those components from their normal role, could interrupt vital cell processes at the biochemical level, and thus lead to damage to the functioning of the cell.

α-Gliadin is not alone in forming such complexes in the brain: both bovine IgG and porcine haemoglobin do this also. Haemoglobin does form ultra-heavy complex in the serum (Hemmings, 1976) but bovine IgG in serum presents only a pattern of BDPs to the right of its origin (Hemmings, 1975c).

The old hypothesis of complete degradation of dietary protein in the gut lumen therefore must be discarded, and the consequences of eating become much more interestingly complex in the light of this information. They can be summarised in outline by Figure 11 where the long arrows represent our large fragments of protein, the BDPs. They are figured entering the enterocytes either by pinocytosis, or directly across the bounding membrane by some process of assisted diffusion. Clearly the mechanism of how such large molecules should enter intact cells is of great importance at all stages of this hypothesis, but it is not part of the present paper to discuss this aspect, beyond mentioning the observation that such markers as ferritin have been frequently observed in the cytoplasm of the enterocyte (Williams, 1976).

Possibly some intracellular degradation of our large arrows occurs in the enterocyte, therefore both small and large arrows are shown leaving it into the lymph: again this is a matter of observation, for ferritin has been figured leaving the cell for the intracellular space in adult rats (Figure 2). A line has

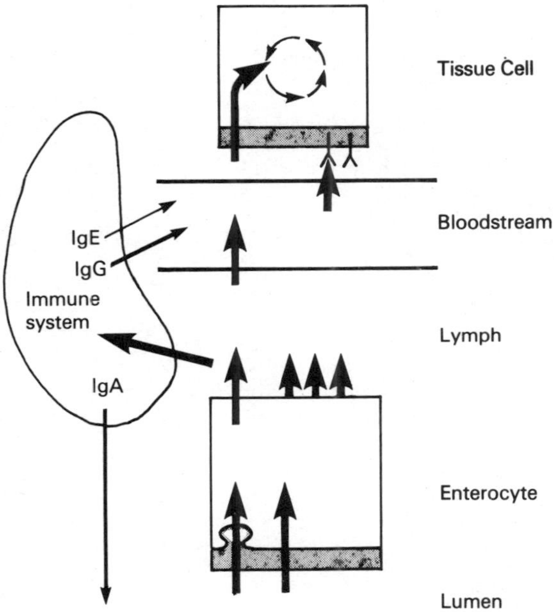

Figure 11 Schematic diagram of the relationships of large molecular weight breakdown products (indicated by long arrows) following the feeding of a protein diet

been drawn between lymph and blood to represent, not a barrier, but the infiltration through the lymph nodes, and indeed the mucosa itself, and the reaction of the immune system summarised separately. This is again a topic separate from this short paper, but is briefly the production of antibody, or alternatively a state of tolerance. We do not yet fully understand how the latter may be induced by gut antigen, but clearly it can (André and Vaerman, 1976). However, if antibody production occurs, it may fall into any or all of three main classes of antibody, IgG, IgA or IgE. IgA primarily is secreted, especially into the gut lumen where it may be expected to influence the absorption and digestion of future meals of the homologous antigen (Green and Freed, 1978). IgG will enter the circulation where it will serve as blocking antibody functioning to clear the antigen from the circulation on future penetration into the blood. IgE antibody will fix to mast cells and so give rise to anaphylactic type sensitivity *vis à vis* the future penetration of the homologous antigen, and hence is responsible for most of the unpleasant symptoms associated with food sensitivity. Finally, at the top of the diagram the long arrow is seen entering the tissue cell and there interfering hypothetically with a biochemical system.

REFERENCES

André, C., Lambert, R., Bazin, H. and Heremans, J. F. (1974). Interference of oral immunisation with intestinal absorption of heterologous albumin. *Eur. J. Immunol.,* **4,** 701

André, C. and Vaerman, J. P. (1978). Biological functions of antigen–IgA antibody complexes: *in vivo* and *in vitro* interference with intestinal absorption and tolerogenic effect. In *Antigen Absorption by the Gut,* W. A. Hemmings, ed. (Lancaster: MTP Press Ltd.)

Ascoli, M. (1902). Ueber den Mechanisms der Albinurie durch Eireiweiss. *Mu. Med. Wochenschr.,* **49,** 398

Bayliss, W. M. (1918). *Principles of General Physiology* (London: Longmans)

Bazin, H., André, C. and Heremans, J. F. (1973). Réponses immunologiques induites par voie orale. *An. Immunol. (Inst. Pasteür),* **124C,** 153

Brambell, F. W. R. (1970). The transmission of passive immunity from mother to young. *Frontiers of Biology,* Vol. 18. (Amsterdam: North Holland)

Brightman, M. W. and Reese, T. S. (1969). Junctions between intimately apposed cell membranes in the vertebrate brain. *J. Cell. Biol.,* **40,** 648

Coons, A. H., Creech, H. J. and Jones, R. N. (1941). Immunological properties of an antibody containing a fluorescent group. *Proc. Soc. Exp. Biol.,* **47,** 200

Croftan, A. C. (1908). *Lancet (Clinic),* **99,** (N.S. 60) 379

Dohan, F. C. (1966). Cereals and schizophrenia: data and hypothesis. *Acta Psychiat. Scand.,* **42,** 125

Ehrlich, P. (1885). *Das Sauerstoff – Bedurfnis des Oranismus* (Berlin: Hirschwald)

Fisher, R. B. (1954). *Protein Metabolism* Chap. 1 (London: Methuen)

Frick, E. and Scheid-Seydel, L. (1958). Untersuchungen mit ^{131}I Markiertem α-Globulin zur Frage der Abstammung des Liquorweisskorper. *Klin. Wochenschr.,* **36,** 857

Green, F. H. Y. and Freed, D. L. J. (1978). Antibody facilitated digestion and the consequences of its failure. In *Antibody Absorption by the Gut,* W. A. Hemmings, ed. (Lancaster: MTP Press Ltd.)

Hammarsten-Mendel (1909). *The Textbook of Physiological Chemistry,* 5th ed. (New York)

Hemmings, C., Hemmings, W. A. and Patey, A. L. (1976a). The fate of oral doses of α-gliadin in suckling and adult rats. IRCS Med. Sci., **4,** 38

Hemmings, C., Hemmings, W. A. and Patey, A. L. (1976b). The fate of oral doses of β and γ-gliadin in adult rats. IRCS Med. Sci., **4,** 152

Hemmings, C., Hemmings, W. A., Patey, A. L. and Wood, C. (1977). The ingestion of dietary protein as large molecular weight degradation products in adult rats. *Proc. R. Soc. B.,* **198,** 439

Hemmings, W. A. (1975a). Degradation products in gut and carcase tissue after injecting labelled ferritin into the ileum of suckling rats. *IRCS Med. Sci.,* **3,** 216

Hemmings, W. A. (1975b). Transport of protein across the small intestine of adult rats following the injection of ferritin to the intestinal lumen. *IRCS Med. Sci.,* **3,** 262

Hemmings, W. A. (1975c). Transport of immunoglobulins across the gut of the adult rat. *IRCS Med. Sci.,* **3,** 282

Hemmings, W. A. (1976). The absorption of haemoglobin from oral doses by adult rats. *IRCS Med. Sc.,* **4,** 393

Hemmings, W. A. and Williams, E. W. (1974). Uptake of labelled ferritin and rat IgG from segments of the gut of the suckling rat. *IRCS Med. Sci.,* **2,** 1450

Hemmings, W. A. and Williams, E. W. (1975a). Transport of ferritin across the ileum of the suckling rat. *IRCS Med. Sci.,* **3,** 215

Hemmings, W. A. and Williams, E. W. (1975b). The attachment of IgG to cell components of transporting membranes.In *Maternofoetal Transmission of Immunoglobulins,* W. A. Hemmings, ed. (London: Cambridge University Press)

Hemmings, W. A. and Williams, E. W. (1976a). The use of direct deposition autoradiography in studies of protein transport. *J. Microscop. (Oxford),* **106,** 131

Hemmings, W. A. and Williams, E. W. (1976b). The transport of large break down products of dietary protein through the gut wall. *Gut*

Hekkens, W. Th. J. M., Haex, A. J. Ch. and Willighagen, R. G. J. (1970). Some aspects of gliadin fractionation and testing by a histochemical method. In *Coeliac disease, Proc. Int. Coeliac Symp.,* C. C. Booth and R. H. Dowling, eds. (London: Churchill-Livingstone)

Hettwer, J. P. and Krix-Hettwer, R. (1926). Further observations on the absorption of undigested protein. *Am. J. Physiol.,* **78,** 136

Hudson, D. A., Purdham, D. R., Cornell, H. J. and Rolles, C. J. (1976). Non-specific cytotoxicity of wheat gliadin components towards cultured human cells. *Lancet,* **i,** 339
Husband, A. J. and Lascelles, A. K. (1974). The origin of antibody in intestinal secretion of sheep, *AJEBAK,* **52(pt5),** 791
Jones, R. E. (1974). Studies *in vivo* and *in vitro* of the transfer of rat IgC and rat albumen across the intestinal walls of young rats. *Biol. Neonate,* **24,** 220
Jordan, S. M. and Morgan, E. H. (1968). The development of selectivity of protein absorption from the intestine during suckling in the rat. *Aust. J. Exp. Biol. Med. Sci.,* **46,** 465
Lee, A. and Foo, M. C. (1978). Natural antibodies and the intestinal flora in rodents. In *Antigen Absorption by the Gut,* W. A. Hemmings, ed. (Lancaster: MTP Press Ltd.)
Mascord, I., Freed, D. L. J. and Durrant, B. (1978). Antibodies to foodstuffs in schizophrenia. *Br. Med. J.,* 1351
Matthews, D. M. (1975). Intestinal absorption of peptides. *Physiol. Rev.,* **55,** 537
Mills, G. A., Dorst, S. E., Mynchenberg, G. and Nakayama, J. (1922). Absorption from the intestine and excretion through the kidney of an unaltered complex protein substance, tissue fibrinogen. *Am. J. Physiol.,* **63,** 484
Morris, B. and Morris, R. (1976). Quantitative assessment of the transmission of label ed protein by the proximal and distal regions of the small intestine of young rats. *J. Physiol.,* **255,** 619
Ratner, B. and Gruehl, H. L. (1934). Passage of native proteins through the normal gastro-intestinal wall. *J. Clin. Invest.,* **13,** 517
Reese, T. S. and Karnovsky, M. J. (1967). Fine structural localization of a blood–brain barrier to exogenous peroxidase. *J. Cell. Biol.,* **34,** 207
Sussman, H., Davidson, A. and Walzer, M. (1928). Absorption of undigested proteins in human beings. III. The absorption of unaltered egg protein in adults. *Arch. Intern. Med.,* **42,** 409
Tschirgi, R. D. (1950). Protein complexes and the impermeability of the blood–brain barrier to dyes. *Am. J. Physiol.,* **163,** 756
Uhlenhuth, P. T. (1900). Neuer beitrag zum spezifischen nachweis von eiereiweiss auf biologischem wege. *Dtsch. Med. Wochenschr.,* **26,** 734
Walker, W. A., Isselbacher, K. J. and Bloch, K. J. (1974). Immunologic control of soluble protein absorption from the small intestine: a gut-surface phenomenon. *Am. J. Clin. Nutr.,* **27,** 1434
Warshaw, A. L., Walker, W. A. and Isselbacher, K. J. (1974). Protein uptake by the intestine: evidence for absorption of intact macromolecules. *Gastroenterology,* **66,** 987
Walzer, M. (1927). Studies in absorption of undigested proteins in human beings. I. A Simple direct method of studying the absorption of undigested protein. *J. Immunol.,* **14,** 143
Wells, H. G. and Osborne, T. B. (1911). The biological reactions of the vegetable proteins. I. Anaphylaxis. *J. Infect. Dis.,* **8,** 66
Williams, E. W. (1976). Uptake and transport of ferritin from the intestinal lumen of the adult rat. Electronmicroscopic and immunological studies. *I.R.C.S. Med. Sci.,* **4,** 214
Winter, L. B. (1944). Anaphylaxis to serum proteins. *J. Physiol.,* **102,** 373

24

Antibodies to gliadin in serum of normals, coeliac patients and schizophrenics

W. Th. J. M. HEKKENS

Following on from our interest in coeliac disease we have been investigating α-gliadin in patients suffering from this disease. During the last months we have elaborated a method of measuring quantitatively the antibodies coeliac patients make in their serum against gliadin, a group of proteins from wheat. We wanted to know if gliadin passes the intestinal wall of coeliac patients in greater quantity than in normals and stimulates antibody production. We used the Enzyme Linked Immuno Sorbent Assay (ELISA) as developed by Engvall and Perlman in Sweden. The technique is illustrated in Figure 1. The alkaline phosphatase activity measured is proportional to the amount of antibody in the serum.

We raised antibodies to gliadin in rabbits and measured the amount in several dilutions. We obtained a curve as illustrated in Figure 2.

Hemmings *et al.* (1976) found that α-gliadin derivatives reached the brain both in suckling and mature rats, and this may be of importance in schizophrenia. There was the possibility that there was a difference in the amount of antibodies formed by these patients. We therefore compared the sera of 26 normals with that of 21 coeliac patients and 20 schizophrenics. The results are summarized in Figure 3.

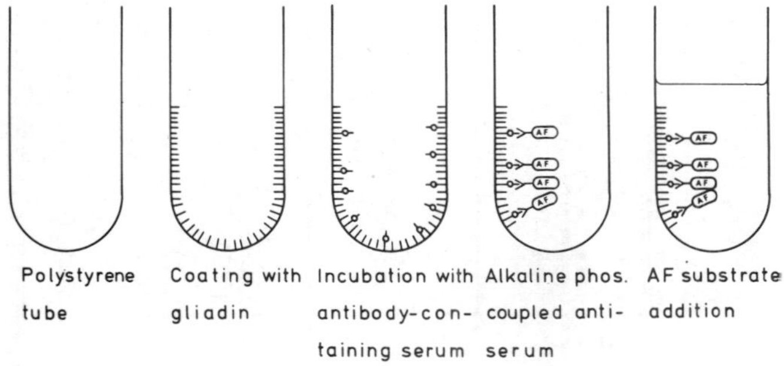

Figure 1 Gluten antibody measurement in serum

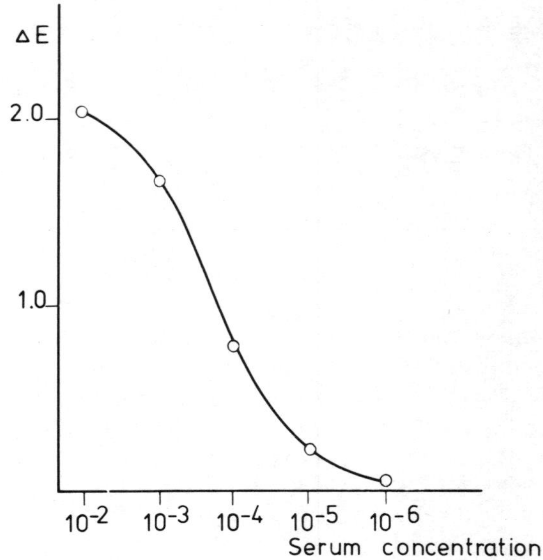

Figure 2 Alkaline phosphatase activity in relation to amount of serum antibodies to gliadin in rabbits

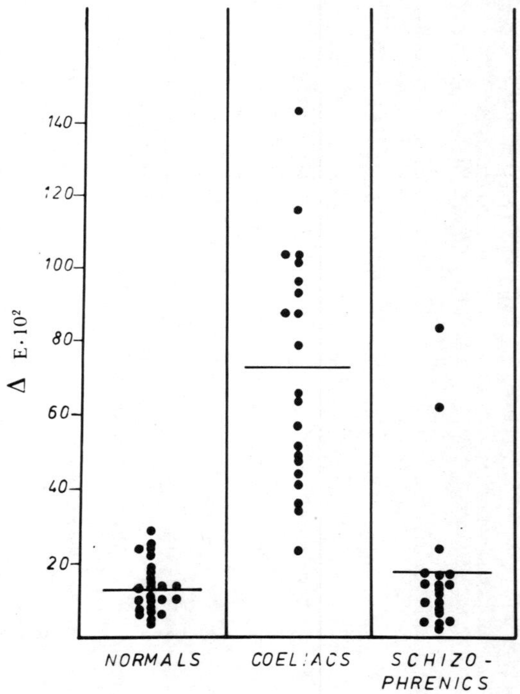

Figure 3 Gliadin antibody levels in normals, coeliacs and schizophrenics

From this figure it can be concluded that in most of the schizophrenics, in contrast to the coeliac patients, the level of antibody is in the range of the normals. Two out of 20 however have a raised level, pointing in the direction of a higher incidence of gluten sensitivity in schizophrenics as postulated by Dohan. This gluten sensitivity in the two patients mentioned has to be proven.

REFERENCES

Engvall, E. and Perlman, P. (1971). Enzyme linked immunosorbent assay (ELISA). Quantitative assay of immunoglobulin G. *Immunochemistry,* **8,** 871

Hemmings, C., Hemmings, W. A. and Patey, A. L. (1976). The fate of oral doses of α-gliadin in suckling and adult rats. *IRCS Med. Sci.,* **4,** 38

SECTION 7:
Alcoholism

25
Screening tests for alcoholism

S. B. ROSALKI

Many workers have suggested an association between schizophrenia and alcoholism. If this is so, the recognition of chronic excess alcohol intake in both disorders is of obvious diagnostic importance. Annual expenditure on alcoholic beverages in the United Kingdom is in excess of £2000 million, and the equivalent of more than 7 l of absolute alcohol is consumed annually per head of population. It has been estimated that more than 2% of the adult population or more than 750, 000 people drink excessively and that more than 10% of admissions to male medical wards have a drinking problem (Hetzel, 1975; Hore, 1977).

The recognition of alcoholism traditionally depends on symptomatology and physical signs. Factors which may suggest alcoholism include at-risk occupations, a history of social difficulties or psychiatric disturbance, and the more overt symptoms of addiction (tolerance, dependence, withdrawal symptoms) or of the diseases traditionally associated with alcoholism (liver disease, psychosis, neuropathy, etc.). Obvious physical signs frequently associated with alcoholism include hoarse voice, puffy face, blood-shot eyes, bruised skin and changes in the palm and nails (Silberfarb, 1976).

These conventional symptoms and signs of alcoholism may be absent or misleading. It is generally recognised that clinical diagnosis of the disorder may present great difficulty, and that an estimated 50% of alcoholics deny heavy drinking (Bailey, Haberman and Steinberg, 1969). There is therefore a need for objective evidence of chronic excess alcohol consumption. Such evidence can be obtained in the vast majority of alcoholics by laboratory procedures.

The most valuable of all laboratory procedures for the detection of chronic excess alcohol intake is measurement of the activity of the enzyme γ-glutamyl-transferase in blood serum (Rosalki *et al.,* 1970; Rosalki and Rau, 1972). Its determination can be used: (1) to detect individuals whose alcohol consumption is excessive, (2) to monitor their condition and (3) to identify liver damage from alcohol.

This enzyme (which I shall abbreviate as GGTP) originates from the liver, where its production is stimulated by alcohol, resulting in increased serum levels. This is an early effect of alcohol excess and precedes abnormal liver function, though with continued drinking, hepato-cellular injury and bilary stasis contribute to serum GGTP elevation and may additionally give rise to elevation of other serum enzymes, especially aspartate transaminase

Since 1969 when I first demonstrated the especial value of GGTP for the detection of alcoholism I have reported studies of 456 alcoholics and heavy drinkers, 347 of whom showed GGTP elevation; an overall incidence of 76% (Rosalki, 1977). Heavy drinking was defined as long-standing alcohol consumption, considered as frankly excessive by the patients' regular medical attendant. Alcoholism was defined as excessive drinking accompanied by alcohol dependence. Out-patient alcoholics and heavy drinkers showed a higher incidence of GGTP elevation (approaching 90%) than hospitalised subjects, illustrating the especial value of the enzyme for detecting early alcoholism. Enzyme values ranged up to 60 times the upper limit of normal, though most were below five times.

Heavy, acute alcoholic consumption in the normal subject produces only a slight and transient effect on the serum GGTP (Rosalki, 1974). A minimum of some three weeks of heavy daily alcohol consumption seems to be required before pathological serum GGTP values are seen.

When an alcoholic stops drinking, GGTP levels usually revert towards normal within days. The majority of patients seen will show a reduction by some 50% within two weeks and near-normal values within five weeks. More persistent elevation is, however, observed in the presence of underlying cirrhosis. Serial measurements are of value in the known alcoholic for monitoring progress and therapy.

GGTP has been used in epidemiological surveys and in case-finding studies in high risk groups. It falls within the definition of a screening procedure as 'a rapid test for the presumptive identification of disease in apparently well persons'. Its sensitivity or the incidence of true positives was found to be 90% in out-patient alcoholics and its specificity or incidence of true negatives was 93% in apparently healthy blood donor controls (Rosalki, 1974).

The especial advantages of GGTP determination in the investigation of alcoholism may be summarised as high diagnostic sensitivity and good specificity for liver, though non-alcoholic liver disease or other hepatic enzyme-inducing drugs may also give elevation. The laboratory determination of GGTP is also exceedingly cheap and simple and is readily automated. The enzyme in serum is also very stable and serum can be stored frozen for several months without deterioration. Enzyme abnormality may provide diagnostic confirmation when excessive drinking is suspected but denied, is useful for demonstrating to the patient the effect of his drinking habits, and is valuable for monitoring progress and alleged abstention from alcohol.

Another procedure which has proved helpful in the laboratory confirmation of suspected excess alcohol consumption is measurement of the erythrocyte mean corpuscular volume (MCV), a measurement which is readily carried out in the haematology laboratory with modern automatic cell counters. Chronic alcohol consumption damages the developing red cell, and gives rise to increased red cell volume reflected by elevation of the erythrocyte MCV (Herbert, Zalusky and Davidson, 1964; Wu, Chanarin and Levi, 1974), though it must of course be remembered that many diseases other than alcoholism can also increase the MCV. The incidence of MCV elevation in alcoholics referred to hospital averages some 50 to 60% (Bagrin *et al.*, 1976).

This incidence of MCV abnormality is significantly lower than that observed for GGTP. In addition, GGTP also shows a greater degree of abnormality and a more rapid and appropriate response to abstinence (Lamy *et al.*, 1976). Nevertheless, the combination of GGTP and MCV measurements may be especially valuable in detection of alcoholics. In a comparative study of hospitalised alcoholics, serum GGTP activity was raised in 75% and erythrocyte MCV values in 60%. Although the majority of alcoholics with elevated MCV value also showed GGTP elevation this was not invariable. In consequence, abnormality of one or other of the determinations was observed in 90%.

A third laboratory procedure which has been reported as frequently abnormal in alcoholism, is the ratio of the plasma levels of the two amino acids, α–amino n–butyric acid and leucine (Shaw, Stimnel and Lieber, 1976). This ratio is increased in more than 70% of alcoholic hospital admissions. A disadvantage of the procedure is the expense and complexity of the determination, which requires specialised apparatus available in only a few hospital centres. The ratio has been described as unaltered in non-alcoholic liver disease, so the method could have special value in the differentiation of alcoholic from non-alcoholic liver disease. In patients with an abnormal GGTP or liver function test value, it could then be helpful in establishing a specific alcoholic aetiology for the abnormality. However a recent study (Morgan, Milsom and Sherlock, 1977) has failed to confirm such specificity.

Though it is chronic excessive alcohol consumption which partially characterises the alcoholic, such patients may also present following recent drinking. Three laboratory procedures are useful in the identification of recent drinking:

(1) The determination of elevated alcohol levels in blood, breath or urine positively identifies alcohol consumption, and has been useful for the identification of intoxication resulting in injury (Rutherford, 1977) and the identification of an alcoholic aetiology in patients attending liver clinics (Hamlyn *et al.*, 1975).

(2) The osmotic effect of alcohol may also result in increased plasma osmolality, and this may serve as a clue to alcohol consumption in suspected intoxication. A blood alcohol level of some 100 mg/dl will increase the plasma osmolality by some 20 mosm/kg (Robinson and Loeb, 1971).

(3) An enzyme procedure, measurement of erythrocyte δ amino-levulinic acid dehydrase (abbreviated as DALD) may also be abnormal following recent acute alcoholic ingestion, and the red cell level of this enzyme is reduced in over 90% of alcoholics with recent alcohol intake (Moore and Goldberg, 1975).

This sensitivity of erythrocyte DALD to alcohol has suggested that it may also be useful for the recognition of chronic alcohol excess. Compared with GGTP it is possibly somewhat more sensitive. In contrast, however, to the gradual elevation of GGTP, DALD is immediately depressed by alcohol ingestion and more promptly returns to normal with abstinence. It is thus a test for very recent alcohol intake. DALD also suffers from the disadvantage that the enzyme is transiently depressed following acute intoxication in the normal subject. In addition, its determination is methodologically far more complex than that of GGTP.

SUMMARY

There are available four laboratory procedures, two of which, serum γ-glutamyltransferase and erythrocyte mean corpuscular volume determination, are simple and two of which, plasma α-amino-butyric acid : leucine ratio and erythrocyte δ-amino-levulinic acid dehydrase determination, are complex, but each of which shows a high frequency of abnormality in patients with high alcoholic intake. By their determination, particularly in combination, objective evidence of chronic excessive alcohol consumption may be obtained, and facilitate the clinical recognition of the alcoholic.

REFERENCES

Baglin, M. C., Bernot, J. L., Bremond, J. L., Lamy, J., Leraux, M. E. and Weill, J. (1976). Efficacité comparés du volume globulaire moyen (VGM) et de la gamma-glutamyltransferase (γGT) serique comme tests de triage des buveurs excessifs d'alcool. *Clin. Chin. Acta*, **68,** 321

Bailey, M. B., Haberman, P. W. and Steinberg, J. (1969). *Millbank Memorial Fund Quarterly*, **47,** 235. Quoted by Hamlyn A. N. (1975). Blood ethanol in liver disease. *Lancet*, **ii,** 991

Hamlyn, A. N., Brown, A. J., Sherlock, S. and Baron, D. N. (1975). Casual blood-ethanol estimations in patients with chronic liver disease. *Lancet*, **ii,** 345

Herbert, V., Zalusky, R. and Davidson, C. S. (1964). Correlation of folate deficiency with alcoholism and associated macrocytosis; anemia and liver disease. *Ann. Intern. Med.*, **58,** 977

Hetzel, B. S. (1975). Tobacco and alcohol. *Medicine*, **II, 5,** 224

Hore, B. D. (1977). Clinical features of alcoholism. *Br. J. Hosp. Med.*, **August,** 106

Lamy, J., Aron, E., Bernot, J. L. and Weill, J. (1976). GGTP activity as a test for the diagnosis of excessive alcohol intake. In (G. Siest, and D. S. Young). (eds.) *Drug Interference and Drug Measurement in Clinical Chemistry*, pp. 42–47. (Basel: Karger)

Moore, M. R. and Goldberg, A. (1975). Some biochemical responses to ethanol in man. *INSERM/MRC Symposium Franco-Brittanique sur l'Alcoolisme*, **54,** 101

Morgan, M. Y., Milsom, J. P. and Sherlock, S. (1977). Ratio of plasma α-amino-n-butyric acid to leucine as an empirical marker of alcoholism. *Science*, **197,** 1183

Robinson, A. G. and Loeb, J. N. (1971). Ethanol ingestion – commonest cause of elevated plasma osmolality. *N. Engl. J. Med.*, **284,** 1253

Rosalki, S. B. (1974). Détermination de la gamma-glutamyltranspeptidase chez les alcooliques et chez les buveurs d'habitude. Proceedings Symposium. Dépistage precoce de l'intoxication alcoolique à l'aide d'um test biologique: le dosage de la gamma-glutamyl-transpeptidase. (Paris:Boehringer Mannheim)

Rosalki, S. B. (1977). Enzyme tests for alcoholism. *Rev. Epidemiol. Med. Soc. Sante Publique*, **25,** 147

Rosalki, S. B. and Rau, D. (1972). Serum γ-glutamyl transpeptidase activity in alcoholism *Clin. Chim. Acta*, **39,** 41

Rosalki, S. B., Rau, D., Lehmann, D. and Prentice, M. (1970). Determination of serum γ-glutamyl transpeptidase activity and its clinical applications. *Ann. Clin. Biochem.*, **7,** 143

Rutherford, W. H. (1977). Diagnosis of alcohol ingestion in mild head injuries. *Lancet*, **i,** 1021

Shaw, S., Stimmel, B. and Lieber, C. S. (1976). Plasma alpha-amino-n-butyric acid to leucine ratio: An emperical biochemical marker of alcoholism. *Science*, **194,** 1057

Silberfarb, P. M. (1976). Recognising alcoholism early by physical signs. *Postgrad. Med.*, **59,** 79

Wu, A., Chanarin, I. and Levi, A. J. (1974). Macrocytosis of chronic alcoholism. *Lancet*, **i,** 829

Index